The
BEST WAY
to Say Goodbye:

A Legal Peaceful Choice
at the End of Life

Your Reading Choices

This book is *about* choices. It also *offers* you choices in reading: Start at the beginning and read everything, or if you prefer. . .

A) Read the *book-within-a-book*. Page 4 explains how to skip *flagged* portions to reduce the number of pages to just over 300.

B) Focus on *Patient Stories and Legal Cases* for discussion, *Humorous Stories* for fun, or *Guidelines and FORMS* for personal planning. Pages xxv through xxx at the end of the Table of Contents list all the Titles. Page 4 illustrates how to recognize each form of writing.

C) For a quick overview, read ten pages: "She revised her Advance Directives from age 16 to 86," and "Which documents do I need when?" on pages 383-389; and *The Seven Principles of Good End-of-Life Decision-Making* on 427-429. View thirst-reducing products on 104.

D) Delve into such general topics as the *medical, legal, religious,* or *family* aspects of end-of-life planning. The Table of Contents can guide your choice of chapters.

E) Implement a **legal alternative to Physician-Assisted Suicide. You can avoid prolonged unbearable pain and suffering** at the end of life as long as you are mentally competent. Read the answers to questions D, & numbers 1-9, 16, 19, 20, 32, 34, 36, 38, & 40.

F) **Prevent years of indignity & dependency from Alzheimer's disease, vegetative states, or persistent unconsciousness.** Learn how to set the stage now so others will honor your wishes in the future, if you no longer can speak for yourself. Read Chapter 3 and the answers to questions numbers 20-22, 25-31, 40, 41, and 43-45.

G) Expand your knowledge. Consult the book's back material including the Medical References and Legal Citations, the Glossary, the Index, and Further Resources. Also visit www.BestGoodbye.com, www.ThirstControl.com, and www.CaringAdvocates.org.

The mission: To promote a culture of extended quality of life

Life's greatest irony is that the freedom to control *when* we die, can—and often does—lead to choosing to *live longer*. In contrast, the greatest end-of-life tragedy is to believe that our only choices are to die illegally, violently, or prematurely—based on the fear that those in power will otherwise force us to endure months or years of unbearable pain and suffering, or to merely exist as our indignity and dependency increase.

The mission of this book is to promote *a culture of extended quality of life*, to maximize enjoyment of whatever time remains. To quell our end-of-life fears, we must be assured that others will honor our Last Wishes if some day, we can no longer speak for ourselves. Yet the challenges to controlling our future are daunting: We will suffer *more pain*—if laws criminalize doctors for prescribing medications at doses that non-medical regulators "judge" as intentional overdoses to hasten dying. Our private conversations around our kitchen tables will receive *less respect*—if States pass new laws that require higher standards of evidence to accept our family's sworn testimony as our enduring end-of-life wishes. The risk of being forced to exist indefinitely after we have lost the essence of what make us human—our greatest fear—*will increase* if judges presume we all want to "err on the side of life."

What can you do? Compose strategically effective Living Wills and Proxy Directives using **The *BEST WAY* to Say Goodbye** as your guide. Modify your State's free form, add lines to such popular forms as "Five Wishes," or complete the forms in this book. Then add such recommended attachments as an "Empowering Statement for My Proxy," a page to designate a "Living Will Advocate," or an "Acceptance Agreement" that all your Proxies sign. Such diligence will dramatically increase your ultimate chance of **success**.

Beyond pragmatism, **The *BEST WAY* to Say Goodbye** considers the only subject that will definitely affect us all... first with our loved ones and then for ourselves. The book considers the *process of dying*, not death itself, from the practical, psychological, clinical, religious, ethical, moral, legal, and political perspectives.

Embracing and then transcending the personal-centered, high-profile political controversy of *autonomy* (freedom to choose **not** to prolong your suffering or indignity) versus *faith-based discipline* (freedom to follow the teachings of your religious leader), the book is the first to ask readers to view Advance Directives as *moral documents* by introducing this noble goal:

*To honor the sanctity of **many** lives.*

Read the praise of others »

Praise for **The *BEST WAY to* Say Goodbye: a Legal Peaceful Choice at the End of Life**

"A comprehensive, insightful, and surprisingly entertaining guide through the maze of end-of-life decisions. It calms our greatest fear: that complete strangers can intrude on our most intimate decisions, and worse—make decisions that we would not make for ourselves. Dr. Terman offers a close to ironclad strategy to preserve control at the end of life, even for those individuals who may ultimately suffer from severe brain damage or dementia. Every pitfall has been considered and solved! It also guides families through the chaos that results from inadequate advance care planning. This book is so good that our organization keeps copies at every office. It is a mainstay of the recommendations we provide our clients. "

Barbara Coombs Lee, PA, FNP, JD; Family Nurse Practitioner and Attorney;
President and Co-CEO, Compassion and Choices;
Chief Petitioner for the Oregon Death with Dignity Act

"If I had only one book to read in the right-to-die field, I would choose this one... I now have renewed interest in this 'BEST WAY' (**Refusing Food & Fluid**). Here is fun reading, despite the seemingly grim subject matter. Its varied style and conceptual ease seems to be designed for 'seniors.' ...a monumental work."

Bill Fagan, Board Member, Hemlock Society of San Diego,
Senior Exit Guide for Final Exit Network

"Dr. Stanley Terman has provided a very insightful analysis of the President's Council on Bioethics' report, *Taking Care: Ethical Caregiving In Our Aging Society*. His detailed suggestions for wording Advance Directives are very important. While it may be utopian to hope, as Dr. Terman proposes, that governmental agencies (such as motor vehicle departments) might require individuals to complete Advance Directives, it would be a major improvement over our present laissez-faire policy of ignoring this issue. I am very supportive of responsible strategies to encourage individuals to complete such documents. The book's final story, *She Revised her Advance Directives from 16 to 86*, clearly illustrates how our views can change as we age and mature, and as our situation changes. Clearly, we need to update our Advance Directives on a regular basis."

Janet D. Rowley, M.D., D.Sc.; President's Council on Bioethics member;
Blum-Riese Distinguished Service Professor of Medicine;
Departments of Hematology and Oncology, University of Chicago;
Albert Lasker Clinical Medicine Research Prize recipient

"An excellent book. Rich with valuable information and compassionate guidance."

Lawrence J. Schneiderman, M.D.
Professor of Family and Preventive Medicine School of Medicine
University of California, San Diego;
Faculty Affiliate of The Ethics Center, San Diego

"Dr. Terman's eloquent and at times deeply personalized account of the challenges of life nearing death offers a unique and useful vocabulary for our emerging national dialogue on end-of-life choices. At last, a comprehensive look at the medical, legal, and spiritual aspects of the dying process that explores the full range of patient options, while highlighting the often-overlooked process of **Voluntary Refusal of Food & Fluid**. The *BEST WAY* to Say Goodbye adds depth and sensibility to an area that is rampant with controversy because of its perceived lack of common ground. This book is that common ground, making it a must-read for all whose diverse views make up the colorful 'right to die' spectrum."

Judith F. Daar, J.D., Professor of Law, Whittier Law School;
Clinical Professor of Medicine;
University of California Irvine, College of Medicine

"People think if they do not die instantaneously in a car accident or from a heart attack, they are going to be caught between two undesirable options—either to be attached to machines for a very long time, often in a state of unconsciousness with no reasonable hope for recovery, or, at the other extreme, to commit suicide or get someone to murder you so that you can end it all more quickly. In a wise, medically well-grounded, and even witty book, Dr. Terman explores the middle course: refusing tube feeding and hydration—a way of dying that is relatively painless, effective, legal, and in keeping with many religious traditions. Critically important for individuals, families, health care professionals, and public policy experts, the book really does point to **The *BEST WAY* to Say Goodbye**."

Elliot N. Dorff, Rabbi, Ph.D., Rector and Distinguished Professor of Philosophy, University of Judaism; author of *Matters of Life and Death: A Jewish Approach to Modern Medical Ethics*

"Dr. Terman has accurately and respectfully presented the Catholic position(s). His chapter on religion has clarity and insight. A valuable resource for those who are seeking greater understanding of end-of-life issues. I agree with the values he holds most dear: 'To do everything possible to learn directly from the patient what she or he wants; and to appreciate that one of life's greatest joys—to be heard and respected—is especially true for needy and vulnerable patients in the last chapter of their lives when their most fundamental values are at stake.'"

John Gillman, Ph.D., ACPE Supervisor of Clinical Pastoral Education;
VITAS Innovative Hospice Care, San Diego, California

"The goal of peaceful dying includes acceptance of death as part of life, to which it gives enhanced meaning. Dr. Terman's approach is in harmony with the goals of Buddhist spirituality, as well as those of Hinduism and Jainism. Here is a balanced presentation of practical facts about the strategic, ethical, moral, religious, and humane aspects of one option to close one's life—**Voluntarily Refusing Food & Fluid**. Many stories enhance the inspirational message and help readers seek their personal meaning. Relevant humor widens the emotional impact of the book that will have great impact on readers of diverse orientations."

The Venerable Mettanando Bhikkhu, M.D., Ph.D., Buddhist monk and physician; educator of medical ethics, hospice care, palliative care and meditation; Bangkok's Special Advisor to the World Congress of Religion and Peace, which advises the United Nations

"How dying can be as comfortable, as dignified, and as humane as possible. The pros and cons of **Voluntary Refusal of Food & Fluid** are compared to Physician-Hastened Dying. If people were better educated about **Voluntary Refusal of Food & Fluid**, and it would take the fight out of the 'pro-life' position since patients can do this on their own—without getting into quasi-legal methods or new laws. 'Pro-life' arguments such as, 'Doctors shouldn't kill,' and 'Do no harm,' would then be irrelevant. An important book for terminally ill patients, their loved ones, and the professionals devoted to helping them."

C. Ronald Koons, MD, FACP; Clinical Professor, Radiation Oncology and Medicine; Chair, Ethics Committee; University of California Irvine Medical Center

"As an emergency department physician for over 30 years, I have seen a great many people die. What emerges from my clinical experience? Two truths: First, we all must die. Second, some ways of dying are more painful to the patient and cause more suffering to the family than others. That is why Dr. Stanley Terman's contribution is so important. My own father decided to leave this world by **Voluntary Refusal of Food & Fluid**. For him and for his family, it was a peaceful way to say goodbye, and consistent with our Christian values. This book covers every aspect of the subject. The medical aspects are sound, including how to make the process as comfortable as possible, and what to do if you change your mind. Dr. Terman explores the spiritual, religious, moral, ethical, economic, and political aspects. The book includes deeply moving memoirs and humorous tales. Always provocative, it stimulates people to make their lives more meaningful right now."

Richard F. Prince, M.D., former Chairman, Department of Emergency Services and Vice Chief of Staff, Scripps Memorial Hospital, Chula Vista, CA; Fellow and charter member, American College of Emergency Physicians

"You choose to make quality decisions for life, so in parallel you choose to make quality decisions for death... if you are free to choose, of course. After four centuries of understandable distrust, African Americans are wary of 'healers' who make life and death decisions regarding them. Many remember the Tuskegee experiment as a historic example of misplaced trust. Dr. Terman must be commended for examining this specific area in the context of options of life and death. Also, the section of his book on religion is just awesome. It held me spellbound with its depth of understanding of our differences and our commonalities as we debate the issue of life and death. If any work should be required reading, this would qualify. The demand for such a work of excellence will only escalate within this decade and beyond. I have personally used its insights in working with families and seen how they can bring great relief in the struggle to make 'their best' end-of-life decisions."

Cecil L. "Chip" Murray, Rel. D., Tanzy Chair of Christian Ethics, School of Religion, University of Southern CA; Pastor Emeritus, First African Methodist Episcopal Church, Los Angeles, CA

"This book probes deeply into questions concerning the decisions people must make for the terminal stage of their lives. The clarity of its message is illustrated by many memoirs. Highly recommended for both professionals and non-professionals."

Jerome S. Tobis, M.D., Emeritus Chair, Ethics Committee, University of California Irvine Medical Center

"I am a healthy Christian, working full time at 68. **The *BEST WAY* to Say Goodbye** is a godsend. Like holy water in a parched desert, I feel like a preacher getting out the word of salvation. My parents looked like Clark Gable and Grace Kelly. Both were Phi Beta Kappa. Yet my mother's life ended in her 50s after 10 years with Alzheimer's disease; my father's life ended in his 70s after 17 years with Alzheimer's disease. Now my husband has Parkinson's. I know, definitively, what it looks like to wait too long so you can no longer access your once excellent mind to make choices about your end-of-life treatment. Dr. Terman's book provides the background and strategies for successful advance planning."

Eugenia Rush Gerrard, M.A.
Marriage and Family Therapist, Encinitas, CA

"An impressive, well-rounded and helpful addition on end-of-life care. Ground-breaking, **The *BEST WAY* to Say Goodbye** effectively integrates practical advice with research studies and moving personal accounts."

Gary W. Hartz, Ph.D., Geropsychologist, Cupertino, CA; Author of *Psychosocial Intervention in Long-Term Care: An Advanced Guide*

"After Grandpa's massive stroke he could not speak. Some family members argued he'd want 'to join' his recently deceased wife of 74 years and would not want to live so inactive? But others interpreted statements in his Living Will as wanting to live. Using the series of questions from a story in this book, *A Time To Be Sure*, on three occasions, Grandpa shook or nodded his head to indicate he wanted to continue tube feeding. I was surprised. We all felt relief. Now we knew what he wanted."

"**C.C.**", Seattle, Washington

"I conduct Sunday seminars after church services in the San Francisco Bay Area, and I lecture at U. Cal and the Graduate Theological Union in Berkeley to introduce the dying with dignity movement. As the text book to guide and to enlighten humanity, I have chosen Dr. Terman's prodigiously brilliant book, **The BEST WAY to Say Goodbye**, an indispensable authoritative resource of information of end-of- life care. It is a literary masterpiece."

Reverend Dennis Kuby, M. Div.; Former Head, Hemlock of California; Founder, Ministry of Ecology, Inc., Berkeley, CA

"A comprehensive reference for those brave enough to consider the last chapter of their lives. Intellectually provocative, Dr. Terman's knowledge and passion has culminated in a book where the term, 'highly intriguing,' applies to almost every page."

Stephanie Mason, MA, Psy.D. cand. (Psychology) San Diego, CA

"Voluntary dehydration, although always part of natural dying, has only recently been recognized as superior to physician-assisted suicide to end an unreasonable burdensome life under most clinical conditions and current laws. So, my compliments on the wealth of information presented on voluntary dehydration. I totally support this method as minimally offensive to control one's destiny either directly or through an advance medical directive. Its widespread acceptance is preferable to fighting to legalize physician-assisted suicide."

Alan D. Lieberson, M.D., J.D., author of *Advance Medical Directives*, Clark, Boardman, Callaghan, publ., 1992

Regarding Dr. Terman's declaration submitted as an affidavit to Florida Judge George Greer, who presided over the fate of Terri Schiavo:

"Mr. Gibbs and I certainly appreciate medical personnel like you who were willing to stand by Terri [Schiavo]. The pro-death culture is becoming overwhelming in America. I pray that doctors like you will be able to stem the tide in the future. Thank you again for your willingness to help Terri."

Barbara Weller, Esq., attorney for Terri Schiavo's parents, the Schindlers; Gibbs Law Firm, Seminole, Florida

...with appreciation for our many teachers
and with loving memories of our parents:

Anne Regan Terman and Irving Terman
Harry Pokalsky Tillman   Guy S. Gardner
Virginia Gordon Wilson Miller and William Baker Miller
Gertrude Stockton Eckhardt Evans and Donald Sidley Evans

Other books by Stanley A. Terman:

Lethal Choice, a medical thriller

**The *BEST WAY* to Say Goodbye:
A Legal Peaceful Choice at the End of Life**
   is the foundation for a new series of books.

   The following titles are expected in late 2007 and 2008:

**The *BEST WAY* to Prevent Prolonged End-of-Life
   Pain and Suffering**

**The *BEST WAY* to Avoid Lingering in Indignity and
   Dependency of Alzheimer's and Related Dementias**

**The *BEST WAY* to Treat People Who Have Lost Their Minds:
   Should We Change Our Laws to "Permit Natural Dying"?**

**The *BEST WAY* to Fulfill Your Last Wishes: Memoirs and
   Professional Advice for Peaceful Transitions**

**The *BEST WAY* to Preserve Your Wealth from the Threat of
   Alzheimer's and Other Chronic Diseases**

...with appreciation for our many teachers
and with loving memories of our parents:

Anne Regan Terman and Irving Terman
Harry Pokalsky Tillman   Guy S. Gardner
Virginia Gordon Wilson Miller and William Baker Miller
Gertrude Stockton Eckhardt Evans and Donald Sidley Evans

Other books by Stanley A. Terman:

Lethal Choice, a medical thriller

The *BEST WAY* to Say Goodbye:
A Legal Peaceful Choice at the End of Life
   is the foundation for a new series of books.

   The following titles are expected in late 2007 and 2008:

The *BEST WAY* to Prevent Prolonged End-of-Life
   Pain and Suffering

The *BEST WAY* to Avoid Lingering in Indignity and
   Dependency of Alzheimer's and Related Dementias

The *BEST WAY* to Treat People Who Have Lost Their Minds:
   Should We Change Our Laws to "Permit Natural Dying"?

The *BEST WAY* to Fulfill Your Last Wishes: Memoirs and
   Professional Advice for Peaceful Transitions

The *BEST WAY* to Preserve Your Wealth from the Threat of
   Alzheimer's and Other Chronic Diseases

The
BEST WAY
to Say Goodbye:
A Legal Peaceful Choice at the End of Life

Stanley A. Terman, Ph.D., M.D.

with Ronald Baker Miller, M.D.,
and Michael S. Evans, M.S.W., J.D.

Life Transitions Publications

Carlsbad CA 92009

Publisher's Cataloging-in-Publication (Provided by Quality Books, Inc.)

Terman, Stanley A.
   The best way to say goodbye : a legal peaceful choice at the end of life / Stanley A. Terman ; with Ronald Baker Miller and Michael S. Evans. —1st ed.
   p. cm.
   Includes bibliographical references and index.
   LCCN 2005924983
   ISBN 978-1-933418-02-5 (hard cover)
   ISBN 978 1-933418-03-2 (soft cover)
   ISBN 978 1-933418-21-6 (large type, soft cover)

   1. Advance directives (Medical care) 2. Life and death, Power over. 3. Patient advocacy. 4. Medical ethics.   I. Miller, Ronald Baker. II. Evans, Michael S. III. Title.

R726.2.T47 2007   179'.7
                 QBI05-600031

Life Transitions Publications * Post Office Box 130129 * Carlsbad, CA 92009

www.TheBestGoodbye.com   www.LifeTP.com   www.CaringAdvocates.org

First Edition; 2007

Foreword

By Jay Wolfson, DrPH, JD
Guardian *Ad Litem* to Theresa Schiavo

The imminent death of Theresa Schiavo, following the removal of her feeding tube, first captured the world's attention in October 2003. Extraordinary media and political resources then focused on end-of-life issues. Pope John Paul II took a personal interest in Ms. Schiavo. In March 2004, the Pope issued an Allocution about patients in the persistent vegetative state using harsh words: removing artificial hydration and nutrition is "euthanasia by omission." Despite the American Civil Liberties Union briefs in support of Ms. Schiavo's right to self-determination, the Governor of Florida and both houses of that State's legislature actively intervened to pass what (later) became known as the first "Terri's Law." Although ultimately declared to be unconstitutional, this unique Act authorized Governor Jeb Bush to order the reinsertion of Ms.. Schiavo's feeding tube. Six days after the tube had been removed, it was thus reinserted. The Act also authorized additional inquiries into Ms. Schiavo's abilities such as swallowing. Finally, the Act mandated the appointment of a Special Guardian *Ad Litem* for Ms. Schiavo, who would report to the court and to the Governor.

As Theresa Schiavo's Guardian *Ad Litem*, I recognized my goal was to represent exclusively her interests. I thus attempted to maintain balance as I tried to acquire the trust and active input of all parties. In the process, I came to believe that the Schindlers (Theresa's parents), and her husband Michael Schiavo were all honestly motivated by what they perceived as being right and in Theresa's interests. I also learned that Theresa was a very shy and sweet woman who loved her husband and parents. For her, the family breach and public circus would have been an anathema. Her husband resolved not to allow the woman he loved to be subjected to medical treatment that he believed she would have abhorred. In court, her parents made statements that hardened Mr. Schiavo's position. They stated that if it became medically necessary to save her life, they would grant medical consent to amputate all her limbs. Furthermore, they admitted that even if Theresa had executed a formal, written Living Will, they would have fought to have it voided because they did not believe it was consistent with their, or her, beliefs. Finally, they admitted that just having their daughter alive produced joy for them.

xiv   *The BEST WAY to Say Goodbye*

As Guardian *Ad Litem,* I reviewed thirty thousand pages of legal and medical records from Theresa Schiavo's then nearly fourteen years of treatment. I met with her parents, siblings, and husband. I talked to hospice staff, attorneys, and Governor Bush. I visited with Theresa on 20 different days, sometimes for as long as 4 hours. Many of these hours led to personal frustration that was consistent with the findings of the medical experts appointed by both the husband and the court: Theresa Schiavo lacked any ability to respond to her environment. This symptom is the hallmark of the Permanent Vegetative State. Diagnosis was critical since the Florida law that permits the withdrawal of life-sustaining treatment requires the patient be in a PVS. While Florida law requires *clear and convincing* evidence that the patient would have wanted life-sustaining treatment withdrawn, this evidence need not be in written form. After Judge Greer heard oral testimony in Ms. Schiavo's trial, he ruled that the evidence was *clear and convincing.*

On December 1, 2003, I submitted my 38-page report to Governor Jeb Bush. I used the term "stand in her shoes" to refer to the ethical standard known as "Substituted Judgment," where decision-makers have sufficient knowledge about a patient's values and preferences to make the same end-of-life medical decisions that she would have made. I also intended this phrase to emphasize that the outcome of the Schiavo matter affects all of us in many ways—morally, ethically, spiritually, intellectually, and politically. The outcome of her personal saga would reflect the current complex and conflicting social attitudes toward dying in America. It should also provoke all of us to consider how our decisions affect our loved ones and ourselves, as we decide how we want to die.

In March of 2005, Ms. Schiavo's feeding tube was removed for the third and final time—fifteen years after Ms. Schiavo collapsed and lost consciousness. Yet the ten years of expensive litigation did *not* end. The U.S. Congress convened in special sessions a week before Easter, passed the second "Terri's Law," and President George W. Bush flew to the Capital to sign the bill into law.

The Federal judicial system again upheld the removal of Ms. Schiavo's feeding tube. Thirteen days after the tube was removed, she died of dehydration (not of starvation). The conservative and liberal polemics were nearly deafening. The Rev. Jesse Jackson joined Governor Jeb Bush, and Randall Terry (the conservative activist leader of Operation Rescue), to advocate for Ms. Schiavo's parents. In June 2005 however, the results of the autopsy that was conducted by a conservative and meticulous medical examiner, showed that little remained of the part of her brain that is considered essential to respond meaningfully to her environment. This anatomic finding was consistent with the behavioral diagnosis of PVS determined by several neurologists, including Dr. Ronald Cranford.

The Schiavo litigation worried those Americans who wanted to make their end-of-life decisions privately, with their doctors and family. It made them want more certainty that their personal decisions about dying will be honored in the face of powerful political and religious challenges. It illustrated the need for diligently writing Advance Directives that include *clear and convincing* explanations for why they chose certain end-of-life options. Underlying the individual saga were profound implications for how our society must grapple with the use of scarce health care resources. These considerations were highlighted by the President's Council on Bioethics' report, "Taking Care: Ethical Caregiving In Our Aging Society." Published just days before the U.S. Supreme Court ruled on Gonzales v. Oregon in 2005, the report documented that increasingly huge numbers of patients and their families with dementia will present one of the greatest challenges our society has ever had to face. Meanwhile, the Court's ruling, that States can determine the "legitimate use of medications," allowed Oregon's Death With Dignity Act to continue, at least until State or Federal legislation changes.

Economist Robert H. Frank asked, "Do the poor deserve life-support?" His 2006 article referred to a Texas law permitting discontinuing futile life-sustaining treatment that then Governor George W. Bush signed in 1999. Dr. Frank considered the larger moral question: if we fail to seriously consider advance care planning and make public policy on a societal scale, then in the future, we may be forced to make end-of-life decisions dictated by the reality of limited resources.

The *BEST WAY* to Say Goodbye deals directly and comprehensively with all the above challenges. While it emphasizes the individual approach, it keeps societal consequences (including those affecting the medically indigent) in perspective. Dr. Terman explains why we must diligently create carefully worded documents that accurately reflect our well-considered end-of-life wishes. He also provides directives and options about the best way to select, to authorize, and to empower appropriate individuals to advocate our end-of-life decisions. Dr. Terman's definition of success in this endeavor is when others faithfully honor our last wishes.

Dr. Terman's book also provides an explicit description of a legal and peaceful alternative to physician-assisted suicide for those who are suffering unbearably. He presents a comprehensive strategy to help individuals avoid the prolonged indignity and burden of total dependence from dementias such as Alzheimer's disease, since for many of these patients, there is no life-sustaining medical technology to withdraw. Dr. Terman considers this "best way to say goodbye" from numerous pragmatic perspectives. He includes memoirs of those who chose to discontinue nutrition and hydration, provides over 250 medical references and legal citations, and describes his personal experience of a total food and fluid fast.

Dr. Terman's considerations of clinical, legal, ethical, religious, sociological, and philosophical implications of advance end-of-life decision-making are comprehensive. He has broken this complex issue into manageable and readable components. First, he poses relevant questions. Then he provides excellent answers that include specific guidelines that can be adopted for practical use. Lay people will find the material entertaining as well as approachable. End-of-life professionals will appreciate the presentations in related fields. I can imagine many recommending specific portions to their clients. Dr. Terman's success in balancing delicate political and religious perspectives makes the book a valuable and usable resource for people worried about themselves or their parents, even when their beliefs are in conflict. It should also be useful for students and practitioners of medical ethics.

An experienced and published psychiatrist, Dr. Terman joined with two collaborators in medical ethics and law to write this important and timely book about navigating the process of dying with strategic planning. The gentle but firm approach to end-of-life decisions can help terminally ill patients and their families achieve peaceful transitions without the need to change present laws. While some may view this "best way" narrowly, as a means to hasten the process of dying, in fact, Dr. Terman convincingly explains the psychological reasons for the surprising result of the "Oregon experiment." When people are given the choice to have some degree of control over how they die, they not only endure less anxiety and worry; they also frequently decide to live longer. Thus, following the guidelines of this book may lead many people to add quantity as well as quality to the weeks, months, or even years of life that remain. This important conceptual contribution is brought to practical realization by the robust strategic advice in the book. No one expects the controversies surrounding the Schiavo saga to disappear. But this book provides a path to transcend them.

Jay Wolfson, DrPH, JD
Distinguished Professor of Public Health and Medicine
Associate Vice President, Health Law, Policy and Safety
University of South Florida, Tampa
April, 2006

Acknowledgments

"2 + 2 = 4"

Ethical arguments can occur only in the context of uncertainty. Few would argue about the validity of the above equation. In contrast, one of the most enduring and profound debates in our society is based on the uncertainty over when life *begins*. Due to advances in medical technology, we also argue about when life *ends*, and what it means to respect the *sanctity of life*.

I would like to thank two colleagues who argued with me for many months, in certain areas, paragraph by paragraph: Ronald Baker Miller, M.D., and Michael S. Evans, M.S.W., J.D. Doctor Ronald Miller is Clinical Professor of Medicine, Emeritus and Director of the Program in Medical Ethics Program Emeritus, at the University of California, Irvine. Attorney (and social worker) Michael Evans has served as legal advisor to four right-to-choose-to-die organizations and provided advice on Advance Directives to hundreds of individuals over the last sixteen years. My colleagues enhanced the multi-disciplinary quality and sophistication of this book, prevented me from making foolish mistakes, and added significant content drawn from their fields. Most important, they convinced me to change my mind... at least sometimes. Two examples: Disheartened by the failure of Living Wills, I had decided to abandon their use, but Dr. Miller convinced me of their value for terminally-ill patients who have a good relationship with their physicians. Initially, I wanted to use the term **Voluntary Refusal of Food & Fluid** for all situations where patients hastened the process of dying by declining nurturance. Discussions with Attorney Evans led me to employ two additional terms: **Refusal of Food & Fluid by Proxy** (via a Proxy Directive) and **Withholding of Food & Fluid** (by a physician as requested in a Living Will).

I am grateful to Dr. Charles von Gunten, Director of the Center for Palliative Studies at the San Diego Hospice and Editor-in-Chief of Journal of Palliative Medicine. He was the first to inform me that **Voluntary Refusal of Food & Fluid** can be comfortable. He also edited my first published papers on the topic.

I thank the following people for their substantial contributions: Rabbi Moshe Levin helped me write about the Jewish views, and the Venerable Mettanando Bhikkhu commented about on the views of eastern religions, on **Voluntarily Refusing Food & Fluid**. Richard Lederer of the PBS radio show, "A Way with Words," commented on my proposal to rename "Physician-Assisted Suicide." Barbara Coombs Lee, Rabbi Elliot Dorff, John Gillman, and Peter Ditto provided detailed comments on various sections of the text. Christina M. Trent, J.D., researched several topics and helped write some end-material. Mark Janssen did bibliographic research, proofreading, and copy-editing. Dr. Jeffrey Abrams functioned as a volunteer researcher by alerting me to medical and news articles.

James Park offered existential and copyediting comments. The hand of Donna Blochwitz followed my instructions to create two cartoons. Simon Warwick-Smith shared his vast experience in what was for me, the new world of book publishing.

I particularly wish to thank all the named and anonymous contributors of articles in the book. I deeply appreciated the authors of journal articles and attorneys who responded to my requests, sometimes within hours, by e-mails and further willingness to correspond by phone.

Thanks to the Orange County's Bioethics Luncheon Discussion Group (BELDG) for giving me a forum to discuss several of the book's topics, and similarly to the members of the San Diego County Coalition to Improve End-of-Life Care.

Thanks to my wife, my sons, and my daughter—who put up with my long obsession to write and rewrite, often to the exclusion of some family events and just "hanging out"—for more years than I care to admit.

I now wish to acknowledge my mother. Although my father was a physician it was she who deliberately introduced me to her concept of death when I was very young. Anne Regan Terman stated this distinction with as much conviction as a universally accepted truth: "Death is not something any one need be afraid of," she would say. "It is peaceful. What I fear is suffering a long time before I die." She did not realize that she was paraphrasing Henry Fielding (1707-1754), who said, "It hath been often said that it is not death, but dying which is terrible."

This book deals only with the process of dying, not death. Grief is an important theme, but the book deals with it in the context of its magnitude, and the depressed mood it creates, depend on how well our loved ones die. When we feel we have done all that we could—to care enough to respond effectively to how our loved ones wanted to die—then we can feel less guilt and less depression, although we will still feel a great loss when someone we have loved is gone.

My mother told me the story of her mother's dying. She was dependent on my mother as her willing caregiver for seven years. During this time, my mother put her own life on hold. I never met my grandmother, but my mother told me that her suffering included self-loathing. In the first half of the Twentieth Century, she explained, end-stage kidney disease had no specific treatment. Excruciating itching could only be partially relieved by eating a low protein diet. My mother's physical and social burden was thus intensified by witnessing her mother's suffering every day, and by feeling helpless to relieve her mother's suffering.

So my mother emphatically wished for a quick and painless death. The good news is that her wish was granted. The bad news is that she died too young, when she still had much to live for. I lost her when she was only 63, a great loss, even though I could take some solace that she died as she wished—quickly and without suffering. I hope that my writing this book honors my mother and her mother.

Stanley A. Terman, Ph.D., M.D.
Caring Advocates
Carlsbad, CA

Contents

Patient Stories and Legal Cases

Humorous Tales and Cartoons

Forms

Guided Conversations

Guidelines and Warnings

Graph and Tables

Preface

To Exercise Personal Choice, Must We Change Our Laws?

"I know how to stop smoking. I've done it a thousand times."   —Mark Twain

O ver the past two and a half years, I have increasingly identified with this quip of Mark Twain. Here is my personal version:

I know how to finish this book. I've done it dozens of times.

The text seemed complete in January 2005 as I finished writing about The Pope's provocative Allocution of March, 2004. John Paul II was quoted as saying that removing feeding tubes from unconscious patients is "euthanasia by omission."

Then came the case of Terri Schiavo. I became professionally involved in this most public end-of-life controversy when one of the litigating attorneys asked me to submit a declaration (although I did not testify). It was clear that national debate about Ms. Schiavo's fate would help shape the future landscape of medical ethics.

One result of Terri Schiavo's legacy was to change this book's motivating direction. Instead of emphasizing *why* it is so important to write Advance Directives, my passion became instructing readers on *how* they can strive to create "ironclad" Advance Directives to overcome challenges from powerful religious or political forces. Yet the book's definition of *success* never changed:

So others will honor your end-of-life decisions.

As I was again finishing the book, the President's Council on Bioethics published *Taking Care: Ethical Caregiving in Our Aging Society*. In the boldest attack on Living Wills since their introduction, this report advised readers *not* to create Advance Directives and *not* to honor patients' clearly expressed wishes—if such actions would *discriminate* against a future *disabled*, demented self. What was The Council's alternative? Proxies, caregivers, and healthcare providers should be guided by *moral values*; they should provide patients with *their* judgment of what *they*—not the patients—consider to be "best care." Worse, these others should apply even if *their* "moral" treatment decisions disregard *patients'* previously expressed wishes. The Council's position made me feel compelled to explain A) how The Council's arguments were flawed, B) why their recommendations violated patients' Constitutional legal rights and current medical practice, and C) how implementing their recommendations would hasten the demise of Medicare, Medicaid, and Social Security. The current projections are that paying for the long-term care of huge numbers of totally dependent patients will affect most of us. Four out of ten patients will die slowly after years of dependency, and seven out of eight couples whose parents are living can expect at least one parent to become totally dependent.

After I finished writing about The President's Council's report, it seemed prudent to wait to include the U.S. Supreme Court's decision on whether or not the U.S. Attorney General could undermine Oregon's "Death With Dignity Act." In January 2006, the Justices ruled that the Controlled Substances Act of 1970 did *not* empower the U.S. Attorney General to punish physicians who act within the State-defined limits of what is "legitimate medical practice." Yet instead of settling the debate, the stage was set for more heated political battles. In 2007, liberals who championed autonomy were disappointed in their attempts to legalize Physician-Aided Dying: in Vermont, and for the *third* time in *three* years, in California.

Then I wrote about the battle as it got more intense. Conservatives were trying to implement new laws that would legally presume that *all* patients would want tube feeding indefinitely, unless their written Advance Directives *clearly and convincingly* requested otherwise for *specific*—read "arguable"—conditions. As of March 2006, twenty-three States were considering such legislation.

Motivation for creating Advance Directives continued to mount; for example: the estimated increase in the number of Alzheimer's patients by mid-Century was revised upward; *The New York Times* reported that several long-term care insurance companies were not paying deserving beneficiaries; a survey published in *The New England Journal of Medicine* revealed that one out of six doctors admitted they would refuse to offer suffering patients terminal sedation based on the doctors' moral or religious convictions; and the saga of Terri Schiavo stimulated deep considerations of the rights of "formerly conscious human beings."

As I added material on public policy and ethics, I was upset to learn about recent personal tragedies. An 84-year-old man, a devoted husband for sixty years, was sentenced to prison for 12 years for the mercy killing of his wife. She suffered from advanced Parkinson's disease. (See the *Prologue*.) A 74-year-old man who had authored a controversial book about helping his wife die, almost failed in his own suicide attempt due to an unwanted attempt at resuscitation and transporting him to a hospital. (See the *Epilogue*.)

Now that legalizing Physician-Aided Dying remained a distant hope, it was clearly urgent for people to learn while **Voluntary Refusal of Food & Fluid** may seem *revolutionary*, it is really a *conventional* way to die that is *legal* everywhere and that it is *peaceful* as long as thirst is controlled since nature automatically takes care of hunger. This method to hasten dying can help hundreds of times as many patients as Oregon's law, which requires competent patients to have the physical ability to self-administer and swallow the medication. For the vast number of patients who are afraid of future dementia, the confidence that others will honor their Last Wishes after they have created effective Advance Directives can allow them to avoid the tragedy of premature dying. They will not feel the need to die *when they can*, but can instead die *when they want to*. On an individual level, there is no need to join a high profile public battle. One can quietly but strategically *transcend* the conflict.

Someday liberals may consider launching a direct voter referendum to legalize Physician-Aided Dying. In the past such efforts have been associated with gross misinformation. With the exception of Oregon, they have failed after huge manpower and monetary expenses. Since Voluntary Refusal of Food & Fluid has the potential to help many more people, I hope activist leaders will also consider directing some energy toward educating people on this method. I am not opposed to changing laws, but my first choice would be to "Permit Natural Dying" for patients who suffer from Devastating Irreversible Brain States. My next book will expand this theme from personal choice to public policy. Compared to high media attention of young patients who suffer permanent brain damage, patients who suffer from progressive dementia receive little publicity. Yet I must ask, for how many years must we aggressively maintain the biologic existence of patients with end-stage dementia? The evolving answer will reflect our individual and societal approach to what is a most threatening challenge to our economic survival.

Permit me to share a perspective from my clinical practice. As I assess the capacity of people in early dementia to make medical decisions, I am impressed with their conviction to refuse specific treatments if their disease progresses to a certain point, and the consistency with which they can express their preferences. This is critically important since for many individuals who will suffer from advanced dementia, there is no "high technology" to withdraw. Often, **Refusal of Food and Fluid by Proxy** is the only method for them to avoid lingering in a state of progressive indignity and dependency. To set the stage so that their Proxies can successfully exercise this option in the future is more formidable a challenge than for any other end-of-life option, but it can also have the greatest and longest benefit for family members and for society.

The contrast between politicians' expenditure of energy to prolong the life of Terri Schiavo, who had not been able to exert any control over her environment for 15 years, and politicians' inaction prior to and after the devastation of Hurricane Katrina, heralds the need to change the attitude of both individuals and society as a whole. I would love to see a powerful consumer-driven call-to-action based in part on applying the strategies in this book, whose implementation can reduce suffering and preserve the dignity of individuals as society's limited financial and medical resources to areas are directed to where they can do the most good. But time is of the essence. We must reach a *tipping point* in this change of attitude before we fall into an economic *sinking* point, from which compromised position certain decisions may be forced upon us because by then, we will simply have no other choice.

Stanley A. Terman, Ph.D., M.D.
Board Certified Psychiatrist
June, 2007

Explaining the *book-within-a-book* and some conventions:

The end-of-life field profoundly affects several disciplines. Striving for depth in each field led to a book with much information. What might suffice for specialists in one discipline might be "TMI" (too much information) for others. But those who concentrate in one field might wish to learn more about another. Attorneys, for example, may want to learn more about religious aspects, while clinicians may desire more knowledge about politics, and so on. Or, vice versa. Similarly, readers who are not in any of these fields may still have good reasons to delve into detail about any particular subject, even seek the original references and citations, or ask their advisors to do so. So we as authors decided *not* to offer an abridged book for "non-professionals," a term that really applies to all of us. Since we cannot presume what depth of information an individual might desire to read, we use **FLAGS** to indicate which sections (about two dozen totaling 100 pages) are more specialized and may be skipped, if desired, as illustrated below. The chapter titles and subheadings, text that introduces material, and the **Index** [page 476] also can help direct your focus reading. The **Glossary** begins on page 457.

To facilitate selective reading, FLAGS like this signal when you may skip:

✇*SKIP*

You may resume reading when you see:

✇*CONTINUE*

Other formats: The web site, www.LifeTP.com, allows you to create your own **e-book** based on your specific interests, and offers related **audios** and **videos**.

Conventions: A "state" is a medical condition; a "State" is a political entity. I capitalize liberally: Federal, Constitutional, Guidelines, Liberty, Pope, Last Wishes, To Delay, and To Deny. I use the symbol **"&"** in "Food & Fluid." To refer to pages in this work: [page #]; for works of other author: [*Page # (in Italics)*].

Guidelines and Forms are indented and use this Arial font.

Humorous stories are indented and use a Comic Sans font.

Memoirs, **clinical stories**, and **legal cases** begin with a drop letter, use Garamond font, and end with this symbol: ✇✇

Prologue

FROM MURDER/SUICIDE TO PEACEFUL TRANSITIONS

Del Mar, California (35 miles north of San Diego);
October 1999:

The exact cause of Hazel May's death will never be known, but there was never any doubt that Tom, her loving husband of 48 years, had actively ended her life. Hazel had lost the ability to speak due to the progression of Lou Gehrig's disease (ALS), which ultimately causes total paralysis. But she did not succumb to the ravages of this devastating neurological disorder. She died either from the overdose of medications that Tom had pushed through her feeding tube, or from breathing carbon monoxide in their garage whose door Tom had closed after leaving their automobile running.

The police arrested Tom, but they did not detain him long in the county jail. Unfortunately, they did not keep him long enough. As investigators tried to decipher Hazel's cryptic note that made Tom believe she wanted to die, and as the district attorney considered what criminal charges to bring against Mr. Tom May, Tom checked into a small motel near Santa Barbara. There, he committed suicide.

In the OP/ED section of the San Diego Union-Tribune, I wrote, "Hazel could have died a third way—one that Tom, like many people, probably did not know about—a way that would have been far more serene for Hazel." I asked, "Why do lay people hear so little about terminal sedation with dehydration?" [This is the clinical term for what this book calls **Voluntary Refusal of Food & Fluid**.]

After all the news covering the conflict over the fate of Terri Schiavo, I asked my writing colleagues if they would join me in answering two additional questions: How can the nonprofessional person sort out the abundance of passionate but conflicting opinions about removing feeding tubes from people with devastating brain damage? And, where can nonprofessional people turn for clear guidance to plan effectively for what is among the most important decisions in their lives—whether or not to stop life-sustaining treatment if their suffering is intolerable and they are terminally ill?

Soon Maha Vajiralonkorn, Thailand (50 kilometers north of Bangkok);
January 2001:

I met Mettanando Bhikkhu, M.D., Ph.D., a physician and Buddhist monk, in
1999, when he was visiting the San Diego Hospice as the Advisor to a foundation
of Thailand's Crown Prince. His mission was to study hospice management in the
United States.

In January 2001, the Venerable Mettanando invited me to lecture at Thailand's
National Cancer Institute. It was hot outside, but inside the lecture hall it was
uncomfortably cool because the air conditioning was too intense. I moved around
a lot as I addressed their hospice staff on Peaceful Transitions®—our organization
of diverse professionals in San Diego who provide support for terminally ill
patients and their families both before and after they are eligible for hospice. We
were providing emotional, relational, legal, musical, spiritual, and pastoral
support to make the final transitions of life more peaceful for both patients and
their families. Following my lecture, the Director of the institution, Dr. Thanadet
Sinthusek, took me on a tour of their new hospice facility.

We entered a large room that looked like one of the hospital wards for wounded
World War II soldiers that I had seen only in black and white movies. No curtains
separated the straight rows of beds. But it was not the lack of privacy that led to
my oppressive feelings. It was the heat. At both 95 degrees and 95% humidity, I
felt very uncomfortable.

"Don't these patients need air conditioning?" I asked.

The Director replied, "Terminal cancer patients are not like us. They don't
mind heat."

To this day, I still wonder if the Director ever asked those "charity cases" about
their comfort in such a way that they could feel free to answer frankly. (Many
months later, I am told, Dr. Sinthusek did improve the privacy and comfort for
patients on this ward.)

For reasons I will now explain, this hospice scene intruded in my mind after I
sent out an early draft of this book in May 2005. I had expected to relax as I
waited for my coauthors to provide input. Instead, I recalled these two old saws:

• Write about what you know, and
• Information is provided on a "need-to-know" basis.

What was bothering me? It took some reflection to appreciate its source. The book presented **Voluntary Refusal of Food & Fluid** as a legal and peaceful choice. It discussed why it might be the *BEST WAY* for some people at the end of their lives, especially for those who had no other way to reduce their suffering that was both legal and peaceful, or if there was no chance that their conscious awareness would ever return. (No problem for unconscious patients). I had first learned from Dr. Charles von Gunten at the San Diego Hospice that conscious terminal patients found the process comfortable. Subsequently, I collected personal anecdotes and memoirs, and researched the medical literature. One anecdote that seemed to disagree was published in the New York Times (discussed later). Arguably, the cause of discomfort was the inexperience of non-hospice staff in controlling pain. So it was this vicarious process that led me to believe that patients who choose to forgo Food & Fluid did not find the process uncomfortable.

—At least some patients. That point still bothered me. Certainly, cancer patients who were alert often reported a loss of appetite; their thirst was minimized by good mouth care. Food even made them nauseated, bloated, and less comfortable. Patients in congestive heart failure often reported it was much easier to breathe once they stopped receiving fluids. Observing family members had sent me numerous anecdotes. Those not included in the book were posted on www.ThirstControl.com, or as testimonials on www.CaringAdvocates.org. All were consistent: **Voluntary Refusal of Food & Fluid** did not cause observable uncomfortable hunger or thirst in their loved ones as they died.

But scientists are trained to suspect negative results. Maybe the families of patients who did suffer when they **Refused Food & Fluid** just did not send in stories of their experiences. Cancers produce toxins; perhaps terminal patients who had other diagnoses would find **Refusing Food & Fluid** uncomfortable. I could not stop wondering if I had made a classic logical mistake of extrapolation. Was I analogously concluding that, if all queens are women, then all women are queens?

The words of Thailand's director, "These patients are not like us," recurred to haunt me. I was never convinced that terminal cancer patients do not want air conditioning. So why should I assume that all terminal patients do not experience hunger and thirst? My sense of responsibility was aroused: I could not justify recommending **Voluntary Refusal of Food & Fluid** to others—especially to those who cannot communicate if they have discomfort—like patients with advanced dementia—if I had not experienced it myself. Was that reasonable? Although physicians most often treat patients with medications that they have never taken themselves, there is also a history of scientific innovators who took the personal risk by being the first to volunteer for their experimental methods. Of course, **Refusing Food & Fluid** at the end of life is far from new. Prior to the modern era of medicine, many people died that way. Although I was confident that my personal risk was low, I did not reveal my plan to my two writing colleagues until my experiment was almost completed. When I did, they informed my wife, only half in jest, that they had no intention of finishing the book "posthumously."

I spent four days **Voluntarily Refusing all Food & Fluid** so I could experience first-hand, whether or not it was uncomfortable.

Now I must confess: Upon changing my role from a researcher/ writer to a person committed to **Refusing Food & Fluid**, I felt a sudden increased "need to know." I did not want to suffer pain so what could I substitute for the oral medications that my orthopedic doctors had prescribed for my moderate spinal stenosis? This question led me to embark on an intense review of an area of the medical literature that I had previously neglected, one which I thought my readers would find useful—non-narcotic medication for moderate pain that could be administered via the rectum. In addition, I learned so much more about *Comfort Care* to the mouth that I started a new web site, www.ThirstControl.com.

I thus discovered the difference between relying on meager accounts reported in the literature and experimenting on myself to find out what works. By the time my personal experiment ended, I was amazed at how much more information I could share with readers of this book. (For example, the photograph on page 104.)

Most patients who **Refuse Food & Fluid** are offered a few ice chips. Instead, I allowed myself one ounce per day of water for medications that permitted me to swallow two pills that were only available in oral form.

What did I discover?

First, medications per rectum were adequate to control my moderate pain. Second, with adequate attention to the mouth, **Refusing Food & Fluid** is really peaceful. I believe that was partially due to some mild dulling of my mental functioning after a couple of days. Third, as the literature promised, I was hardly hungry at all. Here is more detail:

Consider a "**zero**" to "**10**" scale where "**zero**" means no hunger at all, and "**10**" means feeling the most hungry I could imagine. On that scale, I have often felt a "**5**" in the past; for instance after I intentionally missed breakfast in anticipation of a special afternoon buffet. Throughout these four days, however, my hunger never exceeded a "**2**." Most of the time, I did not think about being hungry nor was I aware that I had not eaten—a **zero**. Only when I asked myself how hungry I felt and thought about it deliberately, did I score higher, and even then it was only a "**1**" or a "**2**."

Thirst was more of a problem. I was frequently thirsty—sometimes as much as a "**5**," which I considered quite uncomfortable. But as I learned which dry-mouth aids worked best to eliminate the feeling of thirst, they eventually worked completely. On pages 102-105, I provide details and offer specific suggestions on how to reduce thirst, pain, agitation, and insomnia without taking oral medications.

La Mesa, California (about 20 miles east of San Diego);
August 2006:

Several months after 88-year-old Marie Yvonne Pollock broke her leg, she stopped taking medication for her advanced Parkinson's disease. Later, her sister said, "She probably wouldn't have lived much longer." Her husband, 84-year-old Albert Pollock of La Mesa, CA, admitted considering their options for several weeks. In the early morning of August 22, 2006, he strangled his wife in their bedroom and then called 911 dispatchers to tell them what he had done.

Albert believed his wife had given up hope and feared having to enter a nursing home. His defense attorney, W. Mark Kirkness, said, "There wasn't any malice involved." Prosecutor Jill Lindberg said, "From what we understand, it was a good marriage. There was no violence," and, "He felt that she wasn't going to get any better. He didn't want to put her in a nursing home. He didn't see any other way out."

Mrs. Pollock's niece, Molly Risak, said her aunt and uncle "were a beautiful, loving couple for 60 years... He took care of her every time she was sick."

While the sentence of 12 years means that Albert Pollock will likely spend the rest of his life in prison, his plea "bargain" enabled prison officials to place him in a minimum security prison, making it easier for his family to visit.

Carlsbad, California (35 miles north of San Diego);
May, 2007:

My heart goes out to Tom and Hazel May, both deceased. I also wonder if Albert Pollock now lives with nightmares and guilt. How sad that the eight years between these events have passed without sufficient education of the public that physician-assisted suicide does not have to legalized to avoid "mercy killings," that dying from dehydration can be not only be comfortable but peaceful, and that it is possible to create strategic documents in the form of diligently crafted Advance Directives that can empower a future Proxy to withhold Food & Fluid to hasten dying even after the patient is no longer capable of making medical decisions (for example, in end-stage Alzheimer's dementia).

Practicing psychiatry for thirty-two years has convinced me that the greatest joy in life is to be heard and respected. This is especially true for needy and vulnerable patients in the last chapter of their lives, when their most fundamental values are at stake. This time is also the last opportunity for us to give kindness and understanding to our loved ones. That is why this book includes more than a legal, peaceful method for terminal patients like Hazel and Marie Yvonne. The goal of the stories and guidelines in this book is to explore ways to do everything possible to learn directly from patients, what they want—whether their wish is to maintain life-support for as long as possible, or to not waste limited medical and economic resources and to avoid unnecessary prolonged suffering and indignity.

When survivors can feel in their hearts that they have done everything they can to make their loved one's final transitions as peaceful as possible, then they need not feel guilt. In my clinical experience, it is when guilt is added to grief from loss that depression occurs.

Another way to prevent loved ones from experiencing years of guilt is to include a few words of "anticipatory kindness" in your Living Will or Proxy Directive. Consider for example, words like these that I included in my own Proxy Directive:

> "I know that asking you to make the decision to stop life-sustaining treatment will not be easy. If my mind could *magically* recover just long enough for me to fully consider my disease condition and my prognosis so I could then make my *own* decision before I returned to a state where I depend on you to see that others will carry out my wishes... it would be very difficult decision for me, too. How could I be sure I was making the right decision? I couldn't. How could I predict that researchers would not announce a cure, two months later? I couldn't. So all I ask of you is to make the best decision you can, with the information you have available. I appreciate that it is not possible to predict every possible situation and that it was *my* responsibility to fully discuss my wishes with you when I still could. So if you are not completely sure, I wish I could have been clearer."

It is always sad to lose a loved one. No one can predict with certainty how he or she will face the various challenges of her own last chapter. But dying need not be tragic. With knowledge and advance planning, our final transitions have the potential to be both meaningful and peaceful.

Chapter 1

A STRATEGY TO ATTAIN YOUR END-OF-LIFE GOALS
...WHETHER YOU WANT TECHNOLOGY TO MAINTAIN YOUR
LIFE, OR YOU WISH TO AVOID UNNECESSARY, PROLONGED
SUFFERING, AND DEPENDENCY AND INDIGNITY

Planning for Dying... the Modern Way

Advances in modern medicine have made it possible for more than seven out of ten of us to slowly die of a chronic illness over months or years. Four out of ten of us will depend on others for our care.

During this process, our mental ability may decline to the point where we can no longer speak for ourselves. Once we are incompetent, we can do nothing further to bring about the honoring of our Last Wishes.

Our fate will then depend upon the diligence of our advance care planning, on how clearly and convincingly we have expressed our wishes, and on how well we have chosen and how effectively we have empowered the right individuals to advocate those wishes.

No plan, or an inadequate plan, can result in months to years of personal suffering while litigation may tear our family apart.

This book explains how to maximize the chance that your Last Wishes, and those of your loved ones, will be honored in a legal and peaceful way.

Whether you believe that it is only in the province of God to determine when your biologic existence will end, or it is your wish to actively avoid unnecessary and prolonged end-of-life suffering and/or dependency on others if you lose your personal dignity, this book provides the clinical and legal background and then makes specific recommendations so that you can decide if you want to follow its suggested strategies to maximize the potential for your success.

In a word, this book is all about choice—YOUR choice—what you decide is *BEST* for you. Briefly, that is what the authors of this book mean by "best."

How can one book present strategies for people with divergent goals? Because the basic strategy to get others to honor your Last Wishes is the same, regardless of what you specifically want. While the book strives to present both sides of the major controversies in a balanced way, I permit myself to express my professional opinions as I offer specific advice based on my experience in psychiatry and end-of-life ethics. The presentation is further broadened by Ronald Baker Miller, M.D., a medical ethicist, and by Michael S. Evans, J.D., M.S.W., an attorney who is also a social worker. Still, the book strives to present more than our consensus of personal and professional beliefs. It also hopes to serve more than a useful guide for readers as they try to meet the challenges of the last chapter of their lives. The book suggests that readers view Advance Directives as *moral documents,* whose effect will have impact on society as a whole. It introduces a new concept, "The Sanctity of *MANY* Lives."

Why We Must Learn from Others

Dying is a unique process that each of us experiences only once.

Unlike other experiences in life, there is no way for us to learn from our own mistakes because there is no next time. So...

If we want to learn how to plan effectively, we must learn from others.

This book presents over fifty clinical stories and legal cases to help you decide what is **BEST** for you.

Few people are eager to deal with end-of-life issues. For reasons my parents might be able to explain if they were alive, I am one exception. My mind seems intrigued with solving a puzzle to extend the ability to control my destiny: What strategies can ensure that others will honor my present wishes after I can no longer express myself? Yet wouldn't many people want to know how to transcend a possible future state of incompetence so that they and their families could avoid years of suffering? If you are one who would like the answer, here it is—in three words: *diligent, strategic planning.*

Since 1999, I have written three books and established Peaceful Transitions®— an organization of diverse professionals whose goal is to make the process of dying more peaceful for families and patients, starting before they are hospice eligible. In 2004, I founded Caring Advocates, whose staff helps people create and implement Living Wills and Durable Powers of Attorney for Medical Decisions. The last few pages of this book (483-489) reveal my experience as well as my personal and professional beliefs about the last chapter of life.

I see much hope for the future. In the past, surveys revealed that only about one in five adults completed their Advance Directives. Yet Americans are becoming increasingly aware of the dire consequences of not making end-of-life plans. A recent survey by the National Academy of Elder Law Attorneys (announced by their web site before the surge of publicity from the case of Terri Schiavo) revealed that about a third of Americans between the ages of 35 to 49, and 43 percent between ages 50 and 64, have some form of an Advance Directive. To increase the willingness of young people to engage in advance planning, this book recommends NO Living Will for people who are medically well. It thus eliminates the morbid experience of having to learn about six to eight end-stage diseases in order to predict what medical treatment they would or would not want in the future—an awesome challenge. Healthy people need only to create a document that appoints another person to make medical decisions for them. But even this task must be done diligently. I suggest that the time for you to focus on what medical treatments you DO want, or do NOT want, is when your physician gives you a serious diagnosis.

Another area of hope is that Alzheimer's disease can be diagnosed years before symptoms emerge, which permits not only effective advance planning, but treatment with medications that may delay the onset as well as slow down the progression of symptoms.

With so many compelling reasons to start planning now, the question to answer is, how can we overcome our resistance to starting?

How Can You Transcend the Tendency to Avoid End-of-Life Planning?

If you are tentative about reading this book, or if you are not sure how you can dialogue with loved ones about their Last Wishes, consider the typical psychological reasons why we all resist dealing with these issues.

It is difficult to face mortality. It is also hard to accept the idea that someday you may no longer be capable of expressing yourself. Yet there is another way to look at the task of advance planning. Some years ago, I bought some life insurance. Every three months, as I write the check to pay the premium, I consciously enjoy writing the check and hope it will be a "waste" of money. Similarly, not everyone loses the ability to make medical decisions as their lives come to an end, but it is a comfort to have created an effective plan so that your life can end peacefully, just in case that plan is needed.

To overcome your mental obstacle to end-of-life planning, try to view the exercise in the abstract, as a problem that once solved will provide you with a bit of cognitive immortality. Effective planning allows you to transcend a possible future period of mental incompetence as you exert enduring control over your destiny, based on your life-long values and preferences.

Some people resist dealing with these issues because they are reluctant to discuss their end-of-life wishes with their close family members and friends. Yet such conversations often stimulate the airing of some fundamental values that are themselves worthy of discussion. I've facilitated family therapy sessions for almost three decades, and found that the conversations surrounding end-of-life issues often provide peak potential for healing and for strengthening relationships. Many families can discuss these issues without professional help. Few regret bringing the subject up. If your reason for not having these conversations is because you are unsure of what exactly to say, you are not alone. Several Guidelines in this book provide a series of suggested questions that cover the critical areas for discussion, step by step.

People from some cultures feel that if you think about death, you will bring it about. Actually, the proposed exercises require you to think about dying as a process, not death itself. In some ways it is like planning a long distance hiking trip. For success, you need a good map and the right equipment. Planning for the "last trip" of your life may not seem as enticing due to the uncertainty about its ultimate spiritual destination, yet the goal of planning is noble: to make the transition as peaceful as possible—both for yourself and for others who care about or love you.

When should you start planning? —As soon as you are old enough to drive a car. How often should you revise your documents? —Every time there is a major change in your life.

Although you cannot legally sign papers until you reach the age of majority (usually 18), you can still write down your wishes. Putting your wishes in writing has never been more important. It has always been hard to win arguments based on oral testimony, but now there is a movement to change State laws so that oral statements will have no effect if they relate to discontinuation of life-support. No one wants to put their family through the agony of public court battles which can last for years, as happened to Nancy Cruzan, Robert Wendland, Terri Schiavo, and dozens of other, less celebrated cases.

Anthony DeWitt suggested two possible "legislative fixes": require Advance Directives when renewing drivers' licenses and before issuing high school diplomas [reported by Buckley and others, 2004]. In July 2005, a law was sent to the Governor of Delaware so that drivers' licenses will have information about people's preferences for life support. In September 2005, a similar bill was introduced to the State Assembly of Wisconsin, where 100 comatose people whose wishes are unknown, are being kept alive at a cost of $6 million per year to the State (in addition to the Federal contribution to Medicaid) [previously linked to the Janesville, WI Gazette, 9-26-05]. Other States are considering new laws to inform all who apply for marriage licenses or divorces about Advance Directives [Asbury Park Press, 2005].

This book includes a fictional story [page 383], the basis for which I hope will become realistic: "She revised her Advance Directives from age 16 to 86." A woman I call "Joyce" lived in a State that hypothetically made the above changes in laws; Joyce responded by following the strategies that this book presents.

Disclaimers

General Legal Disclaimer

This publication is designed to provide information with the understanding that the author and the publisher are not engaged in rendering medical, legal, or other professional services by the sale of this book. If professional advice or assistance is required, readers should consult local experts in their respective fields. This product is not a substitute for medical or legal advice.

Other Disclaimers

First, regarding the use of the title's words **BEST WAY**, we distinguish between **what** and **how**. We readily admit that we do NOT know **what** is *best* for you. Instead, we hope that reading this book will help you decide what is *best* for you, and then show you **how**—the best *way* to achieve your goals. Success is defined as when others honor your Last Wishes.

Second, the authors and publisher of this book explicitly state that it is the responsibility of each reader to consult with qualified professionals for medical advice that meets the standard of care in his or her community, and for legal advice that complies with the laws of his or her State of residence, and which takes into account, his or her specific situations and goals, before the reader makes any medical or legal decision, or signs any document.

None of the information in this book is designed for minors, or for people with serious emotional disorders, or for use for illegal purposes.

Some suggestions in this book are designed for consideration by people who wish to avoid prolonging their dying process, but these suggestions are only directed to patients who are terminally ill or who suffer from an incurable progressive condition that will eventually lead to death, and none of these suggestions should be followed without first discussing them with the reader's personal physician.

Third, I have quoted facts, statements, and others' opinions to the best of my ability; but I suggest that you and your advisors refer to the original *legal citations and medical references* to form your own opinions before you take action. They are listed in alphabetical order near the end of the book. If you are listening to an audio version of this book, please request the printed list of relevant legal citations and medical articles, which will be sent to you by U.S. mail at the publisher's cost. You can also download and print this list for free, from the web site, www.BestGoodbye.com, under the LINK, Legal Citations & Medical References.

Fourth, most of the clinical stories are actually composites of more than one patient. There are two reasons: to illustrate several points with a single story, and to protect the confidentiality of patients and their families (in addition to altering possible identifying facts). Any remaining resemblance of characters to actual persons is purely coincidental.

Fifth, several stories in this book were written by others, and a few were contributed anonymously. Although we had no way to verify the accuracy of the events depicted, we included these stories for their instructive value. We humbly agree with the philosophy of Elie Wiesel, winner of the Nobel Peace Prize, who said, "Some stories are true, even if they never happened."

Sixth, since dying is by nature a difficult subject, we have included several humorous stories. One cartoon is funny; another is poignant, and two are political. If you might be among those people who find jokes inappropriate or offensive, you can easily skip them as they have a distinctive border and type font.

Seventh, I, Dr. Stan Terman, assume complete and sole responsibility for the content and the opinions expressed in this book. When the book uses the pronoun "we," it may refer to Dr. Terman and one or both of his coauthors; however it may also refer to all those who suffer from "the human condition." To distinguish between these different uses of the word, when it is important to be clear, the book will acknowledge where Michael S. Evans, J.D., M.S.W., and/or Ronald Baker Miller, M.D., provided significant input of content or of opinion.

Eighth, this book is not intended for children or their parents, who may face challenging end-of-life decisions. Many States have laws that require additional interventions on behalf of children because they are actually so vulnerable. Older, articulate children who can evaluate burdens versus benefits for themselves, and whose parents may or may not agree, can create complex ethical situations beyond the scope of this book. Specifically, readers should NOT generalize from these two stories: A) newspaper account of Sun Hudson, which makes no attempt to include all significant legal facts, and B) the semi-fictional account of "Yvette," which was based on personal communication from a parent, but intentionally omitted or changed identifying information and did not discuss any efforts to obtain advice from attorneys, ethics committees, or social agencies to further the child's best interests.

Ninth, the field of end-of-life ethics is characterized by controversy in a constantly changing landscape. We consider "**ethics**" as the field of intellectual inquiry that can help people deal with challenges to decide which social, moral, medical, legal, religious, or other right is "most right" in a given situation. Such rights are based on principles on which most people agree in general, yet when it comes to a specific case, polarities emerge as opponents present compelling arguments for why one "right" is more "right" than another "right." We believe it is essential to provide the ethical principles upon which this book's advice is based, and not merely provide a specific "bottom line" that may be currently applicable (depending on the State in which you reside). Specifics may change in unanticipated ways. Clinicians may develop new techniques and revise diagnostic criteria; legislators change laws; public morals change; judges change the interpretations of existing laws; religious leaders modify their edicts; and "experts" in the field of medical ethics change their minds. Quotation marks around the word "experts" humbly indicate that there are no "experts." Hence, we do not believe there is one ultimate human authority. Not only do professionals in the field of ethics typically disagree among themselves (including the three who contributed to the content of this book), they also change their minds. We personally know eminent professionals who reversed their opinions on legalizing physician-assisted suicide—in both directions.

Being with a loved one who suffered or who was at peace as his or her life came to a close can be an enlightening as well as emotional experience. Often, it leads to new insights. But there are few opportunities for us to experience such events directly. That is why this book offers a variety of stories. We hope you will be to learn and to identify with some of them.

Finally, although no one can guarantee success, if you follow the strategies in this book, the probability that your Last Wishes will be honored will increase—compared to using quick and easy standard forms for Advance Directives, or to relying on only oral statements, or to hoping that those who already know you will be successful in advocating your wishes if you never discussed your preferences with them or discussed them only in a casual way.

A Bonus

As you plan the last chapter of your life, you may be surprised to discover that it can be a creative process that offers much satisfaction. You may feel empowered from gaining control over your future. You might expand your view of the process by inviting serious inquiry into significant areas.

As you begin grappling with the legal and clinical details, you may discover that you are drawn into examining the emotional aspects of your relationships, the spiritual meaning of your life, and the ethical, moral, religious, cultural, and social implications of your decisions. You may find the exercise is a provocative opportunity to ponder philosophical and practical questions. For example, what is the essence of being human? Can we define minimum criteria that make life worth living? Should we accept all human life as sacred, or not so judge?

Does our concept of an after-life affect our choices for Last Wishes? Can faith in returning to our Maker lead us to yield more gracefully instead of fighting the inevitability of death by using modern medical technology? Should we take economic factors into consideration? How do we respond if relatives or patients demand expensive medical procedures or indefinitely prolonged treatment when the potential for recovering normal functioning is extremely low?

Many end-of-life decisions are appropriately shared; sometimes between the patient and his or her nuclear family; often between the patient and his or her physician. To understand and navigate through this complicated process, it is helpful to understand the roles and obligations of all parties. But for the most personal and private last event in your life, who should decide what is the **BEST WAY** for you to die? —Your doctors, your relatives, your religious leader, your insurance company, your attorney, someone else's attorney, an institution's ethics committee, a judge, a political leader... or you?

Who Will Find This Book Useful

- Any adult who wishes to plan effectively for the last chapter of life
- Patients challenged by a chronic or terminal illness
- Adult children concerned or worried about their parents
- Any person designated as a Proxy who must make life-determining decisions for another human being
- Attorneys, especially those involved in estate planning and elder-care law
- Physicians
- Psychologists and counselors
- Spiritual and religious leaders
- Social workers
- Nurses
- Hospice and palliative care personnel
- All who worry about the prolonged indignity of Alzheimer's disease
- Politicians and health policy makers

- Administrators of hospitals and long-term care facilities
- Those concerned with medical, life, or long-term care insurance
- Students intrigued by the subject of end-of-life bioethics
- Those willing to explore how to allocate scarce medical and financial resources in the future, especially when the cost increases with relatively little benefit

Planning for the Last Chapter of Life

Beyond reading this book, you are invited to both read and contribute to the online discussion board on www.CaringAdvocates.org. By exchanging stories about our experiences, we can all learn more successful paths to meet end-of-life challenges. Let's view the goal of making dying a peaceful process as a collaborative social experiment. First, we will all learn from the currently available information. Then we will formulate the **BEST** plan we can for our own futures and those of our loved ones. Those of us who survive will be in a position to learn how well our planning worked so that we can then share the results with others, who will in turn then be able to more effectively direct their course.

So... let the process of our community dialogue begin.

Chapter 2

YOUR LIVING WILL MAY FAIL,
YOUR PROXY MIGHT LET YOU DOWN, AND
THOSE WITH POWER MAY SABOTAGE YOUR LAST WISHES

Reject Any "15-Minute Solution"

The final chapter of your life is too important... the issues are too complicated... and the challenges are too awesome... especially in the current political and judicial climate... to rely on boilerplate forms whose virtues are quick, inexpensive, and "user friendly"—to achieve your important goals of having others honor your Last Wishes without challenges and litigation.

The highly politicized death of Terri Schiavo probably did more to increase the public's awareness of the importance of completing Living Wills and/or designating a Proxy than all previous educational efforts combined.

Yet when it comes to honoring your Last Wishes...

• The Living Will you filled out to indicate your health care preferences could fail;

• The person you designated to serve as your Proxy might let you down despite his or her best effort;

• A large cast of characters may wield their power to impose their own moral, personal, and religious values on you or your loved ones, thereby sabotaging the honoring of your Last Wishes.

Avoid Quick and Simple Forms to Prevent Years of Possible Suffering and Litigation

Completing such forms may let you feel now as if you have provided a written record of your Last Wishes, but remember: success will be determined in the future, when critical decisions must be made, and when you can no longer speak for yourself. That is when it will be critically important that the form you completed is unambiguous so it does not become a focus of controversy, that it empowers instead of limits your Proxy's authority to make the decisions you would have wanted.

Success is not hard to define—others will honor your Last Wishes—but sometimes, it is not easy to attain. The reality is that there is large cast of characters, including your relatives, doctors, religious leaders, politicians, administrators, and judges—any of whom may wield their power to prevent the honoring of your Last Wishes. (This book will illustrate some of their typical motivations and fears.) So, while some of these "quick and easy" forms are excellent ways *to begin* thinking about this challenging subject, be forewarned: they may fail miserably when you need them most, just when you can no longer express yourself. Some of the stories in this book document such disappointments. Even some "official forms" provided by the States are inadequate, depending on your specific goals. Before you place confidence in any form, learn its flaws and ask why it has not succeeded in the past. Then you will know why it is necessary to be more diligent.

You can modify and amend standard forms, which is prudent if your State requires using their exact form. Other forms, such as "Five Wishes," have been widely distributed and offer a way to express wishes other than medical treatment. Later in this book, I provide a detailed illustration on how you might feel it is necessary to modify "Five Wishes" to make it more likely that certain specific Last Wishes, such as the reduction of end-of-life pain, will be honored.

The tragedy of Terri Schiavo sent a clear warning about the dangers of inadequate planning. It can tear a family apart and force a patient to linger, to suffer, and to endure years of indignity. Headlines repeatedly stated that if only Terri Schiavo had taken a few minutes to sign some forms to indicate her treatment wishes and to designate her husband as her Proxy, then seven years of litigation over her fate would have been prevented. Is that really so?

Would Signing a Living Will and Designating a Proxy Have Prevented Litigation Over the Fate of Terri Schiavo?

—Not necessarily. Such a quick and simple solution may not have sufficed to quiet the powerful political forces that rallied to try to override her spouse's interpretation of her end-of-life wishes that transformed the controversy into a national debate. To explain...

First, consider what actually happened, as Terri had neither a written Living Will nor a formal Proxy designation:

On February 11, 2000, Judge George Greer ordered Terri's feeding tube removed after he determined at trial, that the evidence was *clear and convincing* that she would not want to live in her current state. The process of dying was expected to take between 7 and 14 days. As almost every knows, she died on March 31, 2005. That was 1877 days later.

Now consider this hypothetical: **SUPPOSE** that in 1989, when she was still competent, Terri had signed an Advance Directive that designated her husband as her Proxy, and that she had stated specifically that she would not want to prolong her existence on machines if she were in a **Permanent Vegetative State**.

THEN attorneys for Terri's parents could still have argued:

1. Yes, Terri (hypothetically) signed a document stating she would not want to be attached to machines if she were in a **Permanent Vegetative State (PVS)**. But we have an expert in neurology who believes she is in the **Minimally Conscious State (MCS)**, about which so little is known that no expert can rule-out the possibility that further treatment might bring about an improvement in her ability to function and communicate. She deserves to be given a trial of specialized treatment for MCS patients to see if she can improve. Florida law does not permit the withdrawal of life-sustaining treatment unless the patient is in a terminal state or in a **PVS**. As attorneys representing the parents of Terri Schiavo, we argue that Terri is neither terminal nor **PVS**.

2. Yes, Terri (hypothetically) signed a document that named her husband Michael as her designated legal Proxy. In his role as her fiduciary, however, Michael Schiavo is bound to uphold Terri's Constitutional right to life by approving routine medical measures to keep her alive until it is clear that all possible life-sustaining measures have been attempted and have failed to provide her a benefit since they opposed his wish to withdraw the feeding tube.

3. Yes, Terri (hypothetically) signed a document that she would not want her life to be prolonged indefinitely under certain conditions. We have argued that the conditions stated in her document have not been met (See Point #1, above). Even if the court were to find that the conditions of her Advance Directive were

fulfilled, the court should consider that Terri would change her mind now if she were conscious since in March 2004, the late Pope John Paul II issued an Allocution that the removal of a feeding tube from patients in the vegetative state is "euthanasia by omission" and therefore a mortal sin. Terri was brought up Catholic, and she practiced her religion, so the Pope's statement would have influenced her to remain alive by having her feeding tube maintained.

4. Michael Schiavo, who as fiduciary must put Terri's interests above his own, is now living with another woman with whom he has fathered two children. Although he denies it, he stands to inherit the balance remaining from $700,000 awarded in her malpractice case settlement. Even if it were proved that he has no monetary incentive, his own interests would naturally favor relieving himself of the burden of overseeing her care. He therefore has a conflict of interest, and the court must realize that he has the awesome power to make a life or death decision. The State has an obligation to protect the weak and vulnerable. Therefore Michael's actions should be reviewed (again) by an independent court-appointed Guardian *Ad Litem* and if it is determined that Michael's decision is not in Terri's best interests, then he should be removed as her legal spokesman.

5. Florida law grants a spouse the highest priority for selection as the court-appointed Proxy to make decisions for an incompetent patient. But this is based on the spouse's presumed interest in the marital partner. And the spouse is not the only person with an interest in a helpless patient; a spouse's interest is not exclusive. The parents of Terri also have an interest that deserves recognition under the U.S. and Florida Constitutions. To eliminate the parents from participation in this decision violates due process protected by both Federal and State Constitutions. Therefore the court must provide a means for the parents—***notice and opportunity to present opposing evidence***—for the parents to prevent Michael from making an irreversible decision that would end all possibility of Terri's further recovery.

Would these arguments have prevailed in the courts? Perhaps not. Several State and Federal courts ruled against Terri's parents when they begged to be given permission to be responsible for her care. Many religious people felt that the judges were more concerned about the letter of the law than the "***sanctity*** of life," by which term they meant whatever the condition of the person, respect for human "life" is absolute as long as medical technology can sustain basic bodily functions.

"The problem with our legal system."

Six days before Terri Schiavo died, the Wall Street Journal *Review and Outlook* Section printed, "The problem here is a legal system that makes it extremely difficult for any appeals court to overturn a trial judge's finding of fact unless there has been an egregious procedural or legal error. Once Judge Greer ruled that Terri's husband Michael showed *clear and convincing* evidence that his wife did not want to be kept alive artificially, her fate was probably sealed... .

"But the biggest failing of our legal system is that it could not accommodate the most humane outcome—to return Terri to the care of her parents and siblings, who [were] willing to provide for her... .

"How can it be morally responsible to let a woman die when there [were] family members pleading to take on the burden of caring for her?"

Deputy Editor of The Wall Street Journal, Daniel Henninger, wrote, "The most morally reprehensible act in this whole drama has been [Judge George Greer's] refusal to simply turn Terri over to her poor mother, whose connection to her child-like daughter is more authentic and earned than anything that existed between Terri and Michael Schiavo."

The National Right to Life Committee provides forms and advice on Will-to-Live Directives. All the offered treatment choices will preserve any sign of life, except that a person can choose whether or not to take enough medication to decrease pain, even if doing so might hasten dying. The alternative is to suffer more and longer, hoping the process will increase the probability of salvation.

In the past, people with such goals could merely avoid signing a Living Will since its original purpose was solely to limit treatment, and they could assume that doctors would always preserve life. But there is an increasing trend for ethics committees to support doctors' orders when their opinion is that it is **futile** to continue treatment—even when the family wants to continue treatment. The ethical argument need not be based on comparing the patient's suffering *versus* his or her potential for meaningful recovery. The decision to withdraw life-sustaining treatment may be based on the burden to society's limited resources. To continue life-sustaining treatment, the only recourses are to transfer the patient to another facility, or to obtain a restraining order from the court, both of which can fail, as in the following examples.

In April 2005, critically ill 5 month-old Sun Hudson was taken off life-support and allowed to die over the objections of his mother. This action was legal in Texas because of a law that then Governor George W. Bush had signed. The 1999 "Texas Futile Care [Treatment] Law" [Health and Safety Code sec. 166.046] permits hospitals to withdraw life support within 10 days, if there is no hope of survival, regardless of the family's wishes. [Please see Disclaimer 8, in Chapter 1.]

This is not an isolated Texas case. In December, 2005, Ms. Tirhas Habtegiris, a 27 year-old woman suffering from incurable cancer was removed from life-support, although she wanted to live long enough for a last visit with her mother, who was in East Africa. Still, after 10 days notice, her ventilator was turned off since the clinical consensus was that further treatment was "inappropriate."

In the darkness of this case, economists Steven Landsburg and Robert Frank debated the meanings of "compassion." Dr. Landsburg argued that the poor should be permitted to choose what they want, which would be milk and eggs rather than ventilator insurance (estimated at $75 per year) [2006]. Dr. Frank countered, "In the wealthiest nation on earth, a genuine cost-benefit test would never dictate unplugging a fully conscious, responsive patient from life support against her objections" [2006].

There are significant differences between Ms. Schiavo and Ms. Habtegiris. Ms. Schiavo had Medicaid health insurance, was a white American, and was raised Catholic. She could live indefinitely with tube feeding so activist organizations considered it worthwhile "investing" in her case; for example, fees from the Christian Law Association to the attorneys who represented the parents were $1.9 million in 2003, alone ["Schedule A, Form 990" appears on *Page* 235 in Eisenberg, 2005]. Litigation transformed her case into a cause célèbre. In contrast, Ms. Habtegiris was a terminally ill, uninsured, black legal immigrant. Yet **compassionate** clinical **care** would have granted Ms. Habtegiris' last request to sustain her life until she could die in her mother's arms, even if continued aggressive **treatment** was deemed "**futile**." A final visit could be meaningful for family members even if the patient were unconscious, according to Dr. Larry Schneiderman [1995], a bioethicist who supports the denial of "futile treatment" but still emphasizes that **compassionate care** should never cease.

Was there any way that Terri Schiavo's parents could have prevailed to sustain her life? Yes! If back in 1989, newly-wed Terri had appointed her parents as her Proxies in a written document. Empowering her parents to make current decisions for her would have allowed them to take into account the Pope's Allocution of 2004 (not providing tube feeding is "euthanasia by omission"). To successfully meet challenges from her husband or others, Terri should have also *clearly and convincingly* explained the reasons for her end-of-life wishes in writing. For example, she could have written that she wanted to be an observant Catholic by preserving "the *sanctity* of her life" and defined what that meant to her: to wait until her God decided to take her home to Heaven after receiving all available modern technology. Had Terri designated her parents and written such statements, she might still be alive today, and her parents might be taking care of her in peaceful privacy. —That is, as long as her Medicaid insurance and the treating facility did not consider her treatment futile.

So... if you want to make sure that your Last Wish to maintain your life will be honored, learn what the potential challenges are, designate Proxies you can trust to vehemently advocate your wishes, and empower them by creating an Advance Directive document with statements that clearly and convincingly state, and then explain, what you want and why you want it.

The Other Side: "To Delay" is "To Deny"

Michael Schiavo and those who supported him repeatedly complained, as in this statement made by his attorney, Mr. George Felos: "To permit endless stays for endless appeals is simply a miscarriage of justice." In other words, **To Delay** is **To Deny** the honoring of Terri's Last Wishes.

The saga of Terri Schiavo included legislators of Florida and then of Congress who hurriedly passed laws that many thought were obviously unconstitutional when first proposed. The courts agreed. Many thought that submitting numerous legal appeals with virtually no chance of success were simply delay tactics. If Terri really did not want to be maintained in her present state, then the title of Al Neuharth's editorial of October 8, 2004 in *USA Today* was appropriate: "Torture of Terri is cruel and inhumane."

The original judge heard three witnesses relate seven conversations about what Terri wanted and then ruled the evidence met the high legal standard called *clear and convincing*. Yet it took five more years of litigation, and withdrawing her feeding tube three times to honor her Last Wish. Meanwhile, outspoken opponents called her husband/guardian an abuser, an adulterer, and a murderer. Threats were made on his life. He received little credit for refusing two separate million-dollar bribes to let her parents keep her alive. Others, including Governor Jeb Bush, repeatedly brought up the possibility of spousal abuse, which had no merit. Many refused to believe there was no money left after medical care and legal fees, and doubted Michael's sincere feeling of obligation to keep his promise to his wife whom he still loved.

Our democratic society should value highly, the ethical principle of **autonomy**—that each person has the right to determine what happens to his or her body—and that their wishes should be durable. Yet some people on the religious right feel they can judge whether the choices of others are "good."

"Take back that bad promise!"

On his television show the day that Terri Schiavo's feeding tube was removed for the third and last time, Larry King asked Pastor John MacArthur of Grace Community Church to assume for a moment that

Terri did in fact ask her husband to promise not to let her live in this state. Then Mr. King posed, "What do you morally owe someone after you've made that promise?"

Without any hesitation, Pastor MacArthur responded, "It's a bad promise. You've got to take that one back. The Bible says you can't take a life. God says, 'I give life and I take life. I am the Lord.'"

When Mr. King asked, "Therefore you're against capital punishment?" Pastor MacArthur replied, "Oh no. God specifically delegated that to society in the scriptures very clearly. Everything else beyond that constitutes murder."

Threats came from several sources. Randall Terry, founder of the organization, Operation Rescue, shouted outside of Terri Schiavo's hospice, "There will be hell to pay if Terri Schiavo dies." After she died, Congressman Thomas DeLay said, "We will look at an arrogant, out of control, unaccountable judiciary that thumbed their noses at the Congress and the President when given jurisdiction to hear this case anew and look at all the facts ... The time will come for the men responsible for this to answer for their behavior."

Democrats, including Senator Edward Kennedy, criticized Thomas DeLay's remarks and warned that his words could incite violence against judges. DeLay apologized, but only for the way he said it: "I said something in an inartful [sic] way. I am sorry I said it that way."

Public sympathy for Terri increased through TV clips. One shown repeatedly had Terri looking lovingly at her mother. Almost no TV anchorperson warned viewers that these video clips represented a few edited minutes selected from many hours of videotaping Terri's behavior, and hence were *not* representative of her overall behavior or her neurological examinations. While it appeared that Terri looked at and then smiled at her mother, the autopsy results released weeks later indicated that Terri was blind based on the degeneration of those areas of the brain related to the function of vision. So smiles at her mother were merely random reflexes.

Polls taken just before Terri's feeding tube was removed for the last time showed that 87% of those responding would not want to exist in a state similar to hers. The relevance of such polls is that one way to decide what is in a person's "BEST INTEREST" is to consider what most people would want in that situation. But the wishes of those people who WOULD want to exist in that condition should also be respected.

ᔥ*SKIP*   (*Explained on* page 4.)

In 2002, Dr. Fried and coworkers surveyed 226 persons who were 60 years or older and whose life expectancy was limited due to cancer, congestive heart failure, or chronic obstructive pulmonary disease. Survey questions presented different combinations of benefits and burdens. People chose treatment if they could expect the benefit of restoration of function, even if the burdens of treatment were high (89%); however nine out of ten people would *not* choose treatment and would accept death—if they would be left with severe impairment in their ability to think.

In August 2005, the Florida State Guardianship Association bestowed its Guardian of the Year Award on Michael Schiavo for carrying out his wife's wishes not to be kept alive artificially. "His unwavering commitment to honoring his wife's wishes in the face of public scrutiny and enmity embodied the professionalism and compassion with which court-appointed guardians quietly carry out their duties every day." University of Miami bioethicist Kenneth Goodman said, "What he said his wife wanted is what most reasonable people want. It's primitive to believe that human consciousness is not important. What most of us value about life is cognition and communication and interaction. We don't value simply not being dead." [Bell, 2005.]

If there had been no sworn testimony about what Terri wanted, even if there were no evidence to the contrary, courts in the U.S. cannot assume that her wishes were similar to the overwhelming majority of competent people: that she would not want to exist in a state of complete unawareness. Judges are reluctant to make the ultimate decision, even when the patient seems to be suffering. In the case of Ms. Schiavo, there was a question regarding her religious observance. Some witnesses testified that Terri did not go to confession or take communion in her last year of conscious life.

To avoid prolonging her existence against her wishes for fifteen years, without knowing in advance what future challenges might thwart her Proxy, Terri would need to designate people as her Proxies whom she could trust to vehemently advocate her wishes with medical decision-makers and others. In addition to informing these Proxies of her wishes, she would need to empower them by supplementing her Proxy Directive with a statement that clearly and convincingly explained what treatment she wanted and why.

❧ *CONTINUE*   (*Explained on* page 4.)

Regardless of your beliefs and goals then, the strategy is the exactly the same: Learn enough about the law and about the motivations of those who may challenge your wishes; then create an effective document to empower the Proxies you trust so that your Last Wishes will be honored. This book presents the details of how to accomplish this.

Fear is the most motivating of all emotions. For example, one component of the unpleasant experience we call pain, is the fear of more intense pain and the fear that the pain will not end. So let me again acknowledge what I learned at an early age from my mother: "Death is not something anyone need be afraid of. It is peaceful. What I fear is suffering a long time before I die."

For over two-thirds of us, we have reason to fear two kinds of dying. Usually, it will be one or the other, but some people unfortunately make the transition from one to the other, as illustrated in the following story. But first, the fears:

Our "Two Greatest Fears" are How We Die

• If our brains have been so devastated by dementia or trauma that we are not aware of our environment and cannot respond to others, we fear being forced to exist in a prolonged state of total dependence and indignity; and,

• If our brains are intact, but there is no hope our bodies will ever function normally, then we fear being forced to endure unnecessary unbearable and prolonged pain and suffering.

Dementia is the global loss of intellect, memory, and personality without loss of consciousness [Clare, 1990]. Other definitions are in the Glossary [page 457].

The Pain Transition

Mr. Carole was a sophisticated, successful, and well-educated man of 74 when he received the diagnosis of cancer and the prognosis of dying in severe pain. He clearly expressed his resolve: "I want *no* heroics. When the pain gets unbearable and there is no hope that I will improve, please don't do anything to extend my existence beyond that point."

His widow told me what happened, two years later. "Towards the end, as his pain kept getting worse, he agreed to any procedure that would reduce the pain, such as radiation. And he never stopped asking for more medication. Amazing, isn't it? How strong his will to live was?"

Out of kindness, I did not share my thoughts with Mrs. Carole, but I did consider another, sad, interpretation for her husband's behavior. The very medications used to reduce unbearable pain can also devastate our brains. Poor Mr. Carole probably made the transition from one great fear, that of unbearable pain, to the other great fear, that of not being able to express his wishes. In about five to fifteen percent of patients, the only way to reduce all pain is total sedation.

By the time Mr. Carole's pain became so intense that the usual treatment no longer worked, his mental abilities had been reduced to a single request. At that point, he no longer had sufficient decision-making ability to make another request, one that he had not specifically asked for previously: *to hasten his dying*.

Perhaps neither Mr. Carole nor his wife knew there was a *legal, peaceful way* to hasten dying. Even if they had known, they might have had to overcome the challenges of others with power who could have denied or delayed the honoring of this end-of-life decision.

☙❧

Given the outcome of several court cases and much clinical experience, these additional fears must be added:

- Our Living Wills may fail. Our written health care treatment directives may be too specific to apply to our terminal condition, or so vague that they delay by opening prolonged argument. Or, our document may be impossible to find just when our doctors must make a critical decision. Or, our future new doctors may deliberately choose to ignore what we wrote if they believe that other factors are more important.

- Our designated Proxies may let us down despite their best efforts. They may not be available due to their own illness or death. Or, they may love us too much to make tough decisions. Or, they may not be well enough informed about medical or legal issues, or strong enough to meet the awesome challenges to achieve success as they argue with others to try to advocate our wishes.

- Our Living Wills and our designated Proxies may be deliberately sabotaged by relatives, religious leaders, and politicians who may not know us personally, who may not care about honoring our Last Wishes, but who are instead motivated by their own emotional, religious, or ambitious agendas. Some physicians may consciously or unconsciously impose their own personal, moral, or religious values on us. Other doctors may deny our wishes instead of taking a perceived risk to their licenses. Whatever their motivation or fears, this large cast of characters has the power to prioritize their interests instead of honoring our Last Wishes.

So... .

If Living Wills can fail...

If our designated surrogates and physicians can let us down... and

If others can wield their power...

What steps can we take to make sure that our Last Wishes will be honored?

To begin, let's consider the various meanings of the word *BEST*:

How to Define "Hoping for Your *BEST*"
When You Face Challenging End-of-Life Decisions

What does it mean to hope for the *BEST* at the end of life? And how reasonable is it to expect your hope will be fulfilled? If you become incompetent, the answer will depend on how well you expressed your wishes while you still had the capacity to make decisions. The less clearly you expressed yourself when you did your advance care planning, the less likely your wishes will be honored in the future. The statements below progress from the most clear and likely to be successful to the least clear and most problematical:

A. If you can still express your preferences regarding what you feel is *BEST* as you near the end of your life, you simply hope that others will have the patience to listen and then honor the wishes you express. Even if you have written a **Living Will** and designated a **Proxy**, as long as you retain decision-making capacity you can still change your mind about what treatments you want or do not want and which individuals you want to designate to speak for you, if you no longer can in the future.

Many couples are in the habit of letting one speak for the other. That tendency can become more pronounced if the less assertive one has a chronic illness that makes it harder or slower to speak, even if the patient can still think well. (Examples include strokes and Parkinson's disease.) When a decision can make the ultimate difference between life and death, it is essential to have as much patience as required to find out from the patient, not the spouse, what treatment that person wants or does not want.

B. What is *BEST* if you have lost the mental ability to make medical decisions? Designate an individual as your Proxy in your **Proxy Directive** (also called a **Durable Power of Attorney for Health Care**) and discuss your specific wishes and general values with them so you can have the realistic hope that they will succeed in the process of decision-making called SUBSTITUTED JUDGMENT, defined as knowing you well enough so that they will make the decisions you would have made. This process requires that your Proxies distinguish their values from yours, if there is a difference. Family members often make decisions for more treatment than you would want, sometimes because they do not want to lose you. A family member may have a moral or religious problem refusing treatment that you would want to refuse. Choose your Proxies carefully. If your physicians have given you a serious diagnosis, involve them in these discussions.

Note: A **Living Will**, which this book calls a **Directive to Physician**, was, in the past, touted to accomplish this goal, but there are many reasons why they have not been effective, and why this book will recommend instead, a strategic document called **Empowering Statements for My Proxy** for people who are healthy—all of which is detailed later.

C. If you wrote your treatment preferences for various mental and medical conditions ONLY in your **Living Will (Directive to Physician)**, you hope that your future physicians will interpret what you wrote correctly so they make decisions you would feel are *BEST*. Your physician must read this document, determine if it applies to your future condition, and then decide if the treatment you previously requested or refused is, in his or her opinion, appropriate. The **Living Will (Directive to Physician)** is NOT a self-enforcing document; it often needs a person who cares about you to make sure the document reaches the physician and to ensure that your physician will read and respect what you have written. (See the cartoon on page 251).

D. If you indicated your end-of-life wishes but only orally, you hope that the people to whom you spoke will accurately recall what you said, and that all concerned— including your Proxy, your loved ones, your doctors, your institution's administrators, politicians, legislators, your religious leader, and if necessary— courts of law—will agree on a decision that you would feel is *BEST*.

If you have orally stated your wishes to your physician, you hope that he or she has recorded them in your medical chart so that they will be legally binding and honored by all. In some States, that process is legally binding, yet not all physicians are aware of that, and you might need to ask your physician to make that important note. In case your physician neglects to make this important note—accurately, or at all—if there are no witnesses, it will be your word against his or hers. Actually, I have never heard of a patient ask the physician to read back what he has written—yet I consider this an essential part of process, comparable to finding two qualified witnesses or a notary public. Once read back, the patient should make this reasonable request: Make copies for those who care about me. (Note: The process of giving oral directions to your physician can also be used to revoke or change a previously written Advance Directive.)

E. If you indicate your wishes to non-professionals only orally, and there are disagreements among others regarding what you really wanted, you hope that a court of law will consider their testimony and ***promptly*** decide what is *BEST* for you rather than have litigation drag on for months to years.

F. If you have never spoken to anyone about your end-of-life wishes, let alone put anything in writing so that your relevant wishes are not known, you hope that others will decide what is *BEST* for you based on their knowledge of what "most reasonable people" would decide in similar situations that take into account your physician's opinion about your condition. Called the BEST INTEREST standard of decision-making, this is not as simple as referring to a recent survey. Frequently there is some tension between the State's interest to preserve life and your Liberty interest to refuse unwanted treatment, which cannot be resolved without reference to other specific factors that relate to your age, medical condition, quality of life, burdens and possible benefits of treatment, and your religion and other demographics. (But the more such factors are considered, the more the decision-making process sounds like Substituted Judgment.)

Two studies indicate that some patients prefer family members and physicians make decisions for them, than to follow their own individual preferences about resuscitation [reviewed by Puchalski and others, 2000]. If this is your preference, make sure your family members will be **available** (which requires that they outlive you), **able** (mentally capable of making medical decisions), and **willing** (since the moral burden can be high). Also indicate if you prefer your decision-maker to be one person, the majority of those concerned, or their choice be unanimous. (Note: both majority and unanimous requirements can be quite problematic, so I recommend neither).

☞ *SKIP*

Sometimes the decisions are dependent on the group of "most reasonable people" referred to, based on typical religious or political views:

Examples of Divergent "Best Interests"

Consider two hypothetical patients. Both are dependent on feeding tubes for nutrition and hydration, and both have a certain diagnosis of permanent Minimally Conscious State with no apparent discomfort. Neither left any indication, oral or written, about their personal end-of-life preferences. "Mr. C" is an observant Catholic who has always followed the teachings of the Pope. "Mr. L" has never been religious. He is a liberal who was formerly interested in such issues as feeding the hungry in Africa. With only this information, how would one guess what decision is in their respective BEST INTERESTS?

For Mr. C, one might assume that he would wish to follow Pope John Paul II's Allocution to maintain life.

For Mr. L, one might assume he would want to decrease how long he would be totally dependent and suffer continuing indignity.

Therefore, Mr. C's feeding tube would be indefinitely maintained, while the Mr. L's feeding tube would be promptly removed.

In some U.S. States, when there is no designated Proxy, there is an established hierarchy for sequencing the people who would make decisions for you. Often your spouse is first, then your parents or your adult children, then siblings, and then others. If you are not married to your domestic partner, in most States it will be crucial to have a written document that designates this person as your legally appointed Proxy, if that is your wish. In some European countries, the practice of medicine could be considered somewhat paternalistic by giving doctors the power to decide what is best for you ("doctor knows best").

✂ *CONTINUE*

The point is, unless you make the effort to specify exactly whom you want to speak for you, a great number of factors (some of which are unpredictable) will determine who will make your medical decisions, and what factors they will consider. In addition, some State laws impose restrictions on making certain kinds of end-of-life decisions; for example, in New York State, even a designated Proxy cannot make decisions about withdrawing tube feeding unless the supporting document grants this specific power.

"On what side should we err?"

Answer # 1: Base it on the patient's BEST INTEREST:

Arthur Caplan, Ph.D., Director of the Center for Bioethics at the University of Pennsylvania, emphasizes that the principles of bioethics require decision-makers to "err on the side of BEST INTEREST"; that is, what seems to be BEST for the patient, as guided by what most reasonable people would want under similar circumstances when there are no other guidelines to indicate what the patient would want.

Answer # 2: Always err on the side of (prolonging) LIFE:

President George W. Bush, when he referred to the "complex case" of Terri Schiavo, espoused the American "culture of life" and stated we should "always err on the side of life."

What's the right answer?

More importantly, how will others decide for you? And that depends on politics and religion, both of which may change between now, and when "that time comes." Many Catholics feel that Pope John Paul II reversed a 500-year tradition of weighing burdens and benefits based on considering the patient and his or her family. Some people feel the true political goal was designed to distract the public from the main event (the Iraq War) by inciting fear about threats from the "culture of death."

While science may advance so that some patients who previously seemed neurologically hopeless will improve after several years or decades. But should society maintain tens of thousands of patients for so many years, in the hope that a few might return to some degree of partial functioning while uninsured others go without basic care?

What's for sure?

Two things: Debate will continue, and **To Delay** is **To Deny**. So, if you want others to honor your end-of-life preferences promptly, it is more important now than ever for you to do your advance care planning— diligently and strategically.

Remember the old saw, "Be careful what you wish for"? We live in an era when we cannot joke about certain things in airports. Similarly, this is not a time for idle remarks about what you will want in terms of your end-of-life wishes. These issues require deep thought after careful consideration of the relevant information and focused discussions about your options with others, including your physician and other professionals.

Consider the remarks that Larry King made on his national TV show.

Larry King's Off-Handed "Living Will"

In discussing end-of-life issues after Terri Schiavo's tube was removed for the last time, Larry King voiced his "Living Will" on national TV: **"As long as I am not in pain, I want to be kept alive."**

I wonder if Mr. King considered a rare clinical state, one that is not painful, but which for him, might be even worse than death. The end stage of Lou Gehrig's disease, also called ALS, is the "locked-in" state, which leaves the mind fully functional, but due to complete paralysis, there is no way to communicate. Totally locked-in patients cannot even move their eyelids to blink once or twice, to indicate "Yes" or "No."

For a TV celebrity who admits how much he enjoys his "great gig" of interviewing people, would Mr. King really want to endure a decade or more of living, connected to a feeding tube and a ventilator—if he could no longer communicate? Even without pain, he might experience great suffering.

Mr. King, as he is now, might also dread a future of irreversible progressive dementia from Alzheimer's disease, even though its end-stage may also have no pain.

Further comments: Mr. King's expressed Living Will incorporated the ethical principles of **autonomy** and the **wish of no harm**. But he may have failed to consider the principle of **benefit**—what good comes from his painless existence—and if his continued existence would be fair to society, in accordance with the principle of **social justice** as he uses its resources.

Those who wish to respect "the **sanctity** of life"—by insisting on prolonging the existence of terminal patients as long as possible—may find the next point ironic: When people know they can exercise control over ending their lives without being forced to endure prolonged pain, suffering, indignity, or becoming a huge burden to others—they suffer less anxiety and worry—and they often enjoy more fully their final days to months. Having control to end their lives **earlier** empowers them to decide that what is **BEST** is to live **longer**.

In Oregon, where it is legal for competent people to end their lives with a prescription from their physician, patients often decide to live longer. Knowing this option is available lessens patients' anxiety so they can feel, "Life is a wonderful thing as long as I've got that string."

Important: Despite the last point, this book does NOT recommend the end-of-life option where physicians prescribe a lethal dose of medication as **BEST**, although a small number of people may prefer it. While the reasons are discussed later, this book favors the option of **Voluntary Refusal of Food & Fluid**, which has two main advantages: 1) many more people can use it, including patients with severe physical limitations and those who suffer from dementia, who could not qualify to receive a prescription under Oregon's Death With Dignity Act. 2) **Voluntarily Refusing Food & Fluid** is reversible; that is, patients who initially refuse sustenance can change their minds and resume intake to continue living.

This book has a comprehensive strategic plan that allows patients to control when their lives will end, if that is their choice. The plan can work for those afflicted with Alzheimer's disease and other dementias. The certainty of knowing that they can avoid years of institutionalization in a state of indignity, that they can trust they will die **when they want to** rather than **while they still can**, may ironically permit many patients to decide to live longer. This knowledge can prevent the tragedy of premature dying.

This book gives four examples of premature dying: Janet Adkins, at 54, might have chosen to live longer instead of becoming Kevorkian's first "patient," just three days after she played tennis with her son. Her story is called, "How much longer might she have enjoyed life?" Judge Robert Hammerman, at 76, might have enjoyed a few more years of life instead of shooting himself. His story is: "Many care about me—but none will take care of me." Bob Stern, the "Self-Made Man," shot himself because he could not trust any family member to terminate his existence if his surgery went poorly. Myrna Lebov allowed her husband to poison her, yet she had just enjoyed an evening at the Cirque du Soleil. (Her story is in the Epilogue.) The point is that each of these people, and many thousands like them, could have lived and enjoyed much more of life, had they been assured that they would not have to live with suffering or indignity.

A method to reduce the duration of demented patients' suffering may have enormous social benefit. Only about three-dozen people used pills to hasten their deaths in Oregon in 2004, although several times that number may have benefited just from knowing the option was available. This number is still small compared to those who suffer from the permanent vegetative state—between 16,000 and 25,000 in America (although some estimates are higher), which is, in turn, small compared to the number who suffer from dementia—now almost five million. Worse, this number is expected to increase three- to four-fold by 2050, unless a cure for Alzheimer's is found.

Without changes in the policy and practice of forced-feeding and tube feeding patients in end-stage dementia, Medicare will most likely be bankrupt years before Social Security, and the needs of an increasing number of such patients will exceed the emotional and energy resources of fewer available workers and caregivers. Someday, society may not be able to sustain this huge burden of unprecedented proportions. How huge? The present annual cost of dementia is about twenty times that of maintaining people in the vegetative state [practical bioethics.org, 2004]. If this increases three times, as predicted, society's resources may not allow us to maintain the lives of the many millions of people in end-stage dementia who have no hope of ever knowing who they are and who have no hope of ever recognizing their loved ones. Unlike the extremely rare patient who comes out of a post-traumatic coma after ten or twenty years, that never happens with irreversible, progressive dementias, as long as the initial diagnosis was correct.

Important: While this book does NOT recommend that patients with impending dementia should terminate their existence if or when their dementia becomes severe, it does describe in detail why people might consider that choice. It sets forth the known and potential hurdles to accomplish this goal and strategic ways to be successful. The book presents the markedly different position of The President's Council on Bioethics' report, "Taking Care: Ethical Caregiving in Our Aging Society," but concludes with the theme, "The Sanctity of *MANY* Lives."

SKIP

Given the several meanings to the word ***BEST*** in the discourse above, some readers may be surprised to see the singular phrase in the subtitle: **A Legal Peaceful Choice**. The reason is that this book focuses on **Voluntary Refusal of Food & Fluid**, which is legal everywhere. Prior to the Terri Schiavo tragedy, this method of dying was not frequently discussed. Yet people often died this way before the current era of modern medicine. Today, technology can sustain biologic existence almost indefinitely. But many lay and professional people under-appreciate and misunderstand, and some opponents further their own agendas by intentionally misrepresenting it.

There are other ways to avoid prolonging unnecessary suffering, but they are either *not peaceful* or *not legal*. It was legal for Robert Hammerman to shoot himself in the chest, but it was not peaceful. For more than 50 years, it has not been illegal for a person in America to attempt suicide or to succeed in that attempt. But assisting a suicide is a different matter.

Providing an overdose of sleeping pills may lead to a peaceful death, but it is illegal to prescribe it except in Oregon and in three European countries (and then, only if the patient meets strict criteria and the data follows specific protocol). This book compares physician-assisted suicide and other methods to hasten dying to **Voluntary Refusal of Food & Fluid**. It also considers the worry that people with disabilities and others have over the slippery slope (a fear that the weak and vulnerable in our society could be encouraged or even forced to end their lives before they want to). The U.S. Supreme Court ruled in favor of Oregon in January, 2006. While the U.S. Attorney General cannot punish physicians in Oregon who comply with that State's Death With Dignity Act, polarization continues. One side is introducing bills to restrict end-of-life options as the other is introducing bills similar to Oregon's in other States. The debate, and the challenges, continue.

✒ *CONTINUE*

The option of **Voluntary Refusal of Food & Fluid** is a kingpin in making end-of-life decisions. If you are competent and you can make the decision to **Refuse Food & Fluid**, it will be easier for you to make choices about other, less symbolic life-sustaining treatments. These include such treatments as ventilator support, cardio-pulmonary resuscitation, antibiotic treatment, blood transfusions, radiation surgery, and dialysis for kidney failure. If you have planned for your Proxy to make this decision for you by discussing what end point you would choose if you became incompetent, and your Proxy knows how to argue persuasively for **Voluntary Refusal of Food & Fluid**, it should be relatively easy to achieve success in honoring your other preferences for end-of-life treatment.

Challenging Topics This Book Covers

1.   Although some popular and official State-approved **Living Wills** may give you peace of mind now, they may ultimately fail to achieve the goal of having others honor your Last Wishes.

2.   Your designated **Proxy** (Durable Power of Attorney for Health care) may—despite the best of efforts—fail to overcome outside challenges to honoring your Last Wishes.

3.   A large cast of characters, including some who mean well, can raise serious obstacles your Last Wishes.

4.   **To Delay** is **To Deny** your Last Wishes, but you can take steps now so that you and your family can avoid legal battles in court. (Note: Even if family members are united, intense battles can occur between a family and the government.)

5.   A simple addition to your Living Will can greatly increase the chance that your physician will recognize its written directives. A simple form that your Proxy can sign can greatly increase his or her standing to speak for you and advocate your Last Wishes.

6.   Written examples and reasons explaining your Last Wishes will empower your Proxies to make it more likely that others will honor the medical decisions they make on your behalf.

7.   Life's greatest irony is: "When people can feel assured that they can die *earlier*, they often choose to live *longer*"; and is worth understanding in psychological depth.

8.   You need not use illegal means, pass new laws, or commit acts of violence to avoid prolonged unbearable pain and suffering.

9.   You can die *when you want to* rather than *when you can*. You need not die prematurely if your prognosis is a dramatic decline in mental ability from Alzheimer's disease or related dementias.

10.   **Voluntary Refusal of Food & Fluid** can be seen as a way of letting Nature take its course.

11.   There are steps you can take to prevent others from sabotaging your Last Wish after you fall unconscious.

12.   There are steps you can take to prevent Emergency Medical Technicians from attempting unwanted resuscitations.

13.   Patients recently diagnosed with possible Alzheimer's disease may still be mentally capable of creating Advance Directives; however, a professional must assess their mental abilities at that time, which may be urgent.

14.   A series of Yes/No questions can indicate whether severely brain damaged patients are aware of their environment, and if they want to continue life-sustaining treatment.

15.   Conflicts can arise between what your Proxy decides currently for your end-of-life medical treatment, and your written Living Will (as others interpret it). Depending on your situation and whom you trust, you may decide which to prioritize ahead of time.

16.   Doctors can make family members and Proxies feel more guilty, or less guilty as they ask them to make end-of-life decisions.

17.   The ideal qualities of a Proxy: someone you trust will be objective, assertive, articulate, and knows or can learn about the legal and health care systems to effectively advocate your Last Wishes.

18.   There are places where you can turn, if you cannot identify an individual and alternates to be your Proxies.

19.   **Voluntary Refusal of Food & Fluid** is consistent with the morals of many people and their religious beliefs.

20.   **Voluntary Refusal of Food & Fluid** is generally comfortable.

21.   For certain types of patients, **Refusal of Food & Fluid** is not recommended.

22.   You can change your mind after you begin to **Voluntarily Refuse Food & Fluid**, which is a great advantage of this option.

23.   Explained: the differences between **Voluntary Refusal of Food & Fluid**... and Terminal Sedation, Physician-Assisted Suicide, Self-Deliverance, and Euthanasia.

24.   Documented: **Voluntary Refusal of Food & Fluid** can be peaceful and healing for families who are losing their loved ones.

25.   Exemplified: Revise Advance Directives as you age and mature, as your situation changes, or as laws or policies change.

26.   Case in point: Change your Advance Directives based on the publication of the President's Council on Bioethics report, "Taking Care: Ethical Caregiving in an Aging Society."

27.   View: Our Advance Directives are "moral documents." As we think deeply about what constitutes personhood, we can ask that future decisions about prolonging our existence consider the *sanctity of many lives.*

Chapter 3

WHY YOU WANT TO STAY OUT OF COURT, AND HOW

Our Ultimate Right to Decide What Happens to Our Bodies

Any adult whose judgment is not disturbed by mental illness may refuse any medical treatment—even if such refusal hastens dying.

Incompetent patients have *similar* rights except that their decisions must be made by their legally designated Proxies; however their decisions must meet Federal and State Constitutional *protections* for the "right to life."

The right to refuse treatment was affirmed as a "Liberty interest" in the U.S. Supreme Court case of Nancy Beth Cruzan [1990]. "Liberty interests" are not absolute, however. As reflected in Federal and State legislation, and in precedents set by appeal cases, they are subject to competing values, such as the government's duty to preserve life. If your end-of-life request is litigated, the courts must conduct a complex analysis to balance their interpretation of your stated interests with the competing principle to protect life. The weighing process may require many hearings over many months or years before the court makes its final decision. **To Delay** can be tantamount **To Deny**. The final decisions in many courts may not reflect what patients really wanted for several reasons.

The Courts Can Set Legal Precedents—Years Before Clinicians Reach a Consensus of Opinion

Neurologists reached consensus in defining the Minimally Conscious State (**MCS**) and distinguished it from the Permanent Vegetative State (**PVS**) only in 2002 [Dr. Giacino and others]. Yet courts of law denied the Last Wishes expressed by lay people in the MCS who had earlier expressed only that they "would not want to live like a vegetable." Consider these two legal cases:

"Vegetative" Versus "Vegetable"

The Cases of Michael Martin and Robert Wendland

Michael Martin's wife testified in a Michigan court proceeding to determine whether to continue his life-prolonging treatment. She claimed that her husband had stated he could not tolerate disability and would rather die than be dependent on people and machines. Two co-workers testified that before his accident, Martin told them he would not want to continue living "like a vegetable." He also asked his wife to promise he would not be put "on machines" in reaction to movies that depicted persons who were vegetative or had terminal illnesses and could not care for themselves. But his request was only oral.

The Michigan judges ruled, "Only when the patient's prior statements clearly illustrate a serious, well thought out, consistent decision to refuse treatment under these exact circumstances, or circumstances highly similar to the current situation, should treatment be refused or withdrawn." [In re Martin (1995) 450 Mich. 204 [538 N.W.2d 399, 409-411.]]

Similarly, in the California case of Robert Wendland, the judges of the State Supreme Court considered the statement Wendland made before his accident, "I wouldn't want to live like a vegetable." The judges were concerned that permitting refusal of treatment would "create a serious risk that the law would be unconstitutionally applied in some cases, with grave injury to [the] fundamental right [to life]."

The California judges cited the Michigan standard from the Martin case, and also pointed out the use of the word "vegetable" did not refer to the **Minimally Conscious State** since Robert Wendland did not use those words to describe his ultimate condition, when he expressed his wishes orally. They insisted his words would apply only to the **Permanent Vegetative State**. The judges thus set a precedent to keep similar **MCS** patients alive even though they might be aware enough to experience suffering [Conservatorship of Wendland (2001) 26 C4th 519; 28 P3d 151].

ॐ *SKIP*

The rulings of the Michigan and California courts assumed that these two men were aware of the difference between the **Permanent Vegetative State** ("being a vegetable") and the **Minimally Conscious State** (although the judges did not use this diagnostic term). These men had expressed their wishes orally but consistently; clearly, but without discussing the specific details with their doctors. Yet even if they had discussed their wishes with a specialist in neurology, it is unlikely that, in the early 1990's, they would have written or expressed their wishes in terms specific enough to meet the courts' criteria. Why? Because it was not until 2002 that medical leaders in this field published a *consensus description* of the **Minimally Conscious State**. Note: The preferred standard to describe an illness is called "**clinical evidence**." However after a group of experts who knew most about this condition spent several years of reviewing and discussing the relevant clinical data, they were still unable to establish criteria for **MCS** using the "clinical evidence" standard. Hence, the article by Dr. Giacino and others [2002] had to resort to a lower standard of clinical description called "consensus." Even in 2005, my informal survey (which will be the subject of future research), showed that few doctors and almost no Advance Directives made this important distinction. Misinformation about the categories of brain damage is rampant; for example, many newspaper reports incorrectly referred to Terri Schiavo's condition as "brain dead."

෨෧

We must ask: if several years of clinical discussion left experts just beginning to distinguish between **PVS** and **MCS**, why did the courts rule *post facto*—as if these lay patients had specified one state but excluded the other?

One possible reason is that judges are human and they were afraid to make a decision that would cause the death of a patient who seemed somewhat conscious at times. Consider what the judges in the Wendland case wrote:

"Certainly it is possible, as the conservator here urges, that an incompetent and uncommunicative but conscious conservatee [Robert, in the Minimally Conscious State] might perceive the efforts to keep him alive as **unwanted intrusion** and the **withdrawal of those efforts as welcome release. But the decision to treat is reversible. The decision to withdraw treatment is not**." And in the Martin case in Michigan, the judges wrote, "If we are to err, however, we must err in preserving life."

So judges in both cases felt it was safer to prolong the patients' existence even if doing so would also prolong their suffering. Too often, the system of justice prolongs existence through the extraordinarily lengthy process of litigation itself.

In the United States, in the absence of clear written documentation to indicate otherwise, doctors will often offer resuscitation and use high-technology medical treatment to prolong your existence—even if your suffering is unbearable and such treatment provides virtually no hope of benefit.

Most medical professionals have no clue about the critical legal implications of distinguishing between **PVS** and **MCS**; and most legal professionals are not aware of the criteria that distinguishes these two clinical states. Yet judges, when asked, must rule. So the lesson is clear: If you do not want your fate determined by a judge, you must be diligent about creating your Advance Directives.

✐ CONTINUE

How common is the **Minimally Conscious State**? Neurologists often emphasize causation, however if we step back from traumatic causes of brain dysfunction and focus instead on behavioral features, then we can heed Dr. Joanne Lynn's warning: "Very severe dementia will become a major cause of the minimally conscious state" [practical bioethics.org, 2004]. Dementia affects 47% of people over the age of 85 [Evans and others, 1989], and the total number of aging baby boomers will increase dramatically. So **MCS** will soon become much more common. Patients in advanced dementia will soon number in the millions, dwarfing the tens of thousands of patients currently in vegetative states.

Can you prepare a Living Will to use in the future, if the "experts" in the field create new definitions of new diagnoses? Even the most diligent attempts may fail. You can pursue two directions: Write a behavioral description of the state for which you would no longer want treatment that is not dependent on a specific diagnosis. (Some examples are given later in this book.) The alternative is to use a **Proxy Directive** to empower your Proxy to make medical decisions on your behalf based on your current condition, however defined, when such decisions must be made. But first you must inform your Proxy about your general values and wishes. Would that be foolproof? Unfortunately, no. Interested parties may still petition the court to hear their arguments that your Proxy is not acting in your BEST INTEREST. So you may choose to take two additional steps. First, provide your Proxy with another document that clearly and convincingly supports your wishes. (Later, I provide more specifics on **Empowering Statements for My Proxy**.) Second, consider signing specific documents with your attorney to prevent your case from ever being reviewed in court. The motivation to take all these steps comes from cases such as the following:

What Should We Learn from Jean Elbaum's Case?

For sixty years, Mrs. Jean Elbaum was medically well. Then she suffered a stroke at her Long Island home. For long-term care, she was eventually transferred to Grace Plaza, a skilled nursing facility in Great Neck, New York. According to her husband and children, she had previously expressed her wish that if she were in a "vegetative like state," she would not want to be kept alive by a ventilator like the then celebrated legal case of Karen Ann Quinlan. Jean Elbaum also said that she did not want to be given antibiotics and tube feeding as her own mother had, who then died slowly from terminal cancer. After Mrs. Elbaum extracted promises from her husband and other family members to honor her wishes, the whole family was united in this commitment.

Three years later, however, to keep their promise, her family members had to testify to all these facts in court.

After Mrs. Elbaum arrived at the skilled nursing facility, her doctors changed her diagnosis to Permanent Vegetative State. To fulfill his promise, her husband requested that her feeding tube be removed. But the Grace Plaza administrator refused, even though all family members consistently and desperately requested the tube be removed. One month after her admission, an anguished Mr. Elbaum warned the nursing home administrator that he would refuse to pay for continuing treatment that his wife definitely did not want.

When Mr. Elbaum tried to transfer his wife to another facility, the administrator blocked his request, explaining that he was not certain if Mr. Elbaum had legal authority to speak for his wife. An unstated but likely reason that the administrator blocked the transfer was the fear that the patient would die given the husband's clear intent to discontinue her tube feeding.

To honor his wife's wishes, Mr. Elbaum was thus forced to file a lawsuit. [Elbaum v. Grace Plaza, 1989.]

Nearly three years after the first request to stop tube feeding, the court sided with the Elbaum family. It ruled that the presented evidence met New York's *clear and convincing* standard that was required to terminate life-sustaining treatment of a vegetative person.

> In a previous case, the same New York court ruled in 1988 that Mary O'Connor had NOT been sufficiently *clear and convincing*, even though she repeatedly stated that she did not want to be a burden to anyone by being maintained by artificial means if she could no longer care for herself. The court still questioned whether her orally stated wishes were durable; that is, the judges wondered if this severely demented 77 year-old lady might now want to change her mind, despite the fact that her dementia was progressive. The court forced this woman to linger on for another ten months. She died with a feeding tube in place.

For Mrs. Elbaum, however, the court ordered the nursing home to permit her transfer to another facility where her wishes could be honored, or to her own home if no such facility could be found. The husband arranged for Jean Elbaum to be transferred to a hospice in New York, where finally, tube feeding was withdrawn. She died peacefully, a few days later.

After four more years of litigation, the highest appellate court in New York State ordered Mr. Elbaum to pay about $100,000 for the medical treatment his wife had received for nearly three years, despite his protesting at the time that his wife did not want these treatments and despite his warning that he would not pay. The Court considered the documents Mr. Elbaum signed on his wife's admission as his promise to pay for his wife's care since he did not then indicate any limitations at that time. Furthermore, they considered the nursing home to have acted properly when it insisted on a Court determination of Mrs. Elbaum's wishes. Since Mrs. Elbaum had never executed a Living Will, the court stated it was impossible for the nursing home administrators to know with certainty what her wishes were. Similarly, since she had never executed a Durable Power of Attorney for Health Care, the court stated it was impossible for the nursing home administrators to know with certainty whom she wanted to authorize to make her medical decisions. Thus it was necessary for the court to become involved. The process of sorting out the facts took time, the court explained, and the nursing home should not be held responsible for the cost of the patient's treatment for the time that the Court needed to decide what level of treatment she wanted and who should be her spokesperson.

The story of Jean Elbaum and her family illustrates the importance of creating **written documents** that are *clear and convincing*. Prolonged litigation drains the family's emotions and finances as it effectively denies the patient's Last Wishes. But we should not be hasty to fault either Mrs. or Mr. Elbaum for not having an Advance Directive. Her stroke occurred in 1986, prior to the U.S. Supreme Court's landmark ruling on Nancy Cruzan [1990] and the Federal Patient Self-Determination Act [1990].

The controversy over Jean Elbaum was not the first where **To Delay** was **To Deny** by requiring court authorization to **Withdraw Food & Fluid**. Paul Brophy suffered a stroke in 1983, which left him in a persistent vegetative state. It took three years for the Massachusetts Supreme Judicial Court to rule that individuals in a persistent vegetative state do not feel pain and that a feeding tube can be "intrusive and extraordinary" and the U.S. Supreme Court to refuse to hear the case, for his feeding tube to be removed so he could die peacefully (eight days later). Yet John Jefferson Davis, Ph.D., wrote in the Journal of Biblical Ethics in Medicine [1987], "the case of the first American to die after court-authorized discontinuation of artificial nutrition and hydration to a comatose patient" [Brophy v. New England Sinai Hospital, 1986] "sets a dangerous precedent which places at risk the lives of a large class of incompetent patients, and which also could erode the ethical integrity of the medical profession." This is when the lines of a controversy that still goes on today, were drawn.

Two decades after the cases of Elbaum, O'Connor, and Brophy, the scenario of **To Delay** is **To Deny is** unfortunately still too common. Now, challenges come from a greater number of sources and are based on a wider range of motivations. Nursing homes charge more for patients on tube feeding than for patients whose feeding is assisted. Physicians have cause to worry about possible lawsuits if they remove life-sustaining treatment based on a request from a family member who has no legal authority to speak for an incompetent patient but who insists that the feeding tube be removed. In such situations, doctors can ask for an ethics committee consultation and/or the court for guidance. Doctors fear that if someone does sue them, it will be one of the survivors, not the deceased patient. So they listen more to them than to the dying person, or to his or her previously expressed wishes.

It is common for family members who feel guilty about not having paid enough attention to their dying relative to suddenly take an active interest in them, although such interest is often misguided. In effect, they follow this unwritten rule: "The farther away they lived from the patient in the past, the greater interest they have in prolonging their dying relative's future."

Doctors are still debating whether or not it is moral to inform patients about the option of **Voluntary Refusal of Food & Fluid**. Yet some people criticize physicians that their real motivation may be their own, not their patients,' religious or personal beliefs. The novel, *Lethal Choice*, considers several types of physician bias.

In all of these challenges, this worrisome theme repeats: Others can wield power by putting their preferences before those of the dying patient. Whether their intrusion on the patient's privacy is unconscious or well-intended, what is at stake is the most important decision the patient can make about his or her life. When patients hear stories that lead them to distrust that others will honor their wishes, they then fear they will be forced to endure a state of prolonged suffering and indignity, and some may decide to end their lives—illegally, violently, and prematurely—the greatest tragedy of all.

A Political Football Named Terri Schiavo

A worsening development is the increasing trend in America for the issues of the dying to be used as political footballs. In October 2003, Governor Jeb Bush asked the Florida legislature to pass "Terri's Law" to permit him to authorize the reinsertion of a feeding tube into Terri Schiavo. With only several hours available to review the facts of the case, Governor Bush concluded that the dozens of judicial hearings held from 1998 through 2003 (almost 30,000 pages of documents) did not satisfy his personal standard of certitude.

In September 2004, the Florida Supreme Court ruled Terri's Law was unconstitutional since it violated the doctrine of separation of powers in the State constitution.

Slow forward to March 2005, when, in an emergency session on Palm Sunday between 9 PM and just after midnight, the U.S. Congress passed what could be called, "Terri's Law-II." By then, more than 15 years had elapsed since she collapsed and suffered severe brain damage. Congress created the power for Federal courts to review the case anew, and five subpoenas were issued for Michael and Terri to appear. —An extraordinary sequence of events.

The U.S. Supreme Court refused to hear the case six times. One day before Terri died, Federal Judge Stanley F. Birch, Jr., of the U.S. Court of Appeals for the Eleventh Circuit, who was nominated by George H. Bush and is considered a consistent conservative, took the last opportunity to comment about "Terri's Law-II," which Congress enacted and President George W. Bush signed. After stating the law was unconstitutional, he criticized the executive and legislative branches as acting "in ways inimical to basic Constitutional principles," specifically, "legislative dictation of how a Federal court should exercise its judicial functions invades the province of the judiciary and violates the separation of powers principle."

Media reporting on the conflict over Terri Schiavo's fate did not seem balanced. The New York Times had only a brief note [2005] quoting a clinical expert in Palliative Care, Dr. R. Sean Morrison, M.D., of Mount Sinai Hospital. He stated the clinical process of Terminal Dehydration was peaceful. In contrast, news coverage often included such inflammatory terms as "judicial murder" and descriptions of the process as "cruel and barbaric starvation." Charles Von Gunten, editor-in-chief of the Journal of Palliative Medicine attacked "the sloganism of starvation" in San Diego's Union-Tribune, stating it "misstates the facts and demonizes those who advocate for withdrawal of hydration and nutrition from dying people as 'evil'... [as if it were] neglect or abuse," which he stated, based on his extensive clinical experience, "It's just not true." Instead, patients like Schiavo "die peacefully." [2005]

Arthur Caplan gave this overview: The "level of grandstanding" from "the pro-life constituency in the House and Senate" to keep Terri Schiavo alive was clearly at odds with the "crystal clear" right of "the closest relative" to refuse or to consent to tube feeding, which U.S. courts consider a medical treatment. [MSNBC, 3-18-05].

Politicians even offered medical opinions. Kansas Senator Sam Brownback was quoted as stating, "The fact that Terri can process food should, by itself, be enough to prove that she is alive." Senator William Frist, M.D., offered his opinion that Terri was "alive" and "not in a coma." Later, others criticized him for unprofessional conduct as a medical doctor since he viewed only edited excerpts of old videotapes of Mrs. Schiavo instead of conducting a current bedside examination, and because his area of medical expertise is heart surgery, not neurology. After release of the autopsy report, his aides "angrily said he had never made a formal diagnosis and thus had nothing to retract" [New York Times, 6-16-2005].

But when Frist made his initial statements, many people of faith were delighted with his intense support as he and others demanded a fresh review of all medical data and the use of new technology and other approaches to determine if Terri Schiavo was really in a Permanent Vegetative State without any hope for improvement.

Arthur Caplan noted the "inexcusable silence" of many medical organizations, disease-affiliated groups, and religious groups whose members commonly exercise the freedom to refuse treatment, and whose professionals know that hospice is a great institution—but who "ducked commentary" by "not weighing in with their thinking" to teach that no "hospice would ever let a person die a miserable, painful death." [2005]

$$\wp\!\!\sim\!\!\wp$$

The bottom line, as stated by Michael Schiavo's attorney, George Felos, and by bioethicist Arthur Caplan, among others, is that now you must fear that Congress might intervene in what in the past, has always been a private matter for families and doctors to decide. The situation could worsen if States pass new laws that would dismiss as irrelevant, your heartfelt conversations around the dinner table as having absolutely no evidentiary value unless your wishes are in writing. Fifteen years previously, after the United States Supreme Court ruled that States could set their own standards of proof in cases where life was at stake, the fate of Nancy Beth Cruzan, a case in which many thousands of words had been written, ultimately came down to just these: "Discovery of new evidence regarding patient's intent" [Colby, 2002]. The publicity of the case brought forward three additional witnesses who had not known her married name. They testified in the Missouri court on what they **heard** Ms. Cruzan say. Their testimony was considered *clear and convincing* so the court ruled to permit Nancy Cruzan's parents to remove her feeding tube.

If States that have adopted the *clear and convincing* standard now legislate that such instructions must be in writing, then many more patients with devastating brain disease will be kept alive indefinitely.

It is more critical now than ever **to write** *clear and convincing* Last Wishes, as your State might pass a law similar to the model law suggested by the National Right to Life Committee [May, 2005]. The "Model Starvation and Dehydration of Person with Disabilities Prevention Act" mandates the presumption that patients want to continue nutrition and hydration unless there are *clear and convincing*

written instructions to the contrary. Twenty-three States were considering similar laws as of March 2006 [Cohen and others].

What can you learn from these scenarios?

When it comes to honoring one's Last Wishes... **To Delay** is **To Deny**.

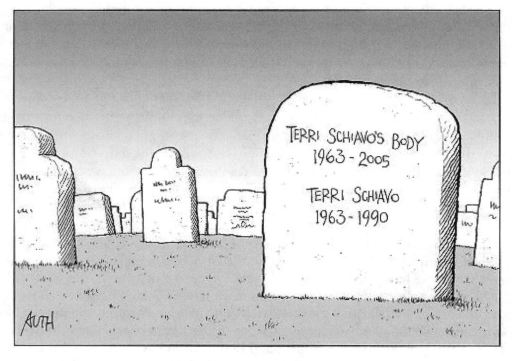

The cartoon above was published before the gravestone was set. When it was, Michael Schiavo added this additional line to the stone: "I kept my promise."

This cartoon also brings to mind the famous epitaph chosen by Nancy Cruzan's parents after their long fight to discontinue her artificial feeding and hydration. Her gravestone has three lines: "Born: July 20, 1957. Departed: January 11, 1983. At peace: December 26, 1990."

We recommend you carefully scrutinize, preferably with your legal and clinical advisors, any quick and user-friendly Advance Directive. Such forms may help you start thinking about end-of-life wishes, but they may, or may not, reflect your personal wishes. They may also not succeed in getting others to honor your wishes. Most forms need your diligent modification. One example is illustrated in Chapter 12, using the popular form, "Five Wishes." Your Proxy may also need additional supportive documents as armamentarium to discourage challenges.

Some people consider consulting an attorney to discuss waiving their right to a court review. In many States, you can simply add a statement to your document that is similar to the example below. Unlike the rest of the Advance Directive, this addendum usually requires your attorney's signature. Before signing such a statement, however, first consider the value of having the protection of the court. Sometimes a Proxy's instructions go against the patient's probable wishes. DO NOT WAIVE YOUR RIGHT TO A COURT REVIEW UNLESS YOU CAN TRUST YOUR PROXY.

Even if you waive your right, your physician may help protect you if your Proxy becomes incompetent or abusive. Dr. Bramstedt [2003] reported that he had to question the decision-making capacity of a patient's relative. The relative first claimed the patient was "mentally simple," and then became agitated. The relative was boisterous, ranted, and veered off topic. The worst was the threat to contact lawyers if the doctors did not immediatelyh terminate life-support. Sometimes, the power of a court is needed to deal with such conflicts, but often the institution's ethics committee will suffice.

In general, the more power you give your Proxy, the more trust you need to have. You may empower your Proxies so their current decisions override what others interpret as your wishes based on your other writing. But the more oversight you ask for, the more possible a future "interested party" can challenge your Proxies, as they try their best to make the decisions you would have made.

Waiver of My Rights to Prevent Court Challenges to Honoring My Last Wishes Since "To Delay" is "To Deny"

The goal of my Advance Directive is to attain a prompt response to my Last Wishes because sometimes, **To Delay** is tantamount **To Deny**, especially if litigation unnecessarily prolongs the process of dying while I suffer from pain and indignity, or creates a further burden to my family or society as my indignity increases.

I want to avoid delays in following my Proxy's decisions if others claim they are not in my BEST INTEREST. To avoid such delays, I hereby waive my right to a court review (if initialed here __ __ __), and to a review by religious leaders (if initialed here __ __ __) regarding what others may consider as being in my BEST INTEREST.

My Proxy may decide however, to request additional medical and legal consultations, or request a court review, a review by an ethics committee, or a review by religious leaders.

My initials here __ __ __ indicate my durable permission to have my Proxy's judgment and decision-making capacity evaluated (if any one believes this is an issue) by two experts—physicians or psychologists—who are qualified to evaluate impairments in judgment and in decision-making capacity. If both experts find my Proxy is impaired, then my next named alternate Proxy should be contacted to serve. If only one expert finds impairment, a third expert should be asked to cast the deciding vote on whether my Proxy is impaired.

I have discussed the risks and benefits of the foregoing choices with my attorney, whose statement and signature are below. I considered his or her advice before I signed below.

My signature: _____

Printed name: _____

Executed this _____ day of _____ , 20__ , at _____

[City, County, State]

My Attorney's Statement:

I am a lawyer authorized to practice law in the State where the accompanying statement about my client's Advance Health Care Directive was executed. _____ (name), was my client at the time he or she executed the accompanying statement about his or her Advance Directive.

I have advised my client concerning his or her rights in connection with the choices made in the foregoing statements, the applicable law, and the consequences of signing or not signing the statements. My client, after being so advised, has executed this document.

I declare under penalty of perjury under the laws of this State that the foregoing is true and correct to the best of my knowledge.

Attorney's signature: _____

Printed name: _____

State Bar number: _____

Executed this _____ day of _____ , 20__ , at _____

[City, County, State]

Caveat

While the strategy above has been thoroughly considered, readers should appreciate that, to our knowledge, it has not yet been tested in the courts.

In such a test, the judge could rule in a way that distinguishes between your rights, and those of close relatives or others. It is legally possible for you to enforce or to waive your own rights and privileges in the above document; but the power to exclude others from participation may not be permitted in some States.

For example, California lists nine different categories of people, including "any interested person," who may petition the court about your medical decisions. But at the same time, California allows a choice by you to limit the categories of people who may petition. You may narrow the field down to these two: Your designated Proxy and your court-appointed conservator.

Caution

DO NOT GIVE UP your right to a court review of your Proxy's decisions UNLESS YOU COMPLETELY TRUST YOUR PROXY.

Do not overlook the protection provided by the courts if your Proxies should become unfit to perform their duties. They may lose their cognitive ability to make medical decisions; they may become temporarily overwhelmed by emotion given the responsibility to let you go; or they may have a conflict of interest.

Discuss with your attorney whether you wish to retain the option of other bases for questioning your Proxies, other than your BEST INTEREST, as opposed to trying to completely block anyone from going to court for any reason. For example, you may wish a court to weigh the high cost of your medical care and its possible benefit to you, compared to allocating those funds from your estate to send your grandchildren to college or for other purposes you feel are important.

Chapter 4

General Questions

Ethics of the American Medical Association:

"The social commitment of the physician is to sustain life and relieve suffering.

"Where the performance of one duty conflicts with the other, **the preferences of the patient should prevail**."

From this point on, we discuss in greater detail, the option of **Voluntary Refusal of Food & Fluid**. We continue to strive to maintain balance in the presentation by revealing the pros and cons, and by suggesting other strategies that may be effective, so you can decide whether or not you would wish this option for yourself or for your loved one. Yet our personal and professional bias is that **Voluntarily Refusing Food & Fluid** can be the **BEST WAY** for many terminal patients (but not all). That is, it is one way to allow Nature to take its course. This method of **allowing**... or of **hastening** the process of dying (depending on your perspective and belief system) is both legal and peaceful.

A. Why Do You Call These "in-Frequently Asked Questions" (i-FAQs)?

We use the term "infrequently" and abbreviate it **"i-FAQ"** to emphasize that these critically important subjects are rarely asked and answered. Most Americans have *not* completed their Advance Directives; of those who have, most have *not* discussed the issues with their Proxies, physicians, or legal advisors; and of those patients who do discuss the issues, most do *not* know enough to ask about **Voluntary Refusal of Food & Fluid**. Similarly, few doctors feel obligated to mention this option, and some feel conflicted about it. The result is that the option of **Voluntary Refusal of Food & Fluid** is rarely discussed. Yet in an increasing number of States, if your Advance Directive does not specifically grant your Proxy the power to invoke this option, your Proxy will not be able to choose this option on your behalf.

What has been more frequently discussed instead? Whatever sells newspapers and increases the ratings of TV news shows. Over the years, the news media has reported on the court trials of Dr. Kevorkian, on several States' attempts to legalize physician-assisted suicide, and on the fate of a few dying people who were turned into celebrities like Terri Schiavo. The issues have served as political footballs for both liberals and conservatives. Yet it is clear that many people are worried. They have reason to be. Consider the sworn testimony [2000] of Father Gerard Murphy, a Catholic priest who testified in court during the initial trial to determine the fate of Terri Schiavo:

"It is not as easy to die as it used to be... [Modern medical technology is] a two-edged sword. God's Will could have been easily done fifty years ago. I think this is a case where the wonderful technology, rather than being an act of health and recovery, has become the obstacle for Nature taking its course... Virtually everyone I know is terrified of a case like this. That is why I believe they would line up to take a pill or shot and go to sleep."

B. Who Should Read the Answers to These "i-FAQs"?

All who want to avoid the risk of prolonged unnecessary suffering at the end of life and the risk of being dragged into prolonged litigation as their rights, their dignity, their financial resources, and their emotions or those of their family, are drained.

The answers to these **i-FAQs** are particularly relevant for:

1. Terminally ill patients who can make medical decisions and want to explore the option of **Voluntarily Refusing Food & Fluid** to avoid prolonging their suffering *now*,

2. People who can make medical decisions now who want to ensure that, if they ever become incompetent, their designated Proxy can choose **Voluntary Refusal of Food & Fluid** for them *in the future*,

3. All who care about, provide care to, or are related to someone who is in one of the above two Categories.

Except for people who are sure that they and their loved ones will never want to **Refuse Food & Fluid** (for example, some observant Catholics and Orthodox Jews), these three categories could include every one. Even religious people may learn from these i-FAQs that **Refusal of Food & Fluid** is permitted when death is imminent, when it causes more suffering, and when nourishment cannot be absorbed.

The reality is that we will all die. And most of us must experience the process of dying several times—first for our loved ones and then ultimately, for ourselves. If we want to make our own final transition as peaceful and as meaningful as possible, then we must learn what we need to know before our last chapter begins. Such learning is also relevant if we are concerned about a loved one who is older or currently ill.

The second group above includes patients with mild **Alzheimer's disease** and related dementias. People recently given these diagnoses have *greater urgency* than those diagnosed with other chronic diseases. Why? Because they must promptly document their wishes while they still have the mental ability to make medical decisions. If they fail to take advantage of their *finite window* to make sure that their designated Proxy can in the future choose **Voluntary Refusal of Food & Fluid** on their behalf—then they and their families may sadly endure many months to years of prolonged suffering and indignity. Such years are often accompanied by huge drains on emotion, energy, and finances.

✋ *SKIP*

Although Alzheimer's accounts for about 60% of dementias, there are other causes: vascular dementia including strokes, Parkinson's Disease, Dementia with Lewy Bodies, Pick's Disease, Huntington's Disease, Alcohol Abuse-Related Dementia (Korsakoff's Syndrome), Creutzfeldt-Jakob Disease, and AIDS. Sadly, these types of dementia cannot be reversed. Yet some medical conditions are reversible and these causes should be ruled out and, if present, treated: vitamin and hormone deficiencies (B12, thiamine, thyroid), depression, over-medication or drug side-effects or interactions, infections, brain tumors, and subdural hematomas.

How long can people live with the diagnosis of Alzheimer's disease? The course is variable and some patients live for 25 years after receiving the diagnosis, but the average is 7 years. [Koopmans and others, 2003.] Most significantly, three-quarters of Alzheimer's patients must be placed in residential facilities within five years of diagnosis due to developing unmanageable psychological and behavioral symptoms. [Hart and others, 2003].

C. What was Your Motivation to Write These i-FAQs?

Americans generally do not like to talk about **their own** death and dying, although they are subjected to blasts of media about new-found celebrities like Terri Schiavo. Despite the controversy and media attention paid to physician-assisted suicide, including a court battle and state referendum to make it legal, when Silveira and others [2000] asked 1000 outpatients in Oregon to complete a questionnaire, of the seven hundred and thirty who responded, only 23% indicated that they knew they could ask for assisted suicide. In addition, only 69% indicated they knew they could refuse treatment, 46% knew they could ask for treatment to be withdrawn, 32% incorrectly thought they could ask for active euthanasia (that was illegal), and only 41% knew that they could ask for enough pain medications to relieve suffering even if it hastened dying. The authors' general conclusions from this survey are relevant to this book: "Greater public knowledge about end-of-life care is needed, and advance care planning must be preceded by education about options in end-of-life care."

✺ *CONTINUE*

More specifically, we believe there are three reasons for the great disparity between what people know, and what they need to know about **Voluntary Refusal of Food & Fluid**. A) intentional and unintentional delivery of *misinformation*; B) *under-informing* due to physicians' reluctance; and C) *over-informing* people about other, highly politicized options.

A.   Misinformation examples: Using end-of-life conflicts as political footballs did not begin with the last round about Terri Schiavo. Demonstrators protested about Nancy Cruzan in 1990. Misinformation also creeps in lower profile ways. In 1995, Ann Landers wrote that, in her opinion, **Refusal of Food & Fluid** was "illegal," "inhumane," "cruel," and "uncomfortable." In 2003, in his effort to encourage the passing of "Terri's Law I," Mr. Joe Pitts (Congressman, R-PA) addressed Florida's State House of Representatives and argued, "Compared to starvation and dehydration, death by hanging, firing squad, or even the electric chair seems humane." And some referred to Terri Schiavo's March 2005 experience as "judicial murder" or "cruel starvation." —Yet **Voluntary Refusal of Food & Fluid** rarely causes death by starvation.

The truth emerged from two recent surveys [Ganzini and others, 2003; Harvath and others, 2004]. In the first survey, they asked experienced hospice nurses to rate the quality of dying for their last competent patient who was capable of drinking fluids but chose **Voluntary Refusal of Food & Fluid**. On average, these patients experienced a **good death** (a score of **8**, where "**9**" was the highest score for "a very good death," and "**0**" was a very bad death). Their **peace** was rated higher, and their **suffering** lower than for patients who opted for physician-assisted suicide. Moreover, 70% of these surveyed nurses would choose **Voluntary Refusal of Food & Fluid** for themselves if they were terminally ill.

✺ *SKIP*

Patients who chose **Voluntary Refusal of Food & Fluid** were rated as "**much at peace**," with an average score of **2**, on a scale where "**0**" denoted very much at peace and "**9**" not at all peaceful. This score of **2** compared to **5** for patients who opted for physician-assisted suicide. Suffering was also lower for those who chose **Voluntary Refusal of Food & Fluid** than those who opted for physician-assisted suicide, although the difference was slight [Ganzini and others, 2003].

The second survey assessed the attitudes of hospice nurses and social workers regarding **Voluntary Refusal of Food & Fluid**. About 85% thought the option should be offered to patients who experienced physical suffering; and 75% thought **Voluntary Refusal of Food & Fluid** should be offered if patients experienced psychological or spiritual suffering. When quizzed about their willingness to care for a patient who chose to hasten his or her death through **Voluntary Refusal of Food & Fluid**, over 95% of the hospice workers would continue, and less than 3% felt that doing so would be immoral. About 70% would consider choosing **Voluntary Refusal of Food & Fluid** for themselves if they were terminally ill [Harvath, Ganzini, and others, 2004].

✎ *CONTINUE*

B.   Under-informing the public: It is not surprising that few lay people know that the option of **Voluntary Refusal of Food & Fluid** exists since it is both under-suggested and under-practiced by the medical profession. The six co-authors in the 2004 article by Harvath and others cited above "could find no research regarding health care professionals' attitudes towards **Voluntary Refusal of Food & Fluid**." In a literature search I performed on December 2, 2004, looking back to 1988 via the National Library of Medicine, there were fewer than 90 articles and letters published on **Voluntary Refusal of Food & Fluid** or its clinical term "terminal dehydration," compared to over 3000 articles and letters published on "Physician-Assisted Suicide." (The search for articles on the term "terminal sedation" was confusing since it overlapped with "Physician-Assisted Suicide.")

✎ *SKIP*

Why might physicians be reluctant to educate and inform the public? In part, because of the controversy stirred by a few vocal doctors over whether or not it is morally right to inform patients of this option. Jansen and Sulmasy argued [2002] that if the patient or the physician believes that physician-assisted suicide is morally wrong, then it is also morally wrong for anyone to collaborate on any action that has an equivalent result. These authors also wrote it was morally wrong for doctors to inform patients about **Voluntary Refusal of Food & Fluid** (if the doctor thought it was morally wrong). Their article stimulated vehement disagreement in several letters subsequently published in the same journal.

Dr. Erich Loewy went one step further in 2001. He wrote that he could accept the practice of physicians who agreed to continue to care for patients who decided **on their own** to ask for **Voluntary Refusal of Food & Fluid**. But he used the word, "macabre," to describe informing patients about **Voluntary Refusal of Food & Fluid** when they "*ask for help in ending their lives.*" His reason: that would be tantamount to "advising them to starve themselves," which he termed "physician-stimulated self-starvation." He argued that its real purpose was solely to "let health care professionals off the legal hook." To support his opinion, Loewy briefly reviewed the cultural benefits of food by noting it "symbolically represents our social acceptance and is an integral part of marriage, burial, and other social practices." He concluded that informing patients about **Voluntary Refusal of Food & Fluid** is "encouraging them to commit **social suicide**." Even worse: "To encourage them to stop eating and drinking *before they truly wish to do so* seems a **cruel act of rejection**." {Emphasis added.}

Before we present other arguments, consider the next story. In a humorous way, it reflects the social significance of ceremonial food:

✎ *CONTINUE*

We Must Save the Strudel

After a long and productive life, Grandpa lay in bed. His children and grandchildren assembled around him. Doctors had pronounced him very near death. For awhile, he was so still that his visitors wondered if he was deeply asleep or in a coma.

Suddenly the old man opened his eyes. "Was I dreaming of Heaven? I could swear that I smelled grandmother's strudel."

"You weren't dreaming," his youngest granddaughter said. "At this very minute, Grandma is downstairs baking strudel."

"How wonderful. As my last wish, since I'll never taste her delicious strudel again, please little one, go down and ask her to cut me a slice, okay?" Expectantly, the old man smiled with joy.

The little girl got up immediately and ran down the stairs. After a few minutes, the muffled sounds from the kitchen became louder and louder.

Eventually, the granddaughter returned. She walked slowly, her head bent down. She was empty-handed.

"Where's the strudel?" asked the old man.

"I'm so sorry, grandpa. I tried arguing with grandma, but she insisted: We have to save the strudel for your wake."

❧ *SKIP*

Certainly, Loewy is correct about the issue of timing: some patients do ask about **Refusing Food & Fluid** *"before they truly wish to do so."* Yet once informed, patients may feel reassurance in knowing they have the option to end their suffering at any future point in time. Obviously, they do NOT need to stop eating and drinking immediately after their doctors provide this information. In fact, one advantage of this method of dying is that patients can even decide to change their mind even *after* they stop eating and drinking by resuming intake.

On the other hand, patients may feel abandoned by their physicians if their doctors refuse to offer information they are desperate to learn. This is especially true when patients ask about *help in ending their lives.*

Dr. Ira Byock [1995] wrote, "In my own practice, while I steadfastly refuse to write a prescription with lethal intent or otherwise help the patient commit suicide, I can share with the patient information that he or she already has the ability to exert control over the timing of death. Virtually any patient with far advanced illness can be assured of dying—comfortably, without any additional physical distress—within one or two weeks simply by refusing to eat or drink. This is less time than would be legally imposed by waiting periods of assisted suicide initiatives. **The discussion and subsequent decision are wholly ethical and legal, requiring no mandated psychiatric evaluations, attorneys, court decisions, or legislation.**" {Emphasis added.}

A key question: How can people make prudent choices if they are not informed about the available options? Physicians who oppose disclosure may be worried about overly influencing their patient to choose **Voluntary Refusal of Food & Fluid**, which in their personal opinion, would be the "wrong" choice. But, we should ask, is not the withholding of relevant information from patients who directly request it, just one way for physicians to impose their personal values on their patients?

Dr. Sherwin Nuland made a frank revelation in his book, *How We Die* [on his *Page 252*, 1994]. He admitted that his own fear of disapproval from fellow surgeons led him to persuade 92-year Ms. Welch to undergo burdensome surgery, which had a low chance of long-term benefit. "I had not been completely forthcoming in predicting the cost" and had "minimized the difficulties of the post-operative period." He confessed, "**I was guilty of the worst sort of paternalism**. I had withheld information because I was afraid the patient might use it to make what I thought of as a **wrong decision**." {Emphasis added.} In terms of Ms. Welch's sad outcome, Dr. Nuland wrote that he suspected his patient's anger at him for his "well-intentioned deception... played a role" in causing her fatal stroke that occurred two weeks later.

✨ CONTINUE

Our motivation to provide the answers to these **i-FAQs**, which provide much information about **Voluntary Refusal of Food & Fluid**, is well expressed by the statement from the American Medical Association that also appears in the box under the chapter title, above. It clearly places a prominent value on every patient's *autonomy*, that each person has the final say over what happens to his or her body: "The social commitment of the physician is to sustain life and relieve suffering. "Where the performance of one duty conflicts with the other, **the preferences of the patient should prevail**." [AMA's Council on Ethical and Judicial Affairs, Document E-2.20, issued December, 1984 and last updated, August, 2005.] Their position on "Withholding or Withdrawing Life-Sustaining Medical Treatment" also states, "There is no ethical distinction between withdrawing and withholding life-sustaining treatment," and it specifically includes artificial nutrition and hydration.

✨ SKIP

Most bioethicists believe that patients' autonomy should rule when it comes to REFUSING treatment. What about the opposite—when patients DEMAND treatment? Aside from considerations of whether the treatment will be more of a burden than a benefit, the fourth principle of medical ethics, the one about social justice, applies. "Individuals [should] have the opportunity to obtain the health care they need on an equitable basis" [Hastings Center, 1987]. Society has an impending economic crisis coming, to pay for the costs of Alzheimer's disease. The way we handle publicized cases that go to court now may determine whether or not we will face this challenge with equity in the future. In medicine, as in law, tough cases can lead to making bad laws. Consider this case:

The British Conflict Over Who Decides

The Case of Leslie Burke

At 45, Leslie Burke had suffered from progressive cerebellar ataxia since he was 23. This neurological disease may some day prevent him from being able to swallow. In 2004, fearing that his physicians might stop administering Food & Fluid artificially when he lost the ability to swallow, he petitioned a trial court to continue to receive this treatment based on the European Convention on Human Rights' protection of right-to-life. Present British guidelines are that doctors may withhold or withdraw life-sustaining treatment, even against the patient's wishes, if doctors deem the patient's condition so severe and prognosis so poor that artificial feeding would be more of a burden than a benefit.

Burke won at the level of the lower court. That ruling entitled him to receive artificially administered Food & Fluid when he became unable to swallow.

But the General Medical Council and the Secretary for Health of the British government jointly appealed. They feared Burke's case might establish a precedent that could threaten the financial resources of the National Health Service, which is chronically underfunded. They argued that physicians must retain the authority to consider the potential benefit of treatment in terms of expected quality of life and the cost of that treatment—to make the final determination on whether the patient receives treatment—regardless of the patient's wishes. They argued that if Burke prevailed, the British system for rationing medical care by the National Health Service and its finances would be threatened if other patients also felt they had the right to demand treatment.

In late July 2005, Britain's General Medical Council won their appeal. They based their claim on the fear that the ruling could eventually force doctors to perform unnecessary or harmful treatment, which treatment doctors considered futile since it would have no benefit, and such a ruling could give other patients the right to make similar demands. The judges stressed that "in the last stage of life" Artificial Nutrition and Hydration—far from prolonging life—may even hasten death.

Lord Justice Nicholas Phillips wrote, "It is our view that Mr. Burke's fears are addressed by the law as it currently stands," and he explained, "For a doctor deliberately to interrupt life-prolonging treatment in the face of a competent patient's expressed wish to be kept alive, with the intention of thereby terminating the patient's life, would leave the doctor with no answer to a charge of murder." But all three Lords agreed: "A patient cannot demand that a doctor administer a treatment which the doctor considers is adverse to the patient's clinical needs."

While Mr. Burke's lawyers said they were pleased, Mr. Burke was still worried: "A doctor is not allowed to refuse me food and water while I remain competent. But when do I become incompetent? When I am no longer able to communicate?" The ruling thus left open possible conflict if Burke disagreed with his doctors when he was still competent.

Britain's Mental Capacity Act is expected to become effective in April 2007. It provides for decisions to be made in the patient's "best interest." The Act provides that no patient can demand that a treatment must be given if doctors judge it to be futile, otherwise the National Health Service could be forced to give futile treatments, which would leave those who may benefit [from beneficial treatments] untreated. This view explains why the General Medical Council, backed by the Department of Health, decided to challenge Burke's original judgment.

❧*SKIP*

Writing about this case in 2005, attorney Wesley J. Smith considered Burke's pleading the most important bioethics case in the world, even surpassing the case of Terri Schiavo. The essential difference, according to attorney Smith was that Mr. Burke was fully competent so there was no dispute about what he really wanted. Mr. Smith felt Burke's case was clearly about money, quality of life, and the right to receive basic care. He cited it as an example of why he was worried about "Futile Care Theory"—a term Smith created and used only by him. Smith warned that the spread of futile care could give physicians and bioethicists the ultimate authority to make decisions about life-sustaining treatment.

❧*CONTINUE*

In contrast, many physicians, including Dr. Robert Orr and Dr. Lawrence Schneiderman believe the term, "futile ***care***" is inappropriate, misleading, and should never be used. They explain, physicians should ***never stop caring*** for their patients, even though the point may be reached for extremely ill patients where ***treatment*** becomes ***futile***. Dr. Schneiderman believes that the goal of medicine is not to sustain life in the Intensive Care Unit, and offered this definition: "If a patient lacks the capacity to appreciate a treatment, or if the treatment fails to release the patient from total dependence on intensive medical care, that treatment should be regarded as futile." [Schneiderman and Jecker, 1995]. For example, Nancy Cruzan was unconscious. So she was "incapable of experiencing, much less appreciating" her treatment [*Page 17*]. "Life-saving treatments are never free and painless. Rather they are by their nature invasive, burdensome, and fraught with serious, lingering harms" [*Page 107*]. Dr.

Schneiderman distinguishes between futile treatment that refers to a treatment that will not benefit an individual patient ***and*** rationing that refers to treatment that may benefit a patient but has limited availability (for example, organs like kidneys, for transplantation). In such cases, society must allocate resources based on the ethical principle of justice. Deciding not to continue life-sustaining treatment is quite challenging, yet many conflicts that arise may be resolved by ethics committee consultations [Schneiderman and others, 2003].

The reality is that finite medical and economic resources may place ethical limits on patients' right to continued sustenance where there is no medical evidence of benefit. Therefore, the family of a person reliably diagnosed as being in a **Permanent Vegetative State** may not have the right to insist indefinitely on endless life-support; e.g., beyond 15 years, in the case of Terri Schiavo. (In the U.S., the **Vegetative State** is typically considered **permanent** after 3 to 12 months, depending on what caused the injury.) Britain's National Health Service is obviously chronically underfunded. In the U.S., however, the financial ramifications are hidden from view. The more fortunate receive treatment, while services for patients on Medicaid are reduced, and an increasing number of people with no health insurance receive grossly inadequate or no care.

C.   The distracting over-informed: Another reason why we wrote the answers to these **i-FAQs**: In addition to those curious or desperate patients who are misinformed, plus the vast numbers of lay people who are under-informed about **Voluntary Refusal of Food & Fluid**, there is a small but active and vocal group of people who are relatively ***over-informed*** about highly politicized options such as euthanasia, physician-assisted suicide, and "self-deliverance." (Derek Humphry introduced the last term in his book, *Final Exit*, first published in 1991.)

Newspapers continue to carry headlines about physician-assisted suicide issue. For example, former Attorney General John Ashcroft resigned on November 2, 2004, and on that same day, his parting shot (publicized a week later) was aimed at doctors who participated in Oregon's Death With Dignity Act. However his successor lost the case before the U.S. Supreme Court, then called "Gonzalez v. Oregon," in January, 2006. Yet that may be only one battle in a long war.

For those who are relatively *over*-informed about physician-assisted suicide, especially those who consider it their only alternative, this book will provide them with a balanced presentation of other options.

How to Bring About Change

To change current practice, the most common non-violent ways are:

1. You can work to create new laws in your legislature and vote for candidates who support change;

2. You can provoke the judicial system to re-interpret old laws;

3. You can re-educate the responsible professionals; and

4. You can inform concerned consumers, the people who are most affected by what options are available, and hope that they in turn will educate their own physicians and get them to change.

We now review all four. As you will see, we put the most faith in the last.

SKIP

1. Create New Laws: It is challenging to create new laws. The "success" of creating Oregon's **Death with Dignity Act** resulted from a combination of factors that are unlikely to recur. As a personal favor to the well-liked Senator Frank Roberts who was at the time dying from painful prostate cancer, the wheel-chaired legislator was allowed to take his bill out of committee to the general session. Frank Roberts was also married to the then governor of Oregon who had on her staff an attorney who was also a nurse practitioner, Barbara Coombs Lee. Still, "Measure 16" passed narrowly (51 to 49%), but that was only the beginning. After a three-year court injunction by opponents to the law, the citizens of Oregon were required to vote a second time—to defeat the repeal of the law they had already passed. This time, the majority in favor of the law was much higher (60 to 40%).

Congressman Henry Hyde (R-Il.) and Senator Don Nickles (R-Ok.) attempted to introduce federal legislation in 1998 and 1999, and then Attorney General Ashcroft tried to use existing laws to accuse and to punish Oregon physicians for misusing controlled medications, to prevent them from following the guidelines of the **Death with Dignity Act**. In February 2005, the U.S. Supreme Court agreed to hear Gonzales v. Oregon (04-623). In October 2005, it was the first case over which the newly appointed Chief Justice Roberts presided. Had Gonzales prevailed, physicians in Oregon could have been prosecuted for prescribing a lethal dose of medication, and lost their license to prescribe other controlled medications for pain, anxiety, insomnia, and controlling seizures. They could even be sent to jail. Striking down Oregon's law could also have induced fear in physicians in all other States, thereby making them reluctant to offer aggressive treatment for pain and anxiety. We mention this because individual States may pass new laws, now that the attempt to prevent choice using the 1970 Federal Controlled Substances Act has failed.

2. Seek Court Rulings: Judges wield power when they interpret the law at the appeal level, which can set precedents. Some people criticize judges for "legislating from the bench" (creating new laws instead of interpreting old ones). For example, the probate code of California does not require evidence to be *clear and convincing* when deciding to remove a feeding tube from persons in the Minimally Conscious State who have no Advance Directive. Yet, in the Conservatorship of Robert Wendland [2001], the California Supreme Court "rewrote" the law by stating [*Page 554*]: "the Legislature cannot have intended to authorize every conceivable application without meaningful judicial review," and "We find no reason to believe the Legislature intended [Probate Code] Section 2355 to confer power so unlimited and no authority for such a result in any judicial decision. Under these circumstances, we may properly construe the statute to require proof by *clear and convincing* evidence to avoid grave injury to the fundamental rights of conscious but incompetent conservatees."

Yet the power of judges may not always be absolute, let alone *expeditious*. Florida Governor Jeb Bush challenged the State appeals court by requesting the Legislature pass a law giving him permission to reinsert Terri Schiavo's feeding tube in October 2003. Although "Terri's Law" was eventually ruled unconstitutional by Florida's Supreme Court since it violated the principle of separation of powers, the litigation still prolonged the patient's existence for over a year.

We might ask, what was Governor Bush's motivation?

Was it noble, to preserve the life of a person who had potential for improvement? —Unlikely, since she showed no signs of improvement *after* 15 years, as expected from the evaluations of most medical experts.

Was it to establish a point of relevant law, as in the California case about Wendland, where the State Supreme Court published its ruling one month after the patient died? —Unlikely, since the law as written, would apply ONLY to one person—Terri Schiavo.

Was it to embrace the religious rights of the patient, given the recent Allocution of Pope John Paul II? —Unlikely, in the words of the attorney George Felos who represented Terri's husband/guardian: "The Schindlers' claim that Terri would choose to be tube-fed for decades because the Pope gave a speech is so frivolous, the court denied their appeal without even asking us for a brief."

Was the goal of Jeb Bush's interest personal and political, to gain power by winning future votes from the religious right? Some people think so and cite his last effort, to reopen the investigation regarding Michael's possible delay in calling 9-1-1 fifteen years ago. Most Republicans agreed to close all related cases once the autopsy report was released. Larry J. Sabato, Director of the Center for Politics at the University of Virginia viewed the governor's action as "a product of his own personal beliefs" but also, possibly, an attempt to win political points. Sabato was also quoted as saying, "Were he interested in running for president or being put on the 2008 ticket as vice president, this would pay dividends" [Goodnough, 2005].

It would be tragic to force a person to linger in an unconscious state for 15 years if the lower court and appeals courts had been correct when they ruled that she clearly and convincingly had told her husband and others that was not what she would have wanted. —Worse, if the motivation was purely political. —Worst, if she were minimally conscious and could experience suffering.

The political basis for motivation was becoming more transparent to the public. Polls revealed that 80% of Americans were against Federal intervention in what they felt should be a private matter best left to individual patients, their families, and their physicians.

Conclusion: It is risky to rely on courts. We should be humbled by their power and motivated to direct enough energy to devise strategies that will effectively avoid litigation.

3. Re-educate Physicians: While much good can be said about such programs as "Educating Physicians about End-of-Life Care"—a Robert Wood Johnson Foundation-funded program, in fact only three hours of the three-day course relate to the general issues surrounding **Voluntarily Refusing Food & Fluid**, according to course director Charles F. von Gunten, M.D., Ph.D. While no funding was provided to support the assessment of outcome data beyond comparing pre- and post-test scores, researchers in education caution in general, that most students can be expected to remember not much more than 10% of what they were taught.

4. Inform Concerned Consumers: This is the challenge of the last alternative: The legal and clinical background must be clearly explained so that non-professionals can appreciate the basis for the proposed strategies. Such attempts, including this book, are worth the effort since consumers have the purest and least selfish motivation.

You care about what end-of-life options will be available for yourself, your spouse, and your parents—not about politics. So your efforts to learn the details in this field can be rewarding in practical terms. And you can derive wisdom from statutes, case law, and personal experiences—wherever you can find useful direction.

For example, one section of California's Probate stature permits you to *exclude* certain people from ever as acting as your agent. Just write their names on the Advance Directive form that the State provides, or one that is similar. While Florida law does not specifically mention that this option is available, there is nothing in Florida law that would seem to forbid a similar statement. Some advisors recommend that Florida residents who fear intervention by politicians include in their document a statement that specifically excludes not only those relatives or friends whose values are different from theirs, but also politicians including the Governor, if he ever proclaimed himself as an "interested party."

✑ *CONTINUE*

Given the lengthy uphill challenge to create new laws, the reasonable fear of the outcome if one goes to court, and the possibility that even those doctors who took special courses may still not be knowledgeable or experienced with **Voluntary Refusal of Food & Fluid**—this book directs its effort to bring about social change by informing the public who are concerned about these issues for themselves or loved ones. Hopefully, they will in turn demand more from their doctors, attorneys, legislators, judges, and other professionals.

To summarize our motivation to write answers to these **i-FAQs**, we quote Dr. Jay Wolfson, Guardian *Ad Litem*, as he concluded his December 2003 report to Governor Jeb Bush: "We remain in Theresa Schiavo's shoes." We can derive two profound implications from this statement: Since we all are mortal, some day we may be at the mercy of others who will be deciding our fate; and, the precedents that our government establishes for one person can ultimately affect us all.

D. How is Voluntary Refusal of Food & Fluid Different From Refusing Other Life-Sustaining Treatments?

1. Food & Fluid have profound cultural significance and are used to celebrate many milestones of life. Wine, and even water have important roles in many religious traditions. Many celebrations occur with feasts, even wakes. The statement that feeding a person is "ordinary and basic" at first glance seems to need no argument or proof. Cultural bias therefore creates resistance to the **Withdrawal or Withholding of Food & Fluid**.

2. **Voluntary Refusal of Food & Fluid** has rarely been observed, which is not surprising since the process of dying by any means is typically hidden in America. One theme promoted by the hospice movement is that no one should die alone. Another is to consider dying at home, not in institutions. Among professionals, surprisingly few have personally observed alert patients **Refuse Food & Fluid**, as Sandra Jacobs wrote [2003]: "... few physicians and nurses... have witnessed such deaths." The minimal opportunity for direct observations makes it easier to popularize myths that go unquestioned such as "denying a person Food & Fluid is cruel and barbaric."

3. **Voluntary Refusal of Food & Fluid** seems final. It is true that once conscious people fall asleep after several days of refusing nutrition and hydration, death is inevitable. But as long as they remain conscious, they can change their

minds by asking for Food & Fluid. Some patients do. In contrast, unconscious patients are at the mercy of others; court orders provoked by politicians can reverse the previous decision to remove a feeding tube, for example, and prolong existence.

4. A point of controversy: Should the administration of Food & Fluid be considered medical treatment? To some, the distinction depends on the method of administration. If surgery is necessary to implant a tube through the skin and a pump is needed to deliver nourishment, then it is medical treatment. Yet the same liquid mixture can be forced-fed with a spoon or poured down the esophagus through a funnel. While some people consider such acts as basic care, others point out that forcing patients to swallow is, in certain circumstances, an unwanted medical intrusion. Below, the term "artificial" will be considered in more detail. Swallowing can be induced as a reflex, and sometimes, spoon-feeding can be forced to the point where it is assault.

Some argue that pulling the plug of a ventilator does not remove the air from a room, so that if a patient can breathe without mechanical assistance, she will. The case of Karen Ann Quinlan is one famous example. A New Jersey court permitted her parents to request that her doctors remove her ventilator in May 1976, but she surprised all by continuing to breath by herself, until June 1985.

In contrast, the removal of a feeding tube, or cessation of assisted feeding denies patients access to life-sustaining sustenance. Yet if bowls of food and containers of fluid, along with spoons and straws, are placed in front of patients who suffer from advanced dementia or who are in the Permanent Vegetative State (**PVS**), these patients—because their brain damage makes them unaware—cannot take in this nourishment that might prolong existence.

Dr. Edward Sunshine, Professor of Theology at Barry University, reflected specifically about Terri Schiavo: "Another moral perspective would see Schiavo's [neurological] condition as lethal, because her brain damage was preventing her from eating and drinking." [2005] To rule that it is moral or legal to withdraw a patient from a ventilator, but that it is not moral or legal to withdraw a patient from a feeding tube makes little scientific sense. Both the ventilator and tube feeding are medical interventions required to maintain biologic existence, although they address different kinds of severe brain deficits.

It is interesting that although Pope John Paul II proclaimed that providing artificially administered nutrition and hydration is "ordinary" care that every human being deserves indefinitely, he did not choose to insert a permanent feeding tube for himself during the last week of his life.

5. In almost 40% of States, legislators have created laws, or judges have ruled on cases in appellate courts to set precedents, which delineate more stringent standards for refusing artificially administered Food & Fluid than for other

potentially life-sustaining treatments [Sieger and others, 2002]. The National Right to Life Committee promoted a "Model Law" in May 2005, which States could adopt to make **Refusing Food & Fluid by Proxy** much more difficult. (This topic is discussed again, in greater detail).

Why the Word "Artificial" is Artificial

The word "artificial" usually means either made by humans (in contrast to natural), or brought about or by caused human-generated forces. Compared to the liquid sustenance that can be swallowed, there is nothing particularly artificial about the material introduced by tube feeding. More correctly, what IS artificial is the method by which sustenance is administered. Due to the bias of culture, laws in many States single out restrictions for Artificially Administered Nutrition and Hydration, but refer to it as "Artificial Nutrition and Hydration." Leaving out the word "administered" makes the term consistent with the commonly used acronym, "ANH." (**AANH** would be more appropriate). In New York State, for example: "Unless your agent reasonably knows your wishes about artificial nutrition and hydration (nourishment and water provided by a feeding tube or intravenous line), he or she will not be allowed to refuse or consent to those measures for you."

In the case of Food & Fluid by mouth, it would seem "natural" for a well person to want to eat and drink, and "artificial" to provide sustenance that bypasses normal desire (hunger and thirst), normal satisfaction (taste and pleasure of chewing), and normal function (swallowing). But patients can have some desire, potential satisfaction, and the physical ability to swallow, but may still find forced feeding an intrusion. How is that possible? Suppose while still competent, they indicated they would not want to continue their existence if they suffered from an irreversible progressive dementia marked by specific "end-points" they considered as loss of their personhood. Then much later, they reach that state so they do not want their biologic existence to be maintained. That's when they would consider forcing Food & Fluid an unwanted intrusion.

The American Dietetic Association's position paper [Maillet and others, 2002] does NOT distinguish between sustenance delivered by artificial versus normal means. This paper considers both oral and artificial means of delivering food and hydration as "medical interventions." It recommends consideration of "whether or not nutrition, either oral or artificial, will improve the patient's quality of life during the final stages of life"—specifically, "whether or not nutrient support, either oral or artificial, can be expected to provide the patient with emotional comfort... "

6. Non-terminal individuals may **Voluntarily Refuse Food & Fluid**. It is easier to understand why a terminally ill patient from end-stage cancer who is toxic and has nausea would **Refuse Food & Fluid**. But followers of the Christian Science and Jehovah's Witness religions who are not terminal cannot be forced to accept medical treatment that their religious teachings oppose. They may suffer from medical conditions for which medical science offers usual treatment with very high rates of survival, yet if these treatments are refused, they die.

Some medical treatments, when refused, have an uncertain outcome; for example some patients survive pneumonia after they refuse antibiotics. But refusal of dialysis in patients with no kidney function, and refusal of blood transfusions in patients with aplastic anemia (who cannot make new blood) are lethal choices just as certain as **Refusing Food & Fluid**. That is why it is so important to make sure that patients who **Refuse Food & Fluid** possess decision-making capacity and are not suffering from mental illnesses that disturb their judgment. [Terman, 2000].

Why have the courts not insisted that the person be terminal to **Refuse Food & Fluid**? Perhaps they were influenced by arguments that being terminal is not the only reason to realistically have no hope for improvement, and that the expectation of a longer life merely sentences the patient to extreme suffering for a longer time. Instead of discriminating against non-terminal patients, the courts allowed them the same rights as terminal patients. Therefore, **any** competent adult may refuse **any** medical treatment because such refusal is a Constitutionally protected right. This example below also illustrates another important point: **Refusal of Food & Fluid** by a competent adult can be reversible.

A Non-Terminal Patient Could Refuse Food & Fluid

The Case of Elizabeth Bouvia

When Elizabeth Bouvia was 26 years old, her doctors said she might live another 20 years on tube feeding. So she was not terminal. Born with severe cerebral palsy, she was nearly quadriplegic and suffered from extreme pain from degenerative arthritis. She petitioned the court to have her feeding tube removed after the institution in which she resided, refused.

In 1986, the California Court of Appeal, 2d District ordered her feeding tube removed after finding that the "right to refuse medical treatment is basic and fundamental," and is "recognized as a part of the right to privacy protected by both the State and federal constitutions... its exercise requires no one's approval... even if the patient is neither terminally ill nor imminently dying." And "it is clear that she has now merely resigned herself to accept an earlier death, if necessary, rather than live by feedings forced upon her by means of a nasogastric tube."

Some experts have interpreted other statements by the lower courts as simply disputing that Ms. Bouvia had a clear intention to kill herself, casting some doubt that the court specifically endorsed the right to refuse life-sustaining treatment, however.

In any case, after her nasogastric tube was removed, Ms. Bouvia decided to live. She accepted other oral means to take in nourishment.

≈≈

The arguments that favor opposing views can also be convincing. Providing Food & Fluid for oral intake is "ordinary care," not a form of medical treatment that can be refused. As caregivers, we should always respect the dignity of our sickest and most dependent fellow human beings. We should never consider a person as merely a "vegetable." Choices about the treatment of individuals whose lives depend on our decisions should never be based on society's economics. The intent to hasten dying when a person can otherwise survive is similar to euthanasia, especially if treatment is withdrawn only because, in someone's opinion, the patient is not dying fast enough.

Yet Oregon and many European countries admit the reality that medical and financial resources are finite, that treating some diseases have priority over others (because of the potential for recovery of function), and that if a line must be drawn due to finite resources, then there will be some diseases below that line for which society cannot afford to provide treatment.

Ethically, the principle of autonomy, that is, of self-determination, gives us the final say over what happens to our bodies, including the right "to let Nature take its course." We are all mortal, but many of us will die slowly and our doctors may not be accurate about our prognosis when they state whether or not we are "terminal." Actually, the prognosis doctors give is disease-dependent. Many cancers can be staged with fairly accurate probabilities of survival, but patients with congestive heart failure embarrassed their doctors: One day before their patients actually died, doctors predicted that almost half of them would live another six months [Lynn, 2000].

 SKIP

The science of medicine not only advances slowly; it is also accepted slowly. Patients with severe end-stage dementia are statistically terminal, even though the science of medicine cannot predict exactly which organ will fail or become the site of a lethal infection as the proximate cause of an individual's death. Yet many professionals still refuse to consider end-stage dementia as a terminal illness. (The statistical view is that one-half of the patients described as "end-stage" will die within a defined period of time—usually six to twelve months.)

The laws in some States do not permit **Proxy's Refusal of Food & Fluid** on behalf of incompetent patients unless they are **PVS** or terminal. But should your right to make future decisions about your body (or your loved one's body) be dependent on the current state of medicine's ability to form a diagnosis or to predict what disease is terminal? Worse, should a judge accept a religious text, to decide that dementia is not terminal? (See the story of Lee Kahan, which is discussed on page 186.)

No doubt, bioethicists and attorneys, clinicians and religious leaders, politicians and consumer-rights advocates will continue to intensely debate the issues surrounding **Voluntary Refusal of Food & Fluid**. We feel there is now sufficient consensus to justify taking a stand on the issue, as expressed in the following answers to the **i-FAQs**. Yet we appreciate that we could not have written this book *twenty-five years ago*. Back then, there was insufficient clinical experience, fewer statutes and little case law. Yet *sixty years ago*, there would have been fewer reasons, let alone compelling ones, to write this book since tube feeding and ventilators had just been introduced and no one expected this technology would someday be used to prolong the lives of permanently unconscious patients. There was still end-of-life suffering, however, and some doctors quietly risked prescribing large doses of morphine for conscious terminal patients with unbearable suffering. Now, we must make prudent, well-informed decisions about what parameters should influence our end-of-life decisions for medical treatment, and for society as a whole to proactively consider how it wishes to allocate its limited resources of medical personnel and technology, as well as its finances.

❧ CONTINUE

So, what is it like, to make the decision for **Voluntary Refusal of Food & Fluid**; that is, to die this way? Author Fran Moreland Johns shared the revealing memoir below. Her story was inspired by a similar case handled by a volunteer for the organization, *Compassion in Dying*, (now called *Compassion and Choices*).

An October Morning

© Fran Moreland Johns

The thought of dying didn't bother Mary Evelyn in the least. It was all those peripheral issues: the crippling osteoporosis, the near-blindness, the heart failure that had left her almost immobilized, the constant pain, and the frustration that no symptom ever got better.

"Everything's gone except my mind, and now, that's going too." It was a grim joke. Not long ago, Mary Evelyn admitted that dementia was creeping in. As the winner of several poetry awards, she found her frequent struggles to remember simple words quite embarrassing.

Mary Evelyn was a small, wiry woman of 84. Her eyes, once the color of the Connecticut sky, had grown cloudy and discouraged.

It was fall in her native New England, the time of year when she had always loved to hike in the woods and watch the migrating birds, to breathe the sharp, shuddering, enlivening air.

Four years earlier, Mary Evelyn had buried her husband of more than half a century. They had lived a robust life together, sometimes contentious but never dull. Their lives were mostly joyful until his last six years, which had been sheer hell. Felled by a major stroke, Walter had lived in debilitating exile beside her, a sudden stranger, captive in a shrinking, non-functioning body.

Mary Evelyn swore, "No long good-byes for me."

When her daughter Roberta tried to argue with her, she'd say, "I mean it. When enough is enough, I want to be able to say so."

Now that time had come. Although Roberta had moved in to be a full-time caregiver, Mary Evelyn said she no longer wanted to be cared for. Instead, she wanted closure for a life she saw as slowly but inexorably slipping away.

Mary Evelyn asked several people about possible help and then one told her about an organization that helps people as they near the end of their lives. They sent over Joan, who talked to Mary Evelyn about her wish to die. But Joan's response was, "I don't know, Mary Evelyn. You look okay to me. I'm a nurse. Perhaps I can help by seeing if you can get better pain medications."

"Well, I'm not okay," Mary Evelyn snapped. "I'm in constant pain unless I take all these pills that keep me groggy. What I have now is not life, not life as I know it. No, I've tried everything. I want you to find a doctor who can help me."

Joan's look was intense. "Physician-assistance to hasten dying is not legal in our State. But I can tell you about another option."

Joan described **Voluntary Refusal of Food & Fluid**.

Mary Evelyn sat up straight in her chair. "Call Roberta in here. I want you to tell her exactly what you've just told me."

Roberta joined them, surprised to learn what was on the meeting's agenda.

Joan said, "It's simple: just stop eating and drinking. Put Vaseline or one of those fancier creams on your lips, and let a few ice chips melt in your mouth from time to time, and your body will shut down. I'll make arrangements for you to get on hospice, since once you refuse all food and drink, you will clearly meet their entry criteria because you will be expected to die within six-months."

"Will she have to go there, to hospice?" asked Roberta.

"No, they'll provide care in your home."

Then Joan called Mary Evelyn's physician so he could talk to Mary Evelyn and meet the hospice nurse at the same time.... .

After discussing the decision at length, the doctor asked Mary Evelyn, "Have we done everything we can?" His next question seemed more reflective, as if he were asking himself. "Am I wrong to allow this, because I can't make you better? Should I try harder to get you to change your mind?"

Regardless of whom the questions were for, Mary Evelyn remained steadfast.

Roberta agonized, "Are you doing this just because you don't want to be a burden? Like Dad was? Haven't I convinced you that I want you here because I love you? Are you saying the only way I can show you that I truly love you is to let you go?"

Joan wasn't sure. "Every dying person is different. I know the available options, but I'm never sure what's best."

Two days later, Mary Evelyn gathered her family and close friends to tell them of her decision to refuse all food and drink. They agreed to support her, including forbidding any intervention unless she changed her mind.

It was a time of gentleness, order and calm, perhaps because Mary Evelyn seemed so totally determined. Although she was constantly offered food and water, she only accepted ice chips, but not many.

Three days later, Joan dropped by for a visit, pleased to find Mary Evelyn smiling and serene, her speech clear and focused. Her face, which had been twisted with anguish before, now seemed calm and peaceful. She lay in the hospital bed the hospice team had brought in. It was turned toward her living room window so she could see the leaves turning gold outside. As Joan joined her looking out, soaring formations of birds were flying south, rising on the chill winds that swept down from the mountains.

After another five days, Joan visited again. Mary Evelyn was surrounded by the people she loved best. Roberta sat in a straight-back chair beside the bed, holding her mother's hand.

When Mary Evelyn asked for her favorite flavor of ice cream, vanilla fudge, hope seemed to rise in the room along with the question, *Perhaps she would change her mind?*

"How delicious," she said. But she took only half a teaspoonful. "I just wanted a taste." Then she smiled and said, "I feel better than I have in a long time."

The next day she fell into a coma.

The following week, on a brilliant October morning, they buried Mary Evelyn on a tree-shaded hillside, near the mountain trails that Walter and she had taken their grandchildren to explore.

⚬❧

E. What Actions Might I Consider After I Read These i-FAQs?

Outside of hospice and palliative care centers, health professionals may not be familiar with certain critical information; some estate attorneys have limited experience with handling end-of-life conflicts; and some religious leaders believe their interpretation of "God's commandments" takes precedence over a human's autonomy.

Whatever your beliefs, you will want others to honor your Last Wishes rather than impose their values on you. So write or revise your **Advance Directives** so that they are *clear and convincing.* And do it NOW! —Even if you are young. Terri Schiavo, Nancy Beth Cruzan, and Karen Ann Quinlan were all in their twenties when they lost consciousness.

To explore your options, consider showing some of the answers to the following **i-FAQs**, stories, and Guidelines to key members of your family, your primary physician, consultants from hospice, your psychiatrist or psychologist, your legal advisors, your religious or spiritual leader, and especially to the individuals you have designated, or will soon designate, to serve as your Proxies for health-care decisions.

To get the most out of these consultations as you finalize your plans, first decide exactly what your end-of-life wishes are, learn about the current and potential future obstacles, and familiarize yourself with the available strategies, and then decide for yourself, what seems ***best*** for you.

—That is what the rest of this book is about.

Chapter 5

A Peaceful Choice

While not the **BEST** way for all, Voluntarily Refusing Food & Fluid is peaceful and relatively comfortable. It allows time for discussions that could promote healing and sometimes, even a change of mind.

---

1. What is Meant by Voluntary Refusal of Food & Fluid? and What is its Purpose?

Voluntary Refusal of Food & Fluid describes a patient's choice to voluntarily cease intake of Food & Fluid, whether by mouth or by a tube, sometimes to deliberately hasten dying. In clinical medicine, the term "Terminal Dehydration" is often used. Competent patients can legally make this choice even if they are not terminally ill. They can also plan for someone else to make this choice on their behalf if, in the future, they become unable mentally to make decisions, provided they have carefully prepared the appropriate documents.

Voluntary Refusal of Food & Fluid is a legal and peaceful way to avoid being forced to endure prolonged or extreme suffering—including psychological and existential suffering of an individual and his or her loved ones. Unconscious, brain damaged, and severely demented patients may have no other expeditious legal choice to shorten their time to suffer. For most people, one of the most precious individual rights is the ability to choose a peaceful dying.

In one study of nurses' perceptions, the most important reasons patients chose **Voluntary Refusal of Food & Fluid** were: "a readiness to die, the belief that continuing to live was pointless, an assessment of the quality of life as poor, a desire to die at home, and a desire to control the circumstances of death" [Ganzini and others, 2003].

We can learn much from family members of patients who were alert before they died. As a son who was also a physician, Dr. David Eddy shared the following story about his mother's peaceful transition.

"I'm still telling others how well this worked for my mother."

© Dr. David Eddy

It's now just over ten years since my mother, Virginia Eddy, died. As I think of her now, I remember the vibrant, independent woman who loved to walk so very much that she would even go out, bundled up, on winter ice. Medically well until her 84th year, she suffered from many medical conditions in her last year of life. But her most challenging obstacle was the struggle to find a graceful and dignified way to avoid prolonging her existence after she made the realistic appraisal of what her continued existence would be like.

While she was certain her time had come, she had no idea how to make that happen. So she turned to me because I was a physician as well as her son. Although I still miss her and I wish that she had been well enough to continue sharing more of our family's lives, I have no regrets about the ultimate decisions she made on choosing when, and how, she died.

My mother's last request was: "Tell others how well this worked for me. I'd like this to be my gift. Whether they are terminally ill, in intractable pain, or, like me, just know that the right time has come for them, more people might want to know that this way exists. And maybe more physicians will help them find it."

My first response to her request was in 1994, when I wrote an article for the Journal of the American Medical Association entitled "A Conversation With My Mother." Since then, I've received hundreds of letters from people around the world telling me how helpful they found my mother's story. Now I continue my promise to her by writing from the perspective of an additional ten years. Briefly, this is her story.

In her 85th year, my mother suddenly and rapidly experienced declining health, including a failed surgery for a painful rectal prolapse. There's no need to list all her medical diagnoses. Suffice it to say she was left bedridden with no prospect of ever taking those walks she had enjoyed so much. She was also anemic, exhausted, nauseated, achy, and itchy. Because her eyesight was failing, she could no longer read. More than anything, she dreaded becoming dependent upon others for care in a nursing home. This fear was much worse than her fear of death. She also did not want to be remembered in what she considered to be a state of indignity.

After her second surgery failed and left her incontinent, she asked me about suicide. Hoping her despondency would be temporary, I convinced her to wait until she had taken some antidepressants. While the medications did help her think more clearly, her resolve only increased. I remember how determined she explained, "My 'quality of life' has dropped below zero. I know there is nothing fatally wrong with me and that I could live on for many more years. I've lived a wonderful life, but it has to end sometime and this is the right time for me. My decision is not about whether I'm going to die—we will all die sooner or later. My decision is about when and how. I don't want to spoil the wonder of my life by dragging it out in years of decay. I want to go now, while the good memories are still fresh." She clearly and persistently asked me to help her find a way...

After some deep reflection while I was alone, I put aside my selfish wish for my mother to live as long as possible. I realized that her conviction that "her time had come" was totally rational. I still enjoyed her company and I loved our conversations, but from her perspective, her life was so burdened with medical concerns that it left little room for anything else. I had to admit that the ultimate decision was hers to make, not mine.

The first option I considered was to ask one of my colleagues to prescribe pills. But the risk was great since physician-assisted suicide was illegal. My mother had previously read the book, *Final Exit*—but she detested the image of suffocating with a bag around her head. She wanted to leave this world in such a way that her dying would be like the ending of a wonderful movie. She wanted it to be a time where good memories would inspire peaceful acceptance.

As I was pondering other possible options, my mother contracted pneumonia. My initial reaction was that this illness would solve my professional dilemma. Yet as I listened to my mother's gurgling sounds as she increasingly struggled for air, I realized that the "old people's friend" of the pre-antibiotic era is not a particularly comfortable way to die. Surprisingly, my mother survived without aggressive treatment. But after that, she was even more discouraged. She felt it was an opportunity that had been lost. That's when she asked me if she could just starve to death.

I was impressed by her determination. From reading about Gandhi she knew that starvation would be neither quick nor pleasant. Like many lay people, she was misinformed about what doctors now call, "terminal dehydration." When I told my mother that she could not live more than several days if she stopped all drinking, as well as eating, her spirits began to lift as she latched on to the idea. After her attending physician demonstrated respect for her clarity and firmness of her decision by responding that her request was legal, my mother's mood changed to a state that came near to delight.

Her physician disconnected her IV, but continued those medications that would keep her comfortable. Coincidentally, the next day was her 85th birthday. She celebrated with friends and family surrounding her and reading her cards. After relishing a piece of chocolate, she stopped all eating and drinking.

In the following four days, she smiled more than she had for almost a year. Her energy remained strong as she greeted several visitors with whom she reminisced about great times in her past and shared stories that made her proud. Between visits, she slept calmly unless we touched her. Then she woke up and enjoyed sharing more memories. If we had questions, she answered them brightly.

On day five, it was more difficult to arouse her. She was too lethargic to communicate at length. On day six, we could not wake her at all. I remember standing over her bed looking at her face in the unusually quiet hospital room, as no machines were running. Her countenance was that of a natural, relaxed smile. Her breathing was uneven but not labored. Overall, she seemed quite peaceful. That morning we had a sense... so instead of talking, we gathered around mostly in silence, and held her hands. Two hours later, she died.

My mother's dying was a "happy dying," although that may sound like an odd combination of words. Her dying was not saddened by years of decline, lost vitality, and loneliness. Instead of a desperate cling to immortality, she accepted death as a part of life, not as a tragedy to be postponed at any cost. She believed dying should be embraced at the proper time, and she chose to bring her life to a graceful close.

The way my mother chose to die spared me the risk of losing my medical license and being charged with a capital offense. She spared herself the anxiety of respiratory distress from suffocating with a plastic bag over her head. She avoided a desperate visit to a "doctor's" office in Michigan disguised in the form of a van filled with bags of lethal IV solutions.

Most importantly, her last few days were among the most engaging and meaningful in her life. She had the opportunity to share intensely. All her good-byes felt complete. If I had been in her situation, even if physician-assisted suicide had been legal in our State, I would not want to miss the positive moments of those four days when she was still alert.

For my mother, for me, and for the rest of her friends and family, it was a "good" death. We cried, of course and we still miss her greatly. But by achieving death at her "right time" and in her "right way," she transformed the experience from a crushing and desolate loss to one where we could be happy because we knew that she was happy.

꧁꧂

If it is remarkable that Dr. Eddy, a fourth-generation physician, initially considered several illegal, less comfortable, and less dignified ways to help his mother die, then it is astonishing that more than a decade later, the option of **Voluntary Refusal of Food & Fluid** is still relatively unknown and has yet to be established as a commonly offered clinical protocol. One indication of the current lack of knowledge is the way Dr. Ganzini introduced her 2003 paper: "Because little is known about the experience of dying among patients who make this choice, we asked hospice nurses... "

How sad that, instead of providing more articles to educate physicians, and informing the elderly and their children about **Voluntary Refusal of Food & Fluid**, our country remains polarized in a liberal-*versus*-conservative conflict, and that our newspapers covered the sport of kicking Oregon's **Death with Dignity Act** like another political football. At least the antics of the morbid exhibitionist, Dr. Jack Kevorkian, have quieted down since he committed euthanasia on national television and was sent to jail. But isn't it time to offer people the substantial documented legal and clinical information they need so they can make prudent choices, choices that can be both legal and peaceful, to avoid unnecessary prolonged suffering at the end of their own lives, or those of loved ones?

How Erich Fromm's "The Art of Loving" Applies to Responding to Loved Ones Near the End of Their Lives

Fromm's classic of the mid-Twentieth Century, *The Art of Loving*, is a tiny volume that offers much wisdom about relationships. Striving to achieve Fromm's "art" in the areas of Knowledge, Respect, Caring, and Respond-ability can also be applied to life's last chapter:

1. Obtain essential **knowledge** about your loved one's end-of-life wishes—by holding frank discussions and by writing *clear and convincing* instructions in your Advance Directives. Acquiring knowledge is a process that has dual responsibilities. The future patient must be willing to share, and the future Proxy (and alternates) must be willing to listen.

2. **Respect** the patient's wishes. People can feel differently yet strongly about what is sacred at the end-of-life. Some wish to prolong life as long as possible by using all that high-technology medicine can offer. Others may wish to leave this world even if their prognosis is not terminal, based on their judgment that their quality of life is so poor.

Similarly, some may defer to the teachings of a religious leader for guidance on making end-of-life decisions while others wish to make such decisions based on what they feel is best for themselves. Serving as a Proxy demands that you show respect by distinguishing between your values and the values of the patient. Ethical principles ask you to put the patient's values ahead of your own, if they differ. That is what "substituted judgment" decision-making requires.

3. **Caring** is a complicated and often conflicting set of emotional feelings that the patient evokes in you. They are typically a mixture of selfish and generous feelings. You may wish that your relative remain alive because you want don't want to miss seeing his or her face, you don't want to go through the grief process, or you still enjoy your conversations. These caring reasons could be considered concerned with self. If you empathize with the patient's pain and suffering and his or her realistic expectation of future indignity, and you are willing to sacrifice by letting him or her go, such caring could be considered generous.

4. **Respond-ability** is the ultimate component of Fromm's Art of Loving, which is one reason why Fromm coined a new word for it. It involves putting the other three components into action. End-of-life examples of respond-ability include making such life-or-death decisions as pulling the plug of the ventilator or discontinuing tube feeding. It also may include aggressively confronting those who wish to sabotage the wishes of the patient. On the other hand, it might involve sacrificing one's career, social life, and financial estate—to devote 24/7 maintaining a brain-damaged person as you follow the teachings of your religious leader.

Dr. David Eddy followed the generous path of *The Art Of Loving*. His mother was not terminal and he still enjoyed her company, yet he intensely explored the means, and then supported her choice, in reducing how long she had to suffer.

In his story, he portrays his mother as being in good spirits during the first four days of her fast. Does her positive mood make it wrong that she still let her life end two days later? Not necessarily, if we consider her whole saga. Prior to her discovery of this legal peaceful choice, she was depressed even though she was being treated with antidepressants and her family's support. But her future was realistically grim, in terms of being able to function. Her mood brightened only after she learned with certainty that she would not be forced to continue to exist indefinitely with her pain, suffering, dependency, and an extremely restricted range of activities.

2. Why do You Use the Word "Fluid" Instead of "Water"? and *What About Tube Feeding?*

Voluntary Refusal of Food & Fluid requires you to cease intake all types of fluid from all sources. Some lines deliver nutrients into veins, which are called intravenous or IV lines. Other tubes deliver nutrients directly into the stomach or lower parts of the digestive tract. If the tube goes through the nose and throat, it is called a nasogastric or NG tube; if it goes directly into the stomach through the skin and abdominal wall, it is called by the name of the minor surgery that created this path: a percutaneous endoscopic gastrostomy or PEG tube. NG tubes are temporary, while PEG tubes can be used for much longer periods of time.

In 2001, Dr. Steven Post conducted an extensive review of tube feeding in patients with advanced progressive dementia. He concluded: "With regard to PEG placement, it is unlikely that a rational person, fully informed of burdens and benefits along the continuum outlined... would choose long-term tube feeding." Dr. Post demythologized the "fictional" benefits of tube feeding (in patients with dementia) by citing the lack of evidence that tube feeding prolongs life, slows down weight loss, mitigates skin breakdown and pressure sores, or prevents the life-threatening illness of aspiration pneumonia. On the downside, tube feeding denies patients the possible oral gratification of taste. Worse, as many as 7 out of 10 tube-fed dementia patients require physical restraints. To these patients, the feeding procedure may seem like an assault. Dementia patients are also at risk for such adverse side effects as tube migration, leakage around the stoma, nausea, vomiting, abdominal distension and cramping, diarrhea, and aspiration (the inhalation of nutrients into the lungs that can cause pneumonia).

For patients with dementia for whom consultations were requested to consider placing PEG tubes, there was no survival benefit for those who did receive PEG tubes [Murphy and others, 2003].

Why would families choose tube feeding? There are several reasons. Many professionals do not fully inform decision-makers of the risks. Worse, some institutions insist on tube feeding *as if* there is no other choice. Why? Tube feeding provides institutions a two-pronged financial incentive. First, it takes far less staff time than the frustrating job of assisted feeding. Second, the reimbursement rate from Medicare is greater for "skilled nursing care" (read: *tube feeding*) than for "custodial care" (read: *assisted feeding*). The hospice option is rarely utilized for demented patients, although it's possible that new guidelines to estimate the expected time until death will increase usage from the astonishing low figure of "less than 1 percent of hospice patients have Alzheimer's disease." Recent data are higher, at 7%. The national average of hospice usage is 22% for all diagnoses of patients eligible for hospice by Medicare guidelines, so many more patients could benefit from this option.

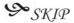*SKIP*

The placement of PEG tubes also does not respect the consensus of patients as revealed by surveys which reveal that 95% of cognitively normal people over 65 would NOT want PEG tubes if they had severe dementia, according to a 1999 paper by Gjerdingen and others. In another study, only 11% of patients of all ages in Boston would want to be tube fed if they were in a state of dementia [Emanuel and others, 1991].

Prior to 1979, inserting a feeding tube into the stomach required major surgery. In that year, Dr. Michael Gauderer and Dr. Jeffrey Ponsky developed the new technique of PEG tubes to temporarily help infants and children who couldn't swallow [reviewed in 2003]. But today, it is used more than 250,000 times a year, is an integral part of end-of-life care, and many feel, is too often used in patients who have no potential for recovery. Dr. Ponsky said, "Once they [PEG tubes] are in, it's so emotionally difficult to take it out and let someone die."

When making a decision that could potentially prolong someone's existence for years, all concerned must realize how difficult it is to assess the degree of pain and suffering experienced by a person who can no longer communicate. In terms of possible benefits, feeding tubes do not always prevent malnutrition, reduce suffering from pressure sores, prevent aspiration pneumonia, provide comfort, improve functional status, or extend life [Finucane and others, 1999]. Yet the burden of feeding tubes in severely demented patients includes high rates of medical complications and an increased need to use physical restraints according to a 2002 paper by Li. No randomized controlled study has provided evidence that tube feeding reduces the risk of aspiration or prolongs life expectancy, on average. Meanwhile, eating may be the patient's last pleasurable activity, as mentioned by Kunz in 2003. For patients in nursing homes, substantial financial incentives may influence decision-makers to favor tube feeding, according to Mitchell in 2004. Fewer than half of surveyed dieticians favored tube feeding for patients who suffer from dementia or who are in a **Permanent Vegetative State**. If they were personally in the same situation, even fewer would want to be tube-fed, according to Healy in 2002. Still, a majority of surrogates reported being satisfied with their decisions to place a feeding tube in their relatives, despite the surrogates' perception that there was no improvement in the patients' quality of life, according to Somogyi-Zalud in 2001.

Surveys show that about 35% of patients in U.S. nursing homes are on feeding tubes, but the figure varies 7 to 10-fold among different States. What accounts for such differences as only 7.5% in Maine but 40.1% in Mississippi? One would hope that it would be clinical parameters or patient preferences. Yet the odds of getting a new tube inserted were nine times higher for African-American patients than overall, even though the average survival for all patients was only six months, according to Meier and others [2001]. Feeding tubes were used more often if the nursing home residents were younger in age, not white, male, and divorced, and worse—if their institution lacked a nurse practitioner or physician assistant on staff, according to Mitchell and others [2003]. Did Advance Directives help? "Specific directives not to provide tube feeding" reduced the odds of having tube feeding 60%, according to Ahronheim and others [2001]. But that may mean that 40% received tube feeding against their wishes. Dr. Ahronheim noted that studies have yet to focus on the influence of "physician characteristics, such as race, attitudes, or knowledge" on the decisions to start tube feeding.

Finally, physicians with less training in end-of-life *Comfort Care* are more likely to over-hydrate their patients and put them at greater risk for developing edema and ascites [Lanuke and others , 2004]. (Edema is the accumulation of excess fluid in the body; it can cause high blood pressure, compromise a failing heart, and make breathing more difficult. Ascites is the accumulation of fluid in the abdominal cavity.)

✎ CONTINUE

In light of much empirical evidence that survival is not prolonged by tube feeding, Debra Lacey [2004] states that health-care providers should refrain from using ***misleading terms*** such as ***"life-sustaining"*** or ***"life-prolonging"*** when discussing tube feeding for patients with dementia. She also suggests these "20th century" terms be removed from Advance Directives. Finally, she questions using the term ***"life"*** when "a person's connection to other human beings and the quality of his or her psychological and spiritual existence" is not extended and ceased to be "an existence that any reasonable person would wish to continue."

✎ SKIP

The paper of Anne-Mei The and her colleagues [2002] offered several useful examples of critical conversations. It found that three criteria were used to decide whether or not to withhold artificial administration of fluids and fluids from dementia patients: the patient's medical condition (administered for an acute medical setback from which recovery is expected); the wishes of the family; and interpretations of the patient's quality of life. In contrast, "Living Wills were helpful, but insufficient." They concluded, "In advanced dementia it is rarely considered beneficial to give fluids and food artificially." They reported respecting the non-verbal expression of "Mrs. N," an 87 year-old suffering from Alzheimer's who turned her head away and closed her lips tightly when nurses tried to feed her orally. After she twice pulled out her IVs, doctors let her go. She died in two weeks.

❧CONTINUE

It is important for all concerned to agree about tube feeding when the time comes. The following story illustrates how it helps to discuss this option prior to when the critical decision must be made.

Dress Rehearsal

© Marjorie Carlson Davis

Six years ago, my mother began to show signs of a devastating Lewy body dementia. First it robbed her of her speech, then her balance, and finally her ability to reason. Now she lies in a wheelchair in a nursing home, her hands clenched tightly under her chin, her nose wrinkled in constant grimace, her eyes unfocused and vacant. Occasionally, when my father, my sister, or I call her name, she groans and her eyes focus briefly, giving us just the slightest signal that the woman we knew and loved still exists there.

Last summer, my mother's health took a turn for the worse: she showed signs of dehydration and for a short time, her death seemed imminent because the nurses could not get enough fluids into her.

As my father was out of town, I had several conversations with my sister about what we should do if mother's situation worsened. We couldn't decide if we would request an IV or feeding tube.

My sister argued, "She's still there; she has to have food and water."

But I wasn't sure. She was so demented, what would it mean to withhold hydration? Yet this was our mother, the woman who gave us life. How could we not prolong her life? I wished I could have known what she would have wanted if she had been aware of her situation, if she could have spoken and simply told us what she wanted.

My father had been traveling but he returned. He gave us copies of mother's Living Will Declaration. "I remember our discussions, more than fifteen years ago," he said. "She definitely would not want her life prolonged artificially." My father made sure the nursing home staff and doctors were aware of her written wishes.

My mother completed her Living Will Declaration when she was in her early fifties and in good physical and mental health. She made her wishes clear.

That summer, my mother's body rallied, as the nurses were able to get her to drink enough liquid. For a time, she became more alert and even began to gain weight.

Though emotionally painful, my family's discussion that summer served as a kind of dress rehearsal for the real thing; we were able to air our feelings about her death, discuss how we would handle her Last Wishes, and how we would cope with that decision.

Through our research, we learned that mother would most likely die from dehydration, or from breathing or swallowing problems. She may die tomorrow, next month, or in a year or more. But now we are clear about her wishes: when it is time to let her go, our decision about using life-prolonging procedures will not be based on our personal difficulty in saying good-bye to a woman we love, nor on some moral or ethical obligation to sustain life. Rather it will be based on her written final wishes, recorded when she was a healthy, happy, mentally sound 54 year-old woman. We feel fortunate that we had this "dress rehearsal," to air all our emotions, questions, and concerns before the end, so we can support each other when the time comes that we must make a tough decision.

৯৹৶

Comment: It is prudent for more than one member of the family to know what the patient wants. In this case, it would have been kind for the father to leave copies of the Living Will with his daughters before he left on a trip.

3. Must I Stop Drinking as Well as Eating? and What About my Medications?

It usually takes between a few days and a couple of weeks to die by dehydration. But if you do not cease intake of fluid, it may take months to die from starvation alone. The more fluid you ingest, the longer you are likely to survive. If you continue to drink or receive fluid by any means—through tubes or by asking for many ice chips, or by eating "solid" or pureed foods (because they are typically about 70% water), then you may considerably prolong how long it takes to die.

Only Water?

A year after her stroke, the physicians caring for Clara Martinez judged she was in an irreversible vegetative state.

Resolved that his wife should not live artificially, her husband, Salvador Martinez, signed a "Do Not Resuscitate" order to keep her from being revived artificially if her heart or lungs were to stop. He also disconnected her feeding machine.

However he continued to provide her with water, perhaps due to uninformed, misdirected kindness.

On the day that her story hit the press, she had survived 30 days without food. By 30 days, virtually all those who also went without fluid would have died.

Pastor Espinoza of the Hispanic Evangelical Church in Chicago was quoted as saying, "It will be an offense against God's principles of ethics," and "It's a sophisticated way of murdering somebody." In response to pressure from publicity in the newspaper, *La Raza*, and several right-to-life organizations, the matter came to the attention of the State of Illinois, Department of Human Services. Soon, her feeding tube was reconnected, despite what her husband said she would have wanted.

৩~ৼ

If you require medication delivered through your veins for you to be comfortable, ask your doctor if he or she can order an alternative to a continuously flowing IV. A *heparin lock* is a short tube that uses a rubber stopper with a small amount of medication that prevents local clotting instead of the continual flow of fluid. (Some physicians just use saline without heparin.) A similar option is the PIC—a percutaneous (through the skin) intravenous catheter (tube).

If you are taking a "water pill" such as the diuretic Lasix, you should probably not stop taking it because doing so may allow fluid to accumulate, which could cause discomfort and prolong the time it takes to die. Also ask your doctor for advice about taking potassium supplements that are prescribed along with some diuretics. Diabetic patients should ask their doctors whether they should continue their insulin or oral medications to control their blood sugar. As you and your doctor discuss such options, keep in mind that some district attorneys might consider it a crime for a physician to provide advice that could be considered assisting suicide, although we know of no physician who was prosecuted for merely counseling, and if you are competent, you have the right to discontinue any medication.

Ask your doctor if there any medications you should not stop because doing so could contribute to your *discomfort*. Continue pain medications, for example.

4. How Long Does the Process Take? and How Does This Time Compare to Other Options?

Death usually comes in several days to a couple of weeks. Ganzini's 2003 study showed that 85% of patients died within 15 days after **Refusing Food & Fluid**. It may seem shorter to patients, however, since most became semi-conscious or unconscious after a few days. If your initial nutritional status is good, however, the process can take longer.

To compare the dimension of time, the end comes in several minutes with *euthanasia*; and in a few to several hours after *ingesting a lethal dose of pills*. Several answers to **i-FAQ**s below compare other aspects of **Voluntary Refusal of Food & Flui**d with *euthanasia* and what is commonly called *physician-assisted suicide*.

As several stories will illustrate, rapidity is not always an advantage. Sometimes the extra time **Voluntary Refusal of Food & Fluid** requires is important: it allows patients to have meaningful visits and deep discussions with family members and friends, as well as to make amends and say good-byes. This time is also important for giving patients the opportunity to change their minds about whether "now" is the right time to maintain their resolve to **Refuse Food & Fluid**.

Next is an example of someone who had to think quickly in order to stay alive:

Quick Thinker

After being injured by a truck whose driver swerved into his line of traffic, a farmer sued for monetary compensation. The case went to court. When he took the witness stand, the attorney for the insurance company handed him a piece of paper. "Please read this statement. It is signed by the policeman who came to the scene of the accident."

The farmer read, "I approached the farmer and asked him how he was feeling. He replied, 'I never felt better in my life.'" The farmer looked up and said, "**But—**"

"Just tell the court, please," said the attorney, "did you or did not you say, 'I never felt better in my life'?"

"Yes, I did, **but—**"

"A simple Yes or No will suffice."

In a low, resigned voice, the farmer said, "Okay."

The farmer's counsel stepped up to the stand. "Please tell the court what happened just before you made this statement."

"Certainly," replied the farmer. "After the accident my horse was thrashing around with a broken leg and my poor old dog was howling in pain. This cop comes along takes one look at my horse and shoots him dead. Then he walks over to my dog, looks at him, and shoots him dead also. Finally, the officer comes straight over to me. His gun was still smoking! So when he asked me how I was feeling, I wouldn't dare say anything else. Would you?"

5. How Does One Die After Refusing Food & Fluid?

After your physician *fully informs* you of your options, and you make a *well-considered, diligent voluntary choice* to allow your existence to end, death can come...

A. from your underlying disease,

B. from dehydration, which leads to an imbalance of critical salts (electrolytes), which the heart needs to function; and to decreased volume of oxygen-carrying blood and low blood pressure so that the heart, brain, and kidneys cannot function; or,

C. from a combination of the underlying disease and dehydration.

Physicians usually list the underlying disease as the **cause** of death, in part because the patient was treated for that condition for the longest time. In 1986, when the Supreme Court of Massachusetts ruled in the case of Paul Brophy, the judges stated, "when such artificial nutrition is removed, the cause of death is the underlying condition." Yet this issue is still confusing. For example, in the autopsy report of Terri Schiavo, Dr. Jon R. Thogmartin wrote: "Cause of Death: Complications of Anoxic Encephalopathy." That means the (original) cause of death was lack of oxygen that caused brain damage. Yet when answering a specific question at a news conference, Dr. Thogmartin replied that Ms. Schiavo technically died of "**marked dehydration**," *not* **starvation**. The legal proximate cause of death was dehydration during her last 13 days, but the medical event that changed the course of her life was lack of oxygen 15 years previously.

We personally have no knowledge of any death certificate that cited the cause of death as "**Voluntary Refusal of Food & Fluid**." It is possible, but we believe unlikely, that any death certificates listed the cause as "terminal dehydration."

If you have been eating and drinking by mouth, your caregivers will continue to offer you Food & Fluid so you have the opportunity to change your mind by resuming eating and drinking. Doing so will honor your autonomy, and may legally protect your caregivers. Sometimes, competent people **do** change their minds... .

She Changed Her Mind Twice: She Was Ready Only After She Had Created Her Loving Legacy

A 43 year-old Utah woman was diagnosed with Lou Gehrig's disease in January 2001. Unfortunately, it was the type that progressed quite rapidly. In May and again in June, she ceased eating and drinking with the intention to hasten her death. But both times, she decided to resume intake of Food & Fluid on the third day.

In late July, after the Utah woman had prepared many years of special gifts and written years of personal loving notes for her young daughter, she again **Refused Food & Fluid**. This time, she maintained her resolve and after a few days, experienced a peaceful transition.

Her husband believes that because his wife knew about and chose the option to **Voluntarily Refuse Food & Fluid**, she did not hasten her life prematurely by taking an overdose of medication. Her additional months of living, though challenging in many ways, were also rewarding. The additional time gave her the opportunity to leave a personal and loving legacy for her daughter.

It is likely that as she began her fast the first two times, she reflected on what possible meaning remained in her life, on what goals she still wanted to accomplish, and on how she would accomplish these goals. So... still conscious after three days, she was able to change her mind—an opportunity that would not have been possible for her, had she chosen "physician-assisted suicide" to hasten her dying. [The clinical portion of this story is based on an account in the editorial comments of Sandra Jacobs, 2003.]

❧

Comment: Friedrich Nietzsche said, "He who has a *why* to life, can bear almost any *how*." This is one way to distinguish pain from suffering. For many people, the closer they are to dying, the more deeply they probe their values and feelings and consider what form they wish to express them as a personal and loving legacy for those we must leave behind [an idea developed in the book by Riemer and Stampfer, 1994]. For this woman from Utah, it may not have been until she experienced her two periods of three-day fasts that she was able to conceive of the form and content of the legacy that she wanted to leave her daughter.

For those of us who consider ourselves *not* near death, if we can break through our denial that we are in fact mortal, that someday we will die, this perspective can motivate us to appreciate even more, how precious life is, and we may be less likely to wait to express our values to our loved ones.

The potential for inner reflection and dialogue with loved ones can be a spiritual turning point for some dying people as they begin **Voluntary Refusal of Food & Fluid**. The ability to change one's mind can be a great advantage; its benefit can transcend to surviving generations. This is one reason why **Voluntary Refusal of Food & Fluid** can be, for some, the *BEST WAY* to say goodbye.

Although most ALS patients can still swallow if someone puts pureed food in their mouths, their usual motivation to stop eating and drinking arises from the typical way the disease progresses: when the muscles that permit them to breathe lose most of their strength, they experience air hunger, one of the most frightening feelings a person can experience. When over-the-mouth-and-nose types of mechanical assistance begin to fail, the patient must make a difficult choice. One option is morphine or an opioid patch to reduce the extreme anxiety from not being able to breathe. The medication causes drowsiness. As the brain gets too little oxygen, the patient eventually dies. The other option is for the patient to go on a ventilator.

If you decide to hasten your dying by **Voluntary Refusal of Food & Fluid** and your current medical condition requires that sustenance be delivered through tubes that are not yet in place, you must decide *not to initiate* tube feeding. If a tube is already in place, you must ask your doctor to write an order to *withdraw* the tube. Most physicians, attorneys, and bioethicists consider *not initiating* a tube that could provide Food & Fluid as ethically and morally equivalent to *voluntarily withdrawing* a tube that is already in place; however some strictly observant religions consider the distinction between withholding and withdrawing as significant.

Religious or not, some lay people (and even some physicians) feel they are "actively doing something" to end a patient's life when they withdraw a treatment that could be life-sustaining. In contrast, they feel they are "passively not doing anything" if they do not initiate the same treatment. For this apparent difference, *not initiating* seems more acceptable than *voluntarily withdrawing*. But there is a practical downside to this point of view: Sometimes treatments are offered to patients to see if their condition will improve even when most experts predict that improvement is unlikely. But if they do improve, it was worth the trial. However those people who believe they cannot remove life-sustaining treatment once started may be far more reluctant to give patients such a final chance.

It is ironic that, if health providers and loved ones can maintain an attitude where they will be willing to withdraw treatment if it ultimately proves to be of no benefit, then the patient may be offered such a treatment trial, and may improve. This is one of the two great ironies in this book. The other will be explained in detail later. Briefly, if patients know they can determine when they will die so they can be sure they will need not to suffer pain or become dependent after loss of dignity, they can live with less anxiety and worry, and often choose to live longer.

6. Is Voluntary Refusal of Food & Fluid Uncomfortable?

No, **Voluntarily Refusing Food & Fluid** is NOT uncomfortable. We base our opinion on six sources:

A. The feelings expressed by those who were alert as the process began. Examples are the stories about Virginia Eddy and "Mary Evelyn."

B. The clinical observations reported by experienced physicians, and nurses. Later in the book, Dr. Ronald Miller relates his story about his mother, Mrs. Virginia Gordon Wilson Miller. Dr. Richard Prince, an emergency department physician, privately told me a similar story about his father, and related it to many patients he treated, as briefly summarized in Praise for this book. Non-medical family members have shared testimonials and observations of the peaceful transition of their loved ones as they **Voluntarily Refused Food & Fluid**. Many compared the patient's peace to the previous level of discomfort or suffering. In contrast, "Our experience has shown that artificial feeding up until death generally increases patient discomfort" [Doctors Schmitz and O'Brien, *Page 36*, 1989]. They continued, "We have not seen evidence that dehydration occurring at the termination of life results in any pain or distressing experience for the patient. To the contrary, even patients who remain quite alert and communicative and become objectively dehydrated are without substantial symptoms when they are treated for dry mouth." Kenneth Bartholomew, M.D., worked with hundreds of dying patients in nursing homes for over 15 years. He "believes that there is very little discomfort, let alone suffering, from a death due to dehydration... their facial countenance does not change. Their reflex activity does not indicate they are in pain... they simply slip deeper and deeper into a coma—the dying person's natural escape from pain and suffering... This is letting go—letting Nature take its course... to die with dignity." [*Pages 46-47*, 1994] "This is what I would do for myself or my own family member [*Page 82*]... When we are talking about humane caregiving, there is only one choice for me. Death due to refusal to be fed and watered... Subsequent dehydration is quick and humane." [*Page 96*]

C. Author Stan Terman's four-day experience [in the summer of 2005] of **Withholding Food & Fluid**, as related in the Prologue.

D. Understanding the basic physiology of over-hydration. According to Schmitz and O'Brien [Lynn and others, *Page 30*, 1989]: "We have noted a reduction of nausea, vomiting, and abdominal pain... . Lessened urinary output means fewer linen changes for incontinent patients and less frequent struggling with commode or bedpan for others. Pulmonary secretions decrease as patients allow themselves to become dehydrated, resulting in less coughing, less congestion, and less shortness of breath. With the decrease in mucous, there is less gagging and choking for those with difficulty swallowing and/or extreme weakness.

Frequently, the need for oral-pharyngeal suctioning is eliminated." Joanne Lynn added that mental confusion is less likely if fluid and nutrition have NOT been maintained prior to the time of death [*Page 53*, 1989]. Dr. Lynn later noted less frequent urination lowers the risk of skin breakdown and bedsores, and less liquid in the circulatory system makes it easier for the patient's heart to pump [1999].

E. Understanding the psychology of dying. Patients often find a new profound sense of peace because they have stopped fighting as they attain acceptance, as Kübler-Ross described [1969]. Schmitz and O'Brien noted, "many patients experience relief and a renewed sense of autonomy from controlling their own intake. When they do not have to force feed themselves to eat under threat that otherwise tube feeding or intravenous fluids will be started, anxiety diminishes" [Lynn and others, *Page 30*, 1989].

Typically, there is increased clarity and satisfaction at the beginning of the process. Over the next few days, calmness progresses to sedation as patients become less aware of their suffering, which may in fact, have decreased.

The bottom line is that few patients report difficulty with maintaining their resolve, and those who decide to resume intake of Food & Fluid usually have reasons other than hunger or thirst. "Caregivers must... recognize that force-feeding or artificial feeding can sometimes be harmful and may thus be contraindicated" [Schmitz and O'Brien [*Page 37*, 1989]. As Lynn and Childress put it [*Page 53*, 1989]: The decision not to maintain artificial nutrition and hydration may "... allow such a patient to live out a shorter life with fair freedom of movement and freedom from fear, while a decision to maintain artificial nutrition and hydration might consign the patient to end his or her life in unremitting anguish."

F. Research studies of patients, such as performed by Linda Ganzini and colleagues [2003], as previously discussed, in which hospice nurses rated the quality of dying as "**8**," on a scale where "**9**" was the best possible.

❧ *SKIP*

Roeline Pasman and colleagues performed the first prospective empirical study to investigate discomfort in patients with severe dementia for whom the decision was made to forgo artificial nutrition and hydration [2005]. Nursing home physicians filled out questionnaires after they estimated discomfort in patients with dementia based on the frequency, intensity, and duration of observed facial expression, vocalizations, and muscle tension. These authors concluded, "Forgoing artificial nutrition and hydration in patients with severe dementia who scarcely or no longer eat or drink is **not associated with high levels of discomfort**," and "An important finding is that the **level of discomfort decreases** in the days after the decision is made to forgo artificial nutrition and hydration. In patients who died within 2 weeks after the decision, the discomfort level decreased until they died." [Emphasis added.]

℘ CONTINUE

For the sake of completeness, we report the one published personal anecdote and one medical opinion about discomfort during **Voluntary Refusal of Food & Fluid**—the only such reports we could find.

Jane Gross wrote about the dying of her 88 year-old mother [2003]: "The last three days were peaceful, an undisputed **9**," she wrote, using the scale of Ganzini, "but the week in the middle was 'harrowing.'" A careful reading of her observations reveals however that it was not the choice of dying by **Refusing Food & Fluid** that led to discomfort. Instead, it was the choice of not having hospice provide care: "My mother chose *Comfort Care* over hospice because she preferred the familiar nurses and social workers to strangers." Her mother's pain was undertreated because, as she wrote: "a nursing home is staffed by people with widely differing views about end-of-life issues... each nurse drew her own conclusion about whether my mother was in enough pain to justify more medication."

Comment: The conclusion to draw from the article by Ms. Gross is that readers should be even more encouraged to choose hospice; however her experience has nothing to say about **Voluntarily Refusing Food & Fluid**.

The one physician whom Attorney Wesley Smith quoted in his article gave no reference to research or to specific patients or any indication of how many patients he had observed [2003]: "St. Louis neurologist Dr. William Burke told me: 'A conscious person would feel it [dehydration] just as you or I would. They will go into seizures. Their skin cracks, their tongue cracks, their lips crack. They may have nosebleeds because of the drying of the mucous membranes, and heaving and vomiting might ensue because of the drying out of the stomach lining. They feel the pangs of hunger and thirst. Imagine going one day without a glass of water! Death by dehydration takes ten to fourteen days. It is an extremely agonizing death.'"

Comment: If a conscious person did feel dehydration was agonizing, wouldn't she ask for more *Comfort Care* to the mouth, or drink something? Yes, diligent care to the mouth and mucous membranes is important. Yes, seizures (usually when the patient is unconscious) can rarely occur. But the process is not agonizing.

The concept of comfort, particularly at the end of life, must be considered in relative terms for those who observe patients in the Minimally Conscious State or in the end-stage of dementia and wonder about their suffering. While pneumonia has been called "the old person's best friend," van der Steen concluded that discomfort was higher shortly before death when pneumonia was the final cause of death than with death from other causes [2002]. Dehydration may be more comfortable. Consider next, this empathic story of a devoted daughter.

"Where's Little Jake?"

© Peg Reiter

It seems like a death march as I walk behind my mother's slow shuffle. The poorly lit hallway smells of yesterday's meals and dirty laundry. I returned to my Mom's home in Iowa this afternoon, and the two of us left immediately to visit Dad on the Alzheimer's Unit. He was admitted three weeks ago. As I follow my mother towards the unit, I feel I will suffocate. I hate the idea that I will soon see the man who is supposed to be my father but no longer is. But I cannot turn back.

My mother enters the secret code and the door opens, permitting us to enter. Dad is sitting on a chair near a table. He is staring into space, his face vacant. I walk up to him, touch his shoulder, and whisper, "Dad, this is Peg." He turns around, repeats my name as if it is a question, looks down, and cries. *Is he embarrassed, ashamed, terrified?*

I hold his hand and place my arm around his shoulder. We hold each other and cry. We choke on words that cannot be said. I so want to run out of this facility and find Dad in the garage back at our home, loading fishing poles and gear into his truck, like he did when I was a kid. We'd climb in his truck with Mom's picnic lunch and drive ten miles to Sportsman's Park. That was the Dad who would bait hooks, tell amusing stories, and joke that he wouldn't clean any of the fish that we kids caught. That was the Dad who, on lazy Sunday afternoons, would spread thick mustard on ham sandwiches, and throw bread crumbs to the fish as we sat on a small, worn dock and dangled our feet in the cool water.

But that Dad is gone, and all that remains is the shell of the man who previously held that spirit.

A woman in a dark blue uniform brings Dad his evening meal on a metal tray. Mashed potatoes, a peanut butter sandwich on Wonder bread, and canned white pears. I don't know why it reminds me of John Lennon's "White" album as I think, *This is Dad's white meal.* He takes a fork and stabs the tan-colored napkin in front of him. He keeps poking and stabbing. He is confused. He does not realize that the napkin is not edible. He cannot distinguish between the napkin and his food.

I guide his hand to the mashed potatoes. His hand shakes as he glides some potatoes on his fork... But on the way to his mouth, he drops the potatoes from the fork and the mess lands on his lap. But now he seems to know what to do, so he tries again. In his lap, again. After one more failed attempt, I lose patience and place my hand on his, pick up some potatoes, and guide the fork to his mouth. He chews and swallows. He drools and I wipe his chin with the poked napkin. We repeat this process over and over until the potatoes are gone. Then it's on to the peanut butter sandwich that I have to cut up and serve with a fork. Finally the slippery pears... .

Now I understand why Mom must visit Dad three times a day. If she is not with him at mealtimes, he will not eat. It takes almost an hour to feed him the "white" meal, a time spent without any real conversation. He is silent as I urge him on. "Chew your sandwich," I say, or, "Drink some juice now." I look around. Other Alzheimer's patients eat and drink in silence. When he is finally finished, Mom and I sit at the table and chat about nothing: the cold January weather, the sweater she is wearing, the furniture in the room... .

We are back in Dad's room when my forty-six year-old brother, Jake, comes in. "Hi Dad. It's Jake." Dad frowns. He looks confused. He turns to my brother and says, "Little Jake? You can't be Jake. Jake's little." My brother sits next to Dad. After a few moments of uncomfortable silence, Dad reaches over and takes Jake's legs in his lap and unties his shoes. *Was Dad acting as a parent for a young child?* Now I chat with my brother about nothing. Mom listens in silence. Later Jake leans over to me. "How old do you think I am in his mind?" he whispers. Then Jake shares that this is a relatively good day for Dad. He explains: "Usually Dad recognizes Mom—not as Mary—but as a helpful and caring person. But when he cries out, 'Where's Mary?' Mom still gets upset even though she won't admit it. Maybe the reason he didn't ask, 'Where's Mary?' today is because you're here. At his best, he seems a few decades behind." Jake raises his voice to get Mom's attention and offers to stay until the nurses get Dad settled for the night. Then, Mom and I can leave.

But as we rise to leave, Dad looks sad he starts to cry. "There was a fire last night and all the children died," he says. I take his hand and ask, "Did you know these children?" Dad looks directly at me. His sobs are deep. "Yes, they were mine."

Mom stands on one side of Dad's chair and I stand on the other. We hold his hands and cry with him. We cry about his imagined loss of children. We cry for the torment that he faces every day. We cry because he lives in a world that no longer includes us. We cry because he no longer lives in our world.

Ironically, his children have died. —At least in his mind.

My father contracted pneumonia a few days after this visit. As a family, we dealt with this challenge by reaching a consensus to support our mother's decision. Mary instructed Dad's doctor not to treat him with antibiotics or to provide him with Food & Fluid. But of course, we wanted him to receive *Comfort Care*. The doctor said he could administer a powerful painkiller that would also reduce his anxiety about breathing—as drops under his tongue.

My father died peacefully, seven days later.

Comment: Had Peg's family decided to pursue aggressive treatment for his pneumonia, her father's dementia would have progressed further. He would have reached the point where he never knew the names of his family members. He might have been more deeply burdened by fears even more horrifying, fears that he could not even express. Feeding him would have taken longer to reduce the possibility of food going down his trachea and causing aspiration pneumonia. As his condition worsened, he might have needed to be strapped down when fed, if he behaved as if he were being assaulted. After experiencing the sharp pain from the insertion of tubes, he might misunderstand his caregivers' intent and dread ordinary care such as turning his body during a sponge bath. If he suffered from severe pain, he would not be able to say so, or indicate where it hurt. Frequent checking for bedsores and infections still would have left many other possibilities for the source of pain. His incontinence of bladder and bowels would progress from often to total, so that he would have to live the rest of his life in diapers. And then, when he lost the ability to swallow, his doctor might have presented the family with this challenging decision: "Do you want to consent to the insertion of a feeding tube?" Most likely, their prudent answer would have been, "No."

So if Peg's family had decided to treat her father's pneumonia, then several months to years later, they might have asked: "What was the point? Where was the value?" As they considered the balance between her father's decreasing ability to enjoy any meaningful human interaction and his personal suffering, plus the anguish of his family members whom he loved and definitely would not want to suffer, they might have wondered, "Were we right to treat his pneumonia?"

Comfort Care for Patients Who Refuse Food & Fluid

Palliative Care usually means aggressive medical care to reduce patients' symptoms. *Comfort Care* can be the same, but may be less intense. There is much that caregivers and nurses can do to make the experience of **Voluntarily Refusing Food & Fluid** peaceful. If necessary, physicians can treat pain and discomfort from the underlying disease by prescribing strong tranquilizers and powerful pain relievers, as detailed in the next **i-FAQ**. Often patients slip into a light sleep that becomes deeper, at which point, all suffering finally ends.

Non-prescription medications may suffice to reduce or eliminate discomfort from hunger and thirst. Many patients report mild euphoria or pleasant light-headedness and a decreased appetite, which is probably due to the increase in *ketones*—the breakdown products of metabolism. Nature's way to ease end-of-life discomfort may explain why dying patients may have less hunger or thirst than healthy people have after they miss only one or two meals. *Ketosis* also explains why overweight people on a diet that contains almost no carbohydrates report little hunger. As noted in the Prologue, I personally felt almost no hunger during my four days without Food & Fluid. Yet thirst was more of a challenge…

Mouth care is critical since that is where we experience thirst. I experimented with a variety of thirst-reducing aids and learned much more than I did from just reading the medical literature. Surprisingly, I liked Lemon-Glycerin Swabsticks (McKesson). At first they seemed like a practical joke—a lollipop with cotton inside—yet two swabs relieved the dryness in my mouth. I also used one or two half-second sprays of Salivart (Gebauer Co.) to refresh my entire oral cavity every hour. Some might prefer instead Oasis (GlaxoSmithKline). A half-inch of Biotene's oral lubricant, OralBalance, spread around my mouth prevented night-time dryness. It may be a good choice for mouth breathers. Chewing two pieces of Biotene's "Dry Mouth Gum," and one or two Listerine FreshBurst Strips (Pfizer) refreshed my mouth in between tooth brushing. Binaca FastBlast spray and Binaca Gel Bursts (Playtex) had an intense flavor that some might find too strong. Patients with mouth sores might welcome a generic "Sore Throat Spray similar to Chloraseptic" (Longs Drugs) containing phenol and menthol. To refresh my whole face, I enjoyed brief sprays of "Rosewater and Glycerin" (Heritage Products). I also used a saline nasal spray (Target Brand) and Lubricant Eye Drops (GenTeal)—other areas that also become dry. I avoided sugary lemon drops since in theory they could awaken my interest in sweets and increase my hunger by increasing insulin levels; but some people might appreciate them. Knowing that the process can be prolonged by too many ice chips, I was pleased to find that I had no need for ice chips. There is one important exception: a small ice chip will help some medications dissolve under the tongue, such as prescription Clonazepam and Lorazepam for anxiety. The material for aromatherapy can be obtained from health stores and may increase comfort and mood. A prescription artificial saliva product, Aquoral spray (Auriga Pharmaceuticals), is now available [2007]. (Note: Ratings, new products, prescription medications, and the opportunity to share personal experiences can be found on www.ThirstControl.com.)

Doctors Schmitz and O'Brien offered these additional recommendations: Viscous lidocaine (a local anesthetic) to alleviate oral discomfort. (Orajel by Del Pharmaceuticals has benzocaine, which is similar.) Half-strength hydrogen peroxide can be diluted with water or normal saline, or with baking soda and water for oral hygiene. Room humidifiers can decrease dryness. Vaseline (or perhaps even better, Aquaphor, by Eucerin) can keep the lips moist [1989].

EXAMPLES OF PRODUCTS THAT REDUCE THIRST

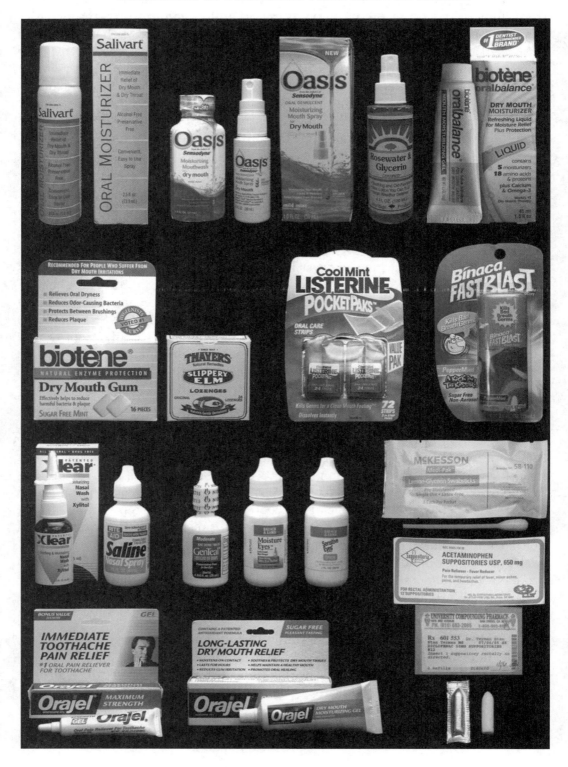

Note: the product sizes on the previous page are not photographed to scale.

I suffer moderate back and leg pain from spinal stenosis so I used two kinds of rectal suppositories: 650 mg of Acetaminophen (Clay Park Labs) and 50 mg of Diclofenac, which I special ordered from a compounding pharmacy although it is also available commercially. Diclofenac required a prescription even though it is similar to medications like Advil and Aleve.I used about three suppositories of each, per day. Many terminally patients will already be on more potent analgesics. Sometimes analgesics by the rectal route are absorbed more slowly and less completely than when they taken by the oral route so if you have pain, insert a suppository before your pain gets bad. Also ask your doctor for his advice on whether you need to use a higher dose. Codeine, for example, must pass through the liver to become an active analgesic, which it does when taken by mouth; when taken by the rectal route, you may need a higher dose. For localized pain, prescription lidocaine patches or ketoprofen transdermal cream can offer relief.

Dr. M. Davis and colleagues extensively reviewed the pharmacology of medications given *per rectum* [2002] and concluded that they are underutilized for palliative care in the United States. While their article appeared in a cancer journal, their suggestions are applicable to all terminal patients. As always, consult your personal physician who knows your medical condition and goals, and can best consider possible drug interactions.

Another component of *Comfort Care* is soothing music. Live harp music can reduce pain and discomfort significantly, the proof of which can be measured by physiological parameters [Terman, 1999]. Some organizations of harp therapists offer their services on a sliding scale according to the family's ability to pay. As an alternative, a music system that plays harp or other soothing music may also help.

A horrific experience? Yes, but for Karen, or Her Mother?

Doctors told Karen Raghavan she could not allow her terminally ill mother to swallow water. The reason they gave was that she might choke to death. Her mother had already indicated these choices: not to have her life prolonged with machines, not to be resuscitated, and not to be fed intravenously.

Karen wrote these words about *her own* experience [2005]: "Watching her waste away was a horrific experience. To see her body reduced to a skeleton, unable to take any nourishment, was shocking. With this also came the delirium, as her mind went... Slowly and painfully you watch, as the person you love finally slips away."

Question: Did **Withholding Food & Fluid** result in a poor outcome and for whom?

Karen was emotionally distressed in part because of how the story began: "Doctors told Karen..." The words sound as if the *doctors had made this decision*, and then justified it as necessary due to her mother's current medical condition (her "Best Interest"). Even though this decision was consistent with all of her mother's previous decisions Karen might have felt less upset if her mother and she had previously discussed and agreed to **Withhold Food & Fluid** in similar situations. It is an act of kindness for patients to discuss these options with their family members so their loved ones can feel more certain they are carrying out their Last Wishes. In this case, the best that could be done was for the doctor to discuss the option with Karen, and to give Karen a greater sense of control of why this important decision was the right one at this time.

In my practice I often say, "Unfortunately, your mother is dying. We want her to have the most peaceful transition possible. While it may at first seem contrary to the usual way we provide nurturing in our culture, there are compelling medical reasons to **Withhold Food & Fluid**. It can will lower the risk of dying from suffocation with choking, or from pneumonia with shortness of breath and fever. Both are far more uncomfortable than dying from dehydation.

Most likely, the ordeal was much harder for Karen than for her mother, who may not have been conscious of her delirium. While Karen complained about *the process of dying*, no doubt the *resulting death* was also hard. It may have been difficult for her to distinguish the two. Karen may also have suffered less had she been informed that **Withdrawal of Food & Fluid** can be comfortable.

Doctors should treat the whole family and educate them about delirium: the patient may not be aware of delirium; the symptoms can be treated; depending on the underlying disease, imminently dying patients may have delirium as a natural part of the dying process even if well hydrated [Dr. James Hallenbeck, cited in Henig, 2005]. Centeno and others [2004] found that of all advanced cancer patients, over 80% eventually experience delirium in their final days.

Sometimes in life, you must decide which alternative is the least bad and also the most certain. Discontinuing medical treatment may not "succeed," depending on your goal, as the next brief story illustrates.

A Failed Attempt to Micromanage Dying

An 88 year-old man suffered from three diseases—hypertension, Parkinson's disease, and kidney failure. He was taking a dozen oral medications and received dialysis three times a week. After due consideration, he decided to stop everything. He assumed he would fall into a coma from kidney failure and have a peaceful death—which he preferred to "the agony of living indefinitely with three chronic, progressive, debilitating diseases."

What happened? His kidneys functioned well enough for him to survive. Three weeks later, he had a stroke that caused paralysis and left him incontinent. He then continued to live and suffered indignity for much longer than he had wanted, and with even greater dependency. He thus failed by experiencing the exact opposite of the more peaceful and quicker dying that he had hoped for. [Adapted from Henig, 2005]

Comment: His advisors might have suggested a contingency plan so that if four diseases (the original three plus the strokes) did not suffice to hasten his dying, he could have authorized his **Proxy to Withhold Food & Fluid** on his behalf.

✎ SKIP

Dehydration to hasten dying does have its downside. It may contribute to delirium, especially for patients taking opioids (morphine-like medications). Cerchietti and colleagues used water containing sugar or salt [2000] as well as an anti-psychotic drug (haloperidol) to reduce symptoms of delirium. (We do not know if the drug alone would have sufficed.) Schmitz and O'Brien [1989] suggested treating the symptoms of increased blood calcium—which can cause twitching, muscle spasms, and altered levels of consciousness—with antispasmodics and sedation instead of water.

The consensus of opinion among researchers is that complaints of the sensation of thirst do not necessarily correlate with "biochemical dehydration." Morita and others [2001] found that terminally ill cancer patients' frequent complaints of thirst are associated with mouth breathing, use of opioids, poor general conditions, and infections of the oral cavity. On the other hand, "no significant correlations were observed between [rating on their] scale for thirst and the blood concentrations of total protein, blood urea nitrogen, creatinine, sodium, osmolality, hematocrit, atrial natriuretic peptide, and biochemical dehydration defined by the levels of BUN, creatinine, sodium and osmolality." In a subsequent study, Morita and others [2004] found that "physicians and nurses in both oncology and palliative care settings frequently observed deterioration of fluid retention symptoms [for example, peripheral edema, ascites and pleural effusions] with limited benefits in alleviating dehydration symptoms by intravenous hydration therapy... so [they] suggested that routine use of artificial hydration therapy should not be recommended."

After Ellershaw and his colleagues [1995] observed "no statistically significant association" between the level of hydration with complaints of "thirst" or "dry mouth" or even the level of respiratory sections in terminal cancer patients, the authors concluded, "Artificial hydration to alleviate these symptoms in the dying patient may, therefore, be futile."

Intravenous therapy in terminal cancer patients during the last two days of life did not improve patients' levels of consciousness [Waller and Adunsky, 1994]. McCann and colleagues [1994] followed 32 conscious terminal cancer patients for a year. For "**all patients,**" they found that "complaints of thirst and dry mouth were relieved with mouth care and sips of liquids far less than that needed to prevent dehydration" (as determined by biochemical studies). Providing *Comfort Care* locally to the mouth effectively reduced complaints of thirst in dehydrated patients, even without restoring body fluids.

✂ *CONTINUE*

Conclusion: **Refusal of Food & Fluid** is usually not uncomfortable in an absolute sense. If it does increase discomfort, this is usually mild compared to the underlying terminal illness. Sometimes, it may increase comfort. At worst, its symptoms can be effectively treated and do not last long, anyway. Compared to other options in the process of dying, for both patients and their family members, it may be "the best way to say goodbye." (There are some types of patients for whom it is *not* best, and some religions do not approve of it, however; see below.)

7. What Medications Can Effectively Relieve Discomfort But Require Minimal Fluid?

The first word to remember about optimal end-of-life care is **hospice.** The staff at hospice has the expertise that comes from their vast experience to reduce many kinds of suffering. Most, but not all, hospices will accept patients if they have decided to **Voluntarily Refuse Food & Fluid** because that commitment makes their condition terminal. We recommend you discuss your options with your personal physician who might refer you to your local hospice. If you discover that one hospice is not willing, then contact another.

Most hospices know it is important for patients to restrict fluids to make the dying process less uncomfortable. But you may encounter some staff members at some hospices who have a moral problem with the explicitly stated goal of intending to hasten dying, even though **Voluntary Refusal of Food & Fluid**. Keep in mind that the goal of hospice is to reduce suffering and make the remaining time at the end of life as meaningful as possible. Schmitz and O'Brien worked at a hospice that did "allow patients to choose what and when they will eat and drink," and these authors stated that "many patients come to hospice having already chosen not to be fed artificially" [1989, *Pages 29-30*].

Out of respect for the goals of hospice, and as a diplomatic way to maximize your success in having your Last Wishes honored, we recommend you consider this "progressive" approach: Enroll in hospice with the sincere hope that their expertise can sufficiently reduce your symptoms of discomfort so that you will want to continue living. After what you consider to be a reasonable amount of time, if their palliative treatment attempts fail to relieve your suffering, you can then state your preference to **cease intake of all Food & Fluid**. This "progressive strategy" may succeed in many hospices.

We now provide some basic information on several medications for sedation and pain relief that can be administered with little or no fluid. **All these medications require prescriptions from doctors who also have licenses from the Federal Drug Administration (FDA) to prescribe controlled substances**. Most physicians who work at hospices know many more options than the few examples we cite below. If you live in rural area far from a hospice and your personal physician has minimal experience in providing *Comfort Care* while restricting fluids, consider asking your personal physician to call the staff of a hospice in your State for some advice over the telephone. Then your own doctor can treat you, taking your particular medical situation and goals into consideration.

To reduce anxiety and insomnia, the brand-name **Klonopin** is available as an oral wafer that quickly dissolves on, or under the tongue. If your mouth is very dry, a small ice chip may be needed. The generic formulation (**clonazepam**) can also dissolve in the mouth, but it takes a little longer, although the taste is pleasant. This Valium-like benzodiazepine provides smooth sedation and overdoses rarely, if ever, depress the drive to breathe. For severe agitation and anxiety, physicians learn what dose you require by repeating a small dose every 2 to 4 hours, until you achieve calmness. The art of medicine is not to give too much, which would make it difficult to remain awake. Since the half-life of clonazepam is long, the initial doses may begin to accumulate. Doctors should also be cautious about the dose of any drug in elderly patients especially if their kidneys or liver are not functioning well. Once the right dose of clonazepam is found, it may be given every 12 hours.

One problem with **Klonopin/clonazepam**: its half-life is long so it remains in your body a long time. You may have to skip more than one dose to regain alertness to visit with a late-arriving relative with whom you have not exchanged goodbyes.

For deeper sedation to treat intractable suffering, Quill and Byock [2000] suggested that physicians consider these medications: Midazolam, Lorazepam, Propofol, Thiopental, Pentobarbital, or Phenobarbital. Palliative care physicians sometimes place a small needle just under the skin, or set the IV to a very slow drip rate, so that minimal fluid is used to deliver these medications.

To reduce pain, **Duragesic/Fentanyl** patches can be applied to the skin to deliver an effective morphine-like medication. It is an alternative to Roxanol, which you take a certain number of drops under the tongue every few hours. Since **Fentanyl** is absorbed slowly, the first patch should start 12 to 24 hours before you stop oral or intravenous narcotics in order to avoid "breakthrough" pain. The patches are available in several sizes based on how many micrograms they deliver per hour. For extreme pain, more than one patch can be used.

Sometimes, families of terminally ill patients must plead with prescribing physicians to persuade them to increase the dose of pain-relieving medications. Some of the signs of discomfort are agitation including thrashing about, waving the hands, gripping the sheets or nightgown, grimacing, and moaning. Since the physicians and nurses who work in hospice have extensive experience recognizing and treating pain, this is the most important reason to consider using hospice. Another reason is that the Medicare hospice benefit offers a full year of support that includes grief groups for the surviving family members. They thus treat another type of "pain": grief.

Duragesic/Fentanyl has several problems. First, the drug can depress the brain center responsible for the drive to breathe so if your doctor prescribes too high a dose, the medication may hasten your dying. Second, the medication is expensive; however most hospices include its cost in their comprehensive care. Third, not only is its half-life is long, but merely removing the patch does not stop drug that has been stored in your skin from continuing to enter your body. Fourth, caution is needed based on recent reports that, in rare instances, the patch inadvertently transferred from a patient to a visitor with a hug. The consequences could be dangerous for children. As with all powerful medications, Duragesic must be used with meticulous care under the supervision of your physician.

An estimated 5 to 15 percent of terminal patients experience extreme suffering that requires **Terminal** (or **Palliative**) **Sedation**. Some professionals prefer the alternate term, **Controlled Sedation for Refractory Suffering**, which I suggested to a committee formed to establish guidelines at the San Diego Hospice in 2000. Defining each word in the term is instructive: "Refractory" means resistant to usual treatments. "Suffering" can be emotional, spiritual, or existential, as well as physical pain. "Controlled" means using a dose of medication that is sufficient only to reduce suffering, not to intentionally hasten dying, to satisfy the ethical requirement of the Double Effect. Even when pain can be controlled, sometimes there are other symptoms that cannot be controlled.

Palliative Sedation puts patients into a deep sleep (mild anesthesia) so they are no longer conscious of suffering. If done close to the time they would die, they do not wake up so the term, **Terminal Sedation**, seems apt. Some patients experience relief from suffering and with rest, renew their motivation to continue living, in which case the term, **Respite Sedation** [Rousseau, 2001] is more appropriate. **Respite Sedation** recognizes it is difficult to deal with emotional, relationship, and existential issues when exhausted and in severe pain. Dr. Rousseau described how several patients, especially those who had been sleep-deprived, could interact meaningfully with others after Respite Sedation. Caution: physicians cannot guarantee you will wake up. Problem: U.S. Senator Sam Brownback, R-Kan., proposed a new Federal bill to punish physicians as criminals if they prescribe these medications, which are also used for Physician-Assisted Suicide [Alvarez, 2006]. If made into law, many physicians would fear being charged for treating severe suffering, so terminally ill patients will suffer more.

If you opt for **Palliative** or **Respite Sedation**, clearly document your desire to **Voluntarily Refuse Food & Fluid** before your doctor initiates sedating and pain-relieving medications which may impair your judgment and cause you to lose consciousness. Put your wishes in writing and sign them in the presence of witnesses. OR, verbally express your wishes to your doctor in front of witnesses and ask your doctor to write down your wishes in a progress note in your medical chart. There are two reasons for these recommendations: You want to make sure that after you lapse into unconsciousness, your doctor does withdraw your IVs or feeding tubes; otherwise, you could exist indefinitely. On the other hand, if you had been eating and drinking by mouth prior to your lapse in consciousness, another person might claim that your physician had committed "**slow euthanasia**" as the induced sedation made it impossible for you to eat or drink.

8. What if I Change My Mind? and How Do I Resume Intake of Food & Fluid?

The sooner you change your mind about resuming intake of Food & Fluid, the less likely you will experience severe medical complications. Try to make all your medical decisions under the care and guidance of a physician who knows your particular medical condition and goals. Discuss your options fully with your physician and those close to you before you start **Voluntarily Refusing Food & Fluid**. Still, the magnitude of the consequences if you maintain your resolve may still lead you to experience an emotional or spiritual epiphany.

There is a risk that changes in your physiology from **Refusing Food & Fluid** will not be reversible, which depends your underlying terminal illness. If you did not consult a psychiatrist or psychologist prior to **Voluntarily Refusing Food & Fluid**, do so as soon as any doubt creeps in. Remember, the time will come when you will no longer be able to change your mind if you become unconscious.

❧ SKIP

We list below some of the laboratory tests that physicians routinely use to assess the consequences of dehydration, for example, when desert hikers run out of water. Note: Some doctors may not agree to suddenly turn aggressive in your medical management after you change your mind, if they feel that *Comfort Care* is still appropriate. Also, laboratory tests are unusual at most hospices.

Whatever state of dehydration you think you might be in, do not underestimate the potential seriousness of your condition. You could die if your heart develops an electrical conduction problem and stops beating; if your kidneys shut down; or if you contract a serious infection.

If you decide to stop **Voluntary Refusal of Food & Fluid**, call your doctor immediately and follow his advice. He may feel it is most important to measure your blood potassium by ordering a blood sample "STAT" (as fast as possible). When the concentration of potassium in blood is too low or too high, dangerous disturbances in rhythm can lead to death. An electrocardiogram (EKG) can check your heart's rhythm. Your doctor may prescribe oral potassium in the form of a pill or liquid, even though some highly concentrated preparations of potassium may irritate the stomach. Your doctor may recommend slowly drinking room-temperature orange juice, Pedialyte, or Gatorade (which all contain potassium), OR if your potassium is not low, water with a teaspoon of salt.

Your doctor may suggest that you begin eating and drinking with watermelon and fruit juice popsicles. Depending on your condition, your doctor may recommend you keep cool by removing excess clothing and loosening other clothing, using air conditioning or fans, staying in the shade if you are outside, and placing a wet towel around yourself or using a spray bottle to deliver tepid water to your exposed skin. He may advise you not to expose yourself to excessive cold or to ice packs, and not to drink very cold drinks rapidly.

The degree of dehydration can be estimated by **signs** (what one can see) and **symptoms** (how you feel). For example, home blood pressure devices measure one symptom: BP is usually slightly lower if dehydration is mild, lower still if moderate, and markedly reduced if severe.

Dehydration is **mild** if you have these symptoms: increased thirst, dry mouth, and a swollen tongue (perhaps not, if you have received good *Comfort Care* to the mouth), feel weak, and have the sensation that your heart is pounding and beating fast. One sign is decreased output of urine, which has a deep yellow color.

Moderate dehydration is marked by symptoms of confusion, being sluggish or weak; not being able to sweat; feeling faint and dizzy when you stand up (due to low blood pressure from decreased blood volume); reduced tears; and some increases in the rates at which your heart beats (pulse) and your lungs breathe (respiratory rate). Your output of urine will be smaller and have a dark amber color. Your eyes may be sunken. Your pulse may be weak and hard to feel. If you pinch the skin under your arm, it may take a while for it to come back to normal.

Dehydration is **severe** if you feel lethargic (find it difficult to remain conscious and to think coherently), feel faint or dizzy even when lying down, your pulse and respiratory rate are markedly increased, your blood pressure is markedly decreased, your pulse is very faint, your eyes are quite sunken, your tears are absent, you have practically no urine output, and you have a fever. If you pinch the skin under your arm, the skin folds may remain tented for a longer while.

You can also note how long it takes for the small veins on the back of your hand to refill. Hold your arm at the level of your heart and compress a vein with your fingertip and then slide it toward your elbow. If it takes less than two seconds for the vein to refill, your dehydration is mild; if between two and four seconds, moderate; and if greater than four seconds, severe.

Laboratory tests: Your urine will have a high specific gravity and contain ketones (breakdown products of metabolism) in increasing amounts. Excessive protein in urine could herald a serious kidney problem. Your blood will have higher concentrations of sodium, potassium, sugar, urea, and creatinine. Blood tests can measure liver damage. A complete blood count may be valuable. As stated above, the most important tests are blood potassium and the heart EKG.

After your doctor listens to your symptoms, examines you, and runs laboratory tests, he or she can decide whether you need to be treated in a hospital or emergency department, or at home, and whether you should be rehydrated by drinking fluids, by intravenous fluids (IVs), or both.

You may have to remain in the emergency department or hospital if you are confused, feverish, and/or your blood pressure, respiration, pulse and temperature are abnormal, or if there is a problem with how well your heart, kidneys, or liver are functioning.

If you were receiving medications like Roxanol or Duragesic patches, you might need temporary mechanical assistance to breathe.

❧ CONTINUE

The bottom line: Obviously, it would be best to consider fully the reasons and consequences of the choice to **Voluntarily Refuse Food & Fluid** BEFORE you begin. However everyone is entitled to change his or her mind. If you do, alert your doctor as soon as possible. This is only one of several important reasons you should always proceed under the supervision of your personal physician.

9. For What Types of Patients is Voluntary Refusal of Food & Fluid NOT the Best Choice?

Sometimes, I begin my lectures with a series of questions modified from those originally posed in lectures by Dr. Joanne Lynn: "How many of you in the audience would like to die of heart disease? Of stroke? Of cancer? Of severe infections? Of accidents or acts of violence including terrorist attacks?" After I pause for the unexpected muffled chuckles, I announce, "Okay, the rest of you will get a Devastating Irreversible Brain State." After some louder nervous laughs, I add that patients who suffer from end-stage dementia usually die of infections.

The opposite tack is to ask the open-ended question, "How *would* you like to die?" From informal surveys, the top preferences are: at home, while asleep, and while doing something productive. The last option is my personal choice. I would re-enact a scene from the film, "The Life of Emile Zola." In the Best Picture of 1937, Paul Muni plays the activist author who is too busy writing to come to bed when his wife requests. Later, he slumps over and dies at his desk—in the middle of a paragraph.

Yet **Voluntary Refusal of Food & Fluid** is not for everyone. Some people have specific clinical, religious or ethical, psychological or social, economic, or logistic reasons for not choosing this method:

1. Clinical. Patients suffering from end-stage liver disease may have large accumulations of abdominal fluid (called *ascites*) that could greatly prolong the process of dehydration and if doctors repeatedly drained off the fluid, others might accuse them of **actively** hastening the patient's dying, even though it could be argued that the reason was to reduce discomfort.

Patients who are obese not only take longer to die, they and others can find the process more unpleasant due to the odor from the breakdown products of fat. While most terminal patients have slowly lost weight, some are overweight, for example those recently diagnosed with a rapidly advancing brain tumor.

Patients who feel it is very important to donate their organs.

Patients receiving **Terminal Sedation** whose medications must be delivered continuously through IVs would not be appropriate for **Voluntary Refusal of Food & Fluid**. Nor would patients who are being sedated as a trial to see if the rest will permit them to enjoy consciousness again. While most medications can be given as a bolus through a heparin lock, some patients, for example those who suffer from constant seizures, require a continuous drip of IV medication.

2. Religious or ethical. People who follow the orthodox teachings of some religions may be opposed to **Voluntary Refusal of Food & Fluid** based on their moral beliefs (discussed further in the next chapter).

Affluent people who wish to hang on to biologic existence may choose to spend their personal funds to prolong the existence of their own, or of a family member's body—after palliative care specialists and ethicists have determined that such efforts are medically futile.

3. Psychological or social. Some patients consider **Voluntary Refusal of Food & Fluid** their second choice due to life-long psychological traits that make them anxious unless they perceive they can exercise exquisite control over the time they will die. They prefer Physician-Assisted Suicide. Once they are assured of this degree of control, their anxiety lessens and they can experience more joy during their last weeks or months of their lives. Some, but not all people in this group, might change their priorities with psychological counseling and further education, however.

Also to be considered are patients' family members. For Karen Raghavan, whose story is recounted above, watching her mother die by **Refusal of Food & Fluid** was an extremely draining emotional experience that further education may or may not have mollified. Some family members are so exhausted by the time the patient decides to die, and have said all the goodbyes possible, that the rapidity of Physician-Assisted Suicide is welcome.

4. Economic. Patients without health insurance might prefer Physician-Assisted Suicide because it costs less and is more expeditious than **Voluntary Refusal of Food & Fluid**, especially if they are currently receiving inadequate treatment for their suffering. The special needs of this population of patients, and some of the moral implications of this suggestion, are discussed later.

5. Logistic. The most tragic people are those who would like to live longer and then exercise the choice of **Voluntary Refusal of Food & Fluid** in the future, but instead they feel they must kill themselves prematurely based on the fear that they will remain stuck in a state of suffering and indignity. (See the stories of Janet Adkins, Robert Hammerman, Bob Stern, and Myrna Lebov, below.) At present, for these millions of people, **Voluntary Refusal of Food & Fluid** does not *seem* to be the BEST choice. Why? Only because society cannot guarantee that their Last Wish will be honored. To be more specific, only because there is no current mechanism to assure these people that an effective Proxy will be available to advocate successfully for **Refusal of Food & Fluid** on their behalf, in the future.

Yet there could be a strategic way to accomplish this goal, which I call **Refusal of Food & Fluid by Proxy**. This important option is discussed extensively in the last quarter of the book.

The logistically challenged group includes two types of people: A) The increasing population of older people who have no competent adult children and whose friends and siblings have already, or may possibly die or become too ill before the time they would serve as their Proxies. B) The increasingly huge number of patients in the early stages of dementia, or those who know they are at high risk for developing dementia, but do not know any individual they can trust to advocate for **Refusal of Food & Fluid** on their behalf if in the future, they reach a certain end-point they have previously defined, in terms of their concept of loss of personhood.

Even people who DO have adult children may fear that they love them too much to let them go. The next "story" alludes to this type of problem.

We Wanted to Wait

Ethel and Morris surprised their friend, a divorce lawyer, when they requested an appointment at his office.

They sat down in front of his desk. In unison they said, "We want a divorce."

Startled, their attorney friend said, "I can't believe it. You two have been married for—it seems forever. My God, you're 94 and 96. Why now, after all these years?"

Ethel started the sentence: "We've always wanted a divorce... "

... which Morris finished: "But we wanted to wait until our children died."

Waiting... Sometimes the advice NOT to wait, whether given explicitly or implicitly, can be tragic. Here, I am concerned about people in the early stages of dementia who wish to engage in advance care planning. They may consult with an organization that teaches "self-deliverance" (discussed below). Afraid of a dismal future, these patients may learn that the organization has nothing to offer them if they reach the late stages of dementia. The reason is that *unassisted suicide* is legal only if patients are competent at the very moment that they end their lives. So these patients may conclude that they must end their suffering, or limit their descent into the indignity and dependency of dementia, by ending their lives when they CAN, instead of when they really WANT TO.

It is tragic when people feel they have no other choice but to end their lives prematurely. Four sad but true stories are recounted in this book. Chapters 9 through 12 provide the strategies for the two alternatives: **Refusal of Food & Fluid** by a Proxy on your behalf, and **Withholding of Food & Fluid** by your physician. Advance care planning must be diligent for this option to succeed, and patients must have confidence in their Proxy or in their physician to risk remaining alive. In reality, success ultimately depends on dealing effectively with formidable challenges. But if the challenges are understood and well planned for, then these patients may experience less worry and anxiety. Then they can choose to continue to enjoy what remains of their precious lives. For some, consulting with professionals who have experience and knowledge about such end-of-life challenges may be the key to the choice to live longer. (See the "Further Resources" section at the end of the book.)

Chapter 6

QUESTIONS ON RELIGION VERSUS SCIENCE

Religion and Science are Not Separable

Religion and science seem to offer different and sometimes opposite ways to view the mysteries of dying and death. Yet some religious arguments use as their premise, current scientific knowledge and medical technology.

The confusing result can lead to intense controversy concerning:

- what is "right" at the end of life;

- the meaning of suffering; and

- what it means to be human or a "person."

---

10. How Do Religions View the Morality of Voluntarily Refusing Food & Fluid? and What About Fasting as a Religious Practice?

Please consider these brief summaries of some views of a few of the world's major religions as introductory. They do not include the wide variety of views of various sects within each religion on end-of-life decisions, nor do they do justice to the personal views of individuals who associate with a specific religion but still maintain their individual beliefs. Furthermore, many of the views are still evolving as religious leaders and their communities grapple with significant recent issues in their attempt to apply their time-honored principles to contemporary situations. (Credit: A portion of the material referred to below began with research compiled by Gerald P. Neugebauer for James Hoefler [2006].)

The Views of Judaism

Jewish Law (*Halakhah*) is based on their Bible (the Five Books of Moses, or *Torah*) and the *Talmud*. While the Orthodox sect endorses the strict tradition as established, Reform and Reconstructionist sects continually update their teaching to reflect modern challenges. The Conservative movement is in unique position for some of its views, clearly expressing two divergent opinions even on its directions to complete Advance Directives.

In addition to this diversity, rabbis have a well-earned reputation for how often they enjoy disagreeing with one another, and this includes the Orthodox. So readers, be forewarned: Do not expect the summary below to lead to a simple guide.

To begin with the most Orthodox, one relevant tractate of the *Talmud* is the *Avodah Zarah* (18a), which contains Laws dealing with Idolatry. They relate to the worship of objects that God did not create, and the respect due to those that He did create.

It is best that He who has given life, shall take it away. No one may hasten his (own) death.

Fundamental to Orthodox Jewish law are the beliefs that God made human beings in His image, that life is the ultimate precious gift of God, and that human beings must respect the **sanctity** of life. The implication is that a person's body is not regarded as his or her possession, but rather as God's possession. Our jurisdiction over our bodies is therefore not total.

Not surprisingly, the Union of Orthodox Jewish Congregations applauded federal intervention in the Terri Schiavo case, noting that "Jewish tradition holds the preservation of human life as one of its supreme moral values." Rabbi J. David Bleich maintained that a feeding tube "is not medicine, it's meals on wheels. It's nothing more than food, and I don't think it is ever appropriate to withhold food." He also stated, "A person who starves to death is committing suicide, as far as Jewish law is concerned," [and] "those who have a duty of care have a duty to provide food and water. You can't withhold it." [Quoted in Ain, 2005]

Conservative Rabbi Avram Reisner explained his position on Terri Schiavo: As a "general rule, I feel that feeding a living person is a requirement. A newborn baby who is not fed won't survive; it is not capable of feeding independently. And if a baby is not fed, [the caregiver] is criminally liable. I would say the same for the disabled who are not able to feed themselves." [Quoted in Ain, 2005]

In contrast, with respect to Terri Schiavo's fate, Leonard Fein, a former director of the Commission on Social Action of Reform Judaism, asked this provocative question: "Is it murder when you reverse an action in the absence of which the person would surely have died?" And Reconstructionist Rabbi David Teutsch said, "You have the right to decide what treatment you want to receive or not" and "most Jewish bioethicists would classify the feeding tube as medicine" [since] eating involves taste, mastication, swallowing and pleasure. None of those are present when a feeding tube is used." [Also quoted in Ain, 2005.]

So there are widely divergent views about this recent controversy.

 SKIP

Traditionally interpreted, the *Talmud* does not permit a patient to refuse potentially life-sustaining treatment, even if the patient is suffering and unwilling, let alone do anything active to hasten his or her death. The additional foundation for this belief is that only God can determine the amount of pain and anguish a person must undergo. For example, if a man's leg is gangrenous and only amputation of the leg would save his life, the leg must be amputated, even against the man's will. Thus, God's will usurps man's autonomy because there is a duty to live.

Rabbi Waldenberg interpreted the *Talmud* in a way that permitted a slightly more liberal and acceptable view for modern Jews, although he expressed it as a negative: Patients in pain may not refuse life-prolonging treatment if the treatment itself will not increase their pain. *If* reverse logic applies, then patients *may refuse* treatment that *will* increase their pain, even if such treatment might prolong their lives, in which view the painful amputation of leg could be refused.

Still more liberal is the view of an Orthodox sage of the last century, Rabbi Shlomo Zalman Auerbach, from Jerusalem's Shaare Zedek Hospital. He differentiated between hastening death and not prolonging death. He stated that when no active hastening of death is involved, the patient has the right to refuse measures to prolong a painful life.

Even the most traditional Orthodox view is that it is wrong to prolong the duration of active or imminent dying since such actions would be considered as opposing the will of God. A famous Talmudic story (although quite condensed) teaches this basic lesson:

Letting God Have His Will

The students of a beloved but very ill rabbi did not want to lose their teacher. They gathered around his bed and engaged in such intense praying that they were able to delay his dying.

The rabbi's servant felt compassion for her master's suffering, left the room, and went to the roof of the home where she received "a message from above." She then returned to the rabbi's room where she intentionally dropped a glass pitcher of water.

In that very instant, as the students were distracted from their prayers, the rabbi died.

In contrast to the view of most bioethicists, Orthodox Jews do distinguish between ***discontinuing*** a life-sustaining treatment (which is never permitted), and ***not initiating*** the same treatment (which is sometimes permitted). In order to avoid the fear of initiating a "trial" that might prolong suffering indefinitely that would lead doctors, patients, and family to decide NOT to initiate a treatment that might have benefit, albeit unlikely—some *authorities* suggest starting a timer as the treatment trial begins, which timer will automatically stop at some predetermined time in the future. Then, if the treatment turns out to be futile, no further human action is required. On the other hand, if the treatment is successful, any action to preserve life is always permitted.

According to Rabbi Eliezer Waldenberg, if a patient is near death (but not actively dying), a doctor may administer medications to reduce severe pain, even if those drugs might hasten death. This modern liberal position is equivalent to the Catholic principle of the Double Effect, discussed below and defined in the Glossary [page 457].

The opposite view, although not mainstream and one that few modern Jews would follow, is summarized below:

Only God can determine the amount of pain and anguish a person must undergo. Suffering serves to increase a person's merit. Therefore to prolong suffering *is a good reason* to prolong life since it can erase sins by allowing patients the opportunity to repent.

In this view, even the inadvertent hastening of dying in order to lessen the physical pain of a terminal patient actually harms that patient's soul.

Some Jews regard the above view as "Christian" since its theme is also found in the traditional Confessional Prayer. In this prayer, the dying person pleads that their earthly suffering can negate eternal punishment they deserve for the sins they committed during their lifetime. While not all Christians believe in the "spiritual benefit of individual suffering," it does reflect the Jewish outlook that prevailed briefly during periods of severe Jewish communal suffering, such as what occurred during the destruction of the Temple in the year 70.

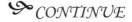 *CONTINUE*

In the strict interpretation of Jewish law, the *Halakhah* does not consider as terminal, patients who are in the Permanent Vegetative State or the end-stage of Alzheimer's disease, yet from a clinical perspective these conditions are irreversible, progressive, and people who suffer from them inevitably die, even though the medical cause might be considered indirect. For example, a severely diseased brain cannot control the muscles required to swallow, so Food & Fluid are aspirated into the lungs, which causes pneumonia, which infection is the proximate cause of death. Nevertheless, continued hydration and nutrition by tubes is considered, according to the strictest rulings, obligatory supportive care and not medical treatment.

Some authorities do permit an exception if a patient must be force-fed or physically restrained. [Breitowitz, 1997.] After analyzing traditional *Halakhic* Judaism, Dr. Gillick [2001] concluded that "withholding nutrition is an inaccurate description of what takes place when a feeding tube is *not* inserted into a person with advanced dementia." In her words: "That person has lost interest in food and will not swallow, or has lost the capacity to eat, as part of his progressive, irreversible dementing illness. When he or she is offered food [and] pushes it away, or takes only a tiny amount, or chokes on it," that person should not be compelled to receive nutrition by tubes since so doing would cause further suffering in a dying individual. Dr. Gillick seems to define "dying individual" medically in terms of a month, as opposed to the traditional Jewish definition of imminent dying (*goses*), often considered as the day before death.

Advance Directives for Conservative Jews: Two Options

According to virtually all Jewish sects, it is strictly forbidden for an individual who is *not* near death and who does not have terminal illness, to do anything that would hasten his or her own death.

Rabbi Bechhofer, in referring to the *original* meaning of "Living Will" that only *restricted treatment*, stated that Living Wills have no intrinsic validity in the (strict) *Halakhic* Jewish Law. Strict Jewish Law can only mandate aggressive treatment, and patients may never be deprived of basic life support, which always includes Food & Fluid, even if they must be artificially administered.

Yet many modern rabbinic authorities agree that it is permissible to let Nature take its course, or to allow dying to happen—for those patients who have an incurable terminal illness and who are suffering or in severe pain. One cannot do anything active to hasten death, but if patients cannot breathe on their own, for example, there is no obligation to initiate life-support by a mechanical ventilator.

Some contemporary rabbinical authorities also permit **Voluntary Refusal of Food & Fluid** for terminally ill patients for whom there is no hope for survival, despite the fact that such an act may possibly shorten life. Among them is Rabbi Elliot Dorff, President of the Society of Jewish Ethics. The Advance Medical Directive of the Rabbinical Assembly of the Conservative Movement includes the following option, in accordance with Rabbi Dorff's interpretation of Jewish law:

> "If there is no reasonable hope of my regaining consciousness, I would want to forgo all treatments and interventions extending my life, including artificial provision of nutrition and hydration, which I consider to be medications. If artificial means of providing nutrition and hydration were used during the period in which my diagnosis was being formed and tested, I hereby ask that the feeding tubes (wherever they are attached to my body) be removed once the diagnosis is confirmed, just as other medications and machines which have proven to be ineffective in effecting my cure may be removed." [1994]

Also in the Conservative Movement's Advance Directive form is Rabbi Avram Israel Reisner's opinion that even for the terminally ill, human life may never be shortened. Rabbi Reisner's view is that unless the patient is imminently dying, we are never permitted to refuse food and hydration because doing so would hasten dying. Implicitly, his definition of **life** includes all existence except *goses*, even if the patient is terminal. The form offers this passage as an alternative:

> "The withholding or withdrawing of medication, nutrition or hydration is prohibited, so long as they are believed to be beneficial for the prolongation of life." [1994]

The form of the Conservative Movement's Advance Directive thus presents two opposing beliefs and suggests precise wording that conform to these two different views. As they complete the form, people are given the explicit option to choose either one. They can therefore make the decision that seems "best" for them.

Rabbi Elliot Dorff considered further the definition of *goses*: "Jewish sources describe a *goses* as 'a flickering candle,' who may not be even be moved." The state of a moribund person applies to dying people for whom mourning can begin as soon as that state is recognized. While some consider "three days" as the actual time frame, it was based on hindsight from learning at what point death could no longer be delayed—as judged by the standards of ancient medicine. Now patients who would have, in the past, died in 72 hours can be sustained for months or years. So others consider the state of *gesisah* as including patients who suffer from incurable, irreversible terminal illnesses, even if their prognosis is a year or more. [Dorff, 1998, *Page 200*.] The appropriate Jewish legal category to describe people with incurable diseases is *terefah* (an imperiled life), according to Rabbi Dorff, who considers it permissible to withhold or withdraw medications and machines as soon as patients enter this state.

Conclusions Possibly Relevant to Many Religions

How can we conclude this brief summary, given the diversity of opinions? An intriguing theme emerges from examining these various Jewish views. Although this consideration can also apply to other religions, the openness of debating different points of view among Jews, in part, permits this theme to emerge. (We know of no other religion that so clearly documents the opinions of two opposing authorities so explicitly, right on their official Advance Directive form.)

The basic undisputed premise is that your body is a precious gift from God, which gift you have accepted since you are alive. Before a *certain point in time*, your obligation from having accepted this gift is to honor God by preserving your life. However, after a certain point in time, you must accept that it is God's will that you die, after which point it would be a sin to prolong the dying process in defiance of His will.

The obvious focal point is: where *exactly* is that point in time? Some would argue after extending existence as long as possible, after every modern technology that medical science now has available has been tried, or until it becomes certain (even though it will become known only by hindsight) that death will inevitably occur within 72 hours. Others argue sooner, pointing out that the time period of 3 days was relevant before medicine developed ventilators, feeding tubes, and dialysis machines, let alone antibiotics and other medicines. Medical science has provided an increase in life expectancy from 46 to 86 years, in just one century. In contrast, the origins of Biblical law go back two millennia.

So the question is, if one religious person says "strictly 72 hours," and another religious person says "as soon as the prognosis is incurable and irreversible, even if it possible to exist for a year or more," *which person is right*? Perhaps they are both right, because God created human beings in His image, and gave them the ability to think and to speak. Or perhaps neither person is right because it has been a long time since God spoke directly to Moses, and they did not cover this particular point, let alone take into account the future advances in medical technology.

Yet another perspective would be for people to resist the tendency to be presumptuous about their ability to interpret the will of God, and to focus more humbly instead on those areas about which human beings do have some direct knowledge. For example, these questions might be more relevant: What are the likely benefits versus the likely burdens for specific medical treatments for specific medical conditions, based on our previously acquired empirical experience, and what do the patient and family want after they are so informed? Some questions to ask, are: Do individuals have the right to decide, or must they follow the Holy Scriptures? Are the scriptures holy, or do they represent the interpretations of man? Do we accept the teachings of our religious leaders, or do we decide for ourselves? Do we consider Christians devout and others as "spiritual" if they follow the interpretation of "the Book" or maintain their "practice," OR, should we note their behavior and ask if they are of responding to the needs of the poor and the sick, according to the fourth principle of bioethics, *social justice*?

The next story provides a transition from the Jewish to the Catholic views:

Tonight? It's Too Dark and Stormy

It was a very dark and very stormy night. Max, whose given name was Moshe, was feeling very thankful. God had granted him a long life. And a good life. He had several children, many grandchildren, and even a few great-grandchildren.

He turned slowly from his position in bed and looked at the loving eyes of his wife. For nearly sixty years, she was by his side. And still was. He sighed. There was no need for him to say anything. She knew and he knew. They both were accepting that his end was near. Someday, she knew, she would join him in the Afterlife.

Sensing some urgency, he took a deep breath, and said, "Call the priest, Sadie, and tell him to come here. Right away."

"The priest? Moshe, are you getting delirious? You must of course mean the rabbi!"

"No," he said. "I do mean the priest. At this point in my life, I should not be a burden to any of God's chosen people. Whom am I, anyway, to disturb our learned rabbi on such a night as this? It's too dark and stormy."

The Views of Traditional Catholicism

Given the recent controversy about Catholic teachings about the obligation to provide tube feeding for unconscious patients, we present key statements in chronological order. The conclusion is that from the Sixteenth Century until 2004, the **doctrine of proportionality** prevailed, where the benefits to the patient were considered along with the burdens to patient, family, and society—to determine whether or not to continue life-sustaining treatments. The late Pope John Paul II stated that, in principle, feeding tubes cannot be removed from even those patients who are unconscious for more than a year, as such acts would be mortal sins; they would be "euthanasia by omission."

༄ SKIP

Francisco de Vitoria, who lived in Spain until 1545, wrote, "If the depression of spirit is so low and there is such consternation in the appetitive power that only with the greatest of effort as though by means of certain torture, can the sick man take food, right away that is reckoned a certain impossibility, and therefore he is excused, at least from mortal sin, especially where there is little hope of life or none at all." [This and the next reference cited by Repenshek and Slosar, 2004.]

Domingo Banez, who lived until 1604, and John de Lugo, who lived until 1660, expanded on this example to distinguish between **ordinary** treatment that God requires, and **extraordinary** treatment that God does not require. De Lugo concluded that one is not obligated to sacrifice by leaving his community to access means to conserve his life, to seek treatment that can be obtained only with great danger or grave inconvenience, or entail intense pain, excessive costs, or intense fear or strong psychological repugnance.

In 1953, Pope Pius XII met with a group of physicians and taught that Catholics are morally bound to respect life and to care for life, but not at all costs. He stated that a Catholic is morally bound only to take advantage of ordinary care, and may refuse care if there is a disproportionate burden compared to the benefit.

In 1958, Pope Pius XII defined **extraordinary** or **disproportionate** means as having excessive expense, pain or other inconvenience OR not offering a reasonable hope of benefit OR involving a grave burden to self or others. Thus the burdens are to be weighed along with the benefits, to decide if they are proportionate included consideration of family and society.

Many consider Pope John Paul II's 1980 "Declaration on Euthanasia" as the standard Catholic reference on end-of-life issues. Among its principles are: It is for the consciences of sick persons, or those qualified to speak in their name, to make these decisions; the principles are that one is never obliged to use **extraordinary** or **disproportionate** means to preserve life still holds good, and that it is wrong to "impose on anyone the obligation to have recourse to a technique which is already in use but which carries a risk or is burdensome."

The Fourth Edition of the *Ethical and Religious Directives for Catholic Health Care Services* [2001] stated, "A person may forgo extraordinary or disproportionate means of preserving life. Disproportionate means are those that, *in the patient's judgment,* do not offer a reasonable hope of benefit, or entail an excessive burden, or impose excessive expense on the family or the community." Excessively burdensome treatment was broadly defined as "too painful, too damaging to the patient's bodily self and functioning, too psychologically repugnant to the patient, too restrictive of the patient's liberty and preferred activities, too suppressive of the patient's mental life, or too expensive."

The U.S. Conference of Catholic Bishops' Committee for Pro-Life Activities [2003] permitted refusing a life-prolonging procedure only if "the real purpose of the omission was to relieve the patient of a particular procedure that was of limited usefulness to the patient or unreasonably burdensome for the patient and the patient's family or caregivers. This kind of decision should not be equated with a decision to kill or with suicide." However, the Bishops *rejected* arguments that **Voluntary Refusal of Food & Fluid** for those in the **permanently unconscious state**, is "the natural dying process which would have occurred without these interventions." Instead they stated, "Decisions about these patients should be guided by a presumption in favor of medically assisted nutrition and hydration." They would only consider permanently unconscious patients, never "patients with conditions like mental retardation, senility [or] dementia."

Bishop Robert Lynch of St. Petersburg, where Terri Schiavo resided, said in 2003, "We are obliged to preserve our own lives, and help others preserve theirs, by use of means that have a reasonable hope of sustaining life without imposing unreasonable burdens on those we seek to help, that is, on the patient and his or her family and community." He added, "It is not clear whether the medically assisted nutrition and hydration is delaying her dying process to no avail, [or] is unreasonably burdensome for her, and contrary to what she would wish if she could tell us."

The Recent Views of Catholicism

In the English translation (from Italian) of his March 2004 Allocution on "Life-Sustaining Treatments and Vegetative State," the late Pope John Paul II said about patients in the **Permanent Vegetative State**: "The administration of water and food, even when provided by artificial means ... should be considered, in principle, *ordinary* and *proportionate*, and as such, morally obligatory, insofar as and until it is seen to have attained its proper finality, which in the present case consists of providing nourishment to the patient and alleviation of his suffering." He explained, "Death by starvation or dehydration is, in fact, the only possible outcome as a result of their withdrawal. In this sense it ends up becoming, if done knowingly and willingly, true and proper euthanasia by omission." In recalling his previous writing in the encyclical Evangelium Vitae, he stated, "such an act is always '*a serious violation of the law of God*, since it is the deliberate and morally unacceptable killing of a human person.'"

Pope John Paul II said it was his "duty to reaffirm strongly that the intrinsic value and personal dignity of every human being do not change, no matter what the concrete circumstances of his or her life. *A man, even if seriously ill or disabled in the exercise of his highest functions, is and always will be a man*, and he will never become a 'vegetable,' [and he] retains human dignity in all its fullness. The loving gaze of God the Father continues to fall upon him."

The late Pope considered the effects on society and the family by stating, "Although the care for these patients is not, in general, particularly costly, society must allot sufficient resources... [and] provide 'breaks' for those families who are at risk of psychological and moral burn-out."

In a Catholic magazine called **America**, two Catholic ethicists commented on the Pope's Allocution from a scientific point of view: Ronald Hamel, senior director for ethics of the Catholic Health Association, St. Louis, MO, which represents 611 hospitals nationwide, and Michael Panicola, Vice President of Ethics of Sisters of St. Mary Health Care, St. Louis, MO [2004]. They stated, "It seems logically inconsistent to classify nutrition and hydration as basic care that is always obligatory even if artificially supplied, while not doing the same for oxygen supplied by mechanical ventilation or other basic elements of care necessary for life. Why does nutrition and hydration merit such a classification? As we see it, the case for doing so has not only not been adequately made; it has not been argued at all."

Shannon and Walter [2004] concluded that the Pope's statement represented a significant departure from the Five-Hundred year tradition that recommended considering the **proportional benefits and harms** to the individual, family, and community "from the mid-1600's through Pope Pius XII and the 1987 *Declaration on Euthanasia*." Challenging end-of-life decisions could even take into account the **financial hardship** or **emotional burden to the family**. But now, they point out, a **deontological principle**, which by definition cannot be questioned, has been invoked. They concluded, "The decision-making process at the end of life is difficult enough... We do not support policies that require medical staff to provide unwanted medical treatment. Such policies might even drive people *toward* euthanasia, by making them feel that they have lost a traditional and sympathetic ally in their final journey."

Repenshek and Slosar [2004] noted that one way to view the Pope's Allocution was to focus on the words "in principle," which they understood "does not mean 'without exception,' but only 'all other things being equal.'" They concluded, "there should be a presumption in favor of providing nutrition and hydration to all patients, *as long as* this is of sufficient benefit to outweigh the burdens involved to the patient," which view permitted them to continue to be guided by Directive 58 of the *Ethical and Religious Directives*. In his lecture [2004], Dr. Hamel also noted this way *to wiggle out* of some of the Pope's message, although he might not have used these exact words.

Cardinal William H. Keeler, chairman of the U.S. Bishops' Committee for Pro-Life Activities, applauded the February 28, 2005, statement of the Catholic bishops of Florida, which applied the Pope's March 2004 teaching to the Schiavo case. The bishops reiterated their plea that Terri Schindler Schiavo "continue to receive all treatments and care that will be of benefit to her."

On the other hand, Professor Edward Sunshine of Barry University [2005] pointed out in the National Catholic Reporter, the difference between the **medical** versus **moral** ways of looking at the extraordinary/ordinary distinction. He wrote, "When the bishops and the Pope teach, they discuss objective norms of morality that apply in general. They do not (indeed, cannot) tell people how to act in conscience because conscience is the domain of the person before God." To repeat his clearly stated view: "**Another moral perspective would see Schiavo's [medical] condition as lethal, because her brain damage was preventing her from eating and drinking**." He explained, "After 15 years of continual deterioration in Schiavo's condition, with no medical prognosis that she would improve, it was **unclear how she would benefit from the machines that were keeping her alive**." Dr. Sunshine concluded, "Catholics... are getting from the bishops of Florida a limited and one-sided picture of a difficult issue, at times tinged with embarrassing rhetoric."

Rev. Kevin O'Rourke is a scholar at Loyola University's Neiswanger Institute for Bioethics and Health Policy. The 78-year-old Dominican priest received his canon law degree in Rome. On matters of end-of-life care, he stated in 2005 that half a millennium of Catholic tradition holds that people have the right to refuse treatments they consider of little benefit or unduly burdensome, even if doing so results in their death. Although a committed Catholic cannot seek death, he can choose to protect his human dignity by refusing medical measures that are too painful, costly, or fundamentally repugnant when the results of that care are of questionable value. "If you're not able to love, think, plan, relate, or consciously direct activity toward God, then just maintaining a physical existence is not beneficial." In affirming autonomy, Rev. O'Rourke said, "Our tradition has always held that it's the people who have the right to make decisions for themselves when their lives are coming to an end, based on their personal circumstances, not the church." [Reported by Judith Graham, Chicago Tribune, 4-29-2005.]

Dr. John Harvey, Catholic theologian, physician, and chair of the Bioethics Committee at Georgetown University, believes there is no hope of recovery after one year in the persistent vegetative state, and that the yearly cost of $80,000 should be considered when weighing the burden of treatment. In 2005, he said on PBS: "Life has great value, of course, but it's not the final value of human life. The final value of human life is life with God in heaven, and when we keep that from happening by treating a futile situation, we're blocking the final 'telos'—as the Greeks say—of human life... The patient is dying because of the illness that he or she has, the physiological change of not being able to eat." [Telos means ultimate goal.]

☙ *CONTINUE*

Many professionals in the areas of medicine and law consider the late Pope's new strict teachings to be in direct conflict with autonomy, and with the secular law since the U.S. Supreme Court upheld the rights of patients to refuse artificially administered sustenance as a medical **treatment**. The new teachings are also in conflict with public opinion. A 2003 Gallup Pole revealed that 80% of those surveyed supported a spouse's decision to allow the painless death of a patient in a **Persistent Vegetative State**. Just before Terri Schiavo's feeding tube was pulled for the last time, 87% of those surveyed indicated that they would not want to remain alive if they were in a state similar to hers.

"Must we all die with a feeding tube?" For Himself, **Pope John Paul II's answer was No!** The question is the title of an article by Arthur Caplan [MSNBC, 4-6-04] in which he wrote that the (late) "Pope was wrong about what confers dignity on the sick and the dying. It is not about artificially feeding them against their will, but about finding ways to let their will be respected... Removing a feeding tube is not a cruel form of euthanasia" (and therefore a mortal sin). See page 133: the Graham family had the same answer.

Summary of the Catholic Positions

Much of traditional Catholic teaching is enlightened and progressive. While Rabbi Wallenberg has been quoted as endorsing the oppressive statement that prolonged suffering is a good way to repent, Catholic ethicists introduced and taught the world about the principle of the Double Effect. With origins back to the Thirteenth Century, this principle allows a patient to receive enough pain medication to reduce suffering even if the foreseen but unintended side-effect would be to hasten dying.

Pope John Paul II still permitted **Refusal of Food & Fluid** if *death is imminent* and cannot be prevented, if the body *can no longer absorb* Food & Fluid, or if continued administration of Food & Fluid is an *extreme burden* and if there is *no hope* that food and water will provide any *benefit*. Followers have interpreted the Pope's teachings to mean that refusal of Food & Fluid is **unacceptable** if the intent is precisely because a patient is not dying quickly enough based on the judgment that the patient's quality of life is so low that it no longer has value. So the Pope would permit **Refusal of Food & Fluid** by cancer patients who lose their appetite and suffer from nausea when they eat, by patients with gastrointestinal problems who feel more pain or discomfort when they try to ingest food and water, and by patients in congestive heart failure who find it easier to breathe if they reduce or stop intake of fluids.

While it may be possible to return to the practice of the traditional Catholic view of proportionality by focusing on a few words such as "in principle" to find exceptions to the Pope's Allocution, it is not easy to ignore his words "euthanasia by omission." As previously noted, it is likely that future debate will focus on which side to err upon in ambiguous, complex clinical situations—the side of PRESERVING life, or the side of what many or a consensus of people (as on an ethics committee) believe is in the patient's BEST INTEREST. One set of arguments is based on the origin of such decisions: is the ultimate source a divinely inspired edict, or is the source the patient's individual conscience and autonomy. The debate within the Catholic Church thus reflects the larger debate in Twenty-First Century America.

Note that the United States is unique for a variety of reasons. For example, in Britain, it is physicians who make life-and-death decisions about terminating treatment, although the recent court decision regarding Leslie Burke may change this. Third-world countries do not have the medical and technological resources to permit considering prolonged extension of lives. Thus when they say, "Let God worry about it," they truly mean that. They do not expect to allocate the resources of their countries' working citizens or the sacrificing of basic medical and other needs to indefinitely keep alive a few people who cannot feed themselves.

The Views of the Religion of Islam

According to Khaleel Mohammed, Ph.D., a specialist in Islamic Studies [lecture and personal communication, 2005], San Diego State University, the God of Islam forbids killing anyone unless there is a just cause. In the Koran, the fundamental text of Islam, Chapter 5 verse 32 values the *sanctity* of life so highly that to indicate its magnitude it states: "If you kill one person it is as if you had slain the entire people, and if you save the life of one person it is as if you have saved the entire people."

The religion of Islam endorses the general principle of choosing the lesser of two evils, that it is better to commit a crime that causes less damage than another crime that would cause more damage. However this principle does NOT apply to the rationing of medical and financial resources because of this specific prohibition: "Do not kill your children for fear of poverty because God will provide for them." Therefore, you cannot allocate resources by removing Artificial Nutrition and Hydration from one unconscious person in order that many others will receive better basic medical care.

Followers of Islam believe in miracles. It is more acceptable to not initiate artificial prolongation of life than it is to stop those means once they have begun. According to Islam, you do not have the right to kill yourself and you therefore do NOT have the right to make a Living Will that says for example, "If I am in severe pain and suffering, or in a persistent vegetative state and there is no hope of recovery, then I want to turn off life support." But it is permitted to not initiate life support if doing so would only prolong your life artificially beyond the point you would have died naturally.

In terms of prolonging the existence of a person where there is absolutely no hope, as in the end stage of a progressive irreversible dementia, at least some followers of Islam would consider such persons to no longer possess the basic attributes of life. They must possess all five basic functions: 1) to be capable of living (with independence); 2) to practice your religion; 3) to have intellect; 4) to reproduce; and 5) to own property. Since patients in end-stage dementia have none of these, they would be permitted to refuse medical treatment, "leaving the consequences up to God."

The Views of Baptists

Baptist/United Churches of Christ Family Groups state, "Prolonging the dying process would be seen as 'playing God' and extraordinary means are not necessary" [http://jmahoney.com/bapfamchurches.htm; 08/14/00]. Southern Baptists encourage followers to "consider the provision of nutrition and hydration by medical means to be compassionate and ordinary care"; however the declarations of organizations within the Southern Baptist Convention are not binding on individual conscience. "Although withdrawing medical treatment from dying patients is morally acceptable to most Southern Baptists, the Trustees of the Christian Life Commission (CLC) have attempted to draw the line at artificial nutrition and hydration, by directing staff to consider the provision of nutrition and hydration by medical means to be compassionate and ordinary care" [see "On Euthanasia and Assisted Suicide," 1992]. Declarations of organizations within the Southern Baptist Convention are not binding on individual conscience according to Simmons [2003]. In contrast, the stand on Physician-Assisted Suicide is clear. C. Ben Mitchell, who serves as bioethics consultant for the Ethics and Religious Liberty Commission of the Southern Baptist Convention wrote [2001], "Instead of abandoning patients, compassionate medicine provides hospice care. Rather than allowing dying patients to suffer, truly humane medicine treats their pain and alleviates their fears. Palliative care must trump the lethal failure of the Oregon medical establishment. Nothing less than our humanity is at stake."

The Views of Mormons

"When dying becomes inevitable, it should be seen as a blessing and a purposeful part of eternal existence. Members should not feel obligated to extend mortal life by means that are unreasonable" [Policy of Church of Jesus Christ of Latter-day Saints, 1998: 1]. "Allowing death to occur is permissible when death is the inevitable and natural outcome and the measures required to postpone it would rob the patient of the ability to relate meaningfully to others or to experience satisfaction with the quality of his or her existence. Such measures include artificially assisted nutrition and hydration" [Durham, Jr. WC, 1992].

A search of such sources as "Mormon News: ALL the News about Mormons, Mormonism, and the LDS Church" revealed no statements about making end-of-life treatment decisions. However Senator Gordon Smith (R-Ore.), an LDS Church member who was once an LDS bishop and also a hospital volunteer in Pendleton, Oregon, stated, "I honestly believe that there is a natural course to living and dying," and "I think we should leave that to God and Nature." He thus explained his vote in 2000, when he supported a Federal bill that did not pass, but would have prohibited the use of Controlled Substances to end a patient's life. Against the majority vote in his state, Smith was quoted as saying that sometimes, following the majority is *not* the right thing to do.

The Views of the United Methodist Church

"For the United Methodist Church, theological and ethical reflection leads to the conclusion that obligations to use life-sustaining treatments cease when the physical, emotional, financial, or social burdens exceed the benefits for the dying patient and the caregiver" [Book of Records: 33; Book of resolutions 1992]. "The family is the proper context for decision-making... government should not intrude in even a surrogate role" [DuBose, *Page 7*; See also United Methodist Church 1996: 90]. "[W]e assert the right of every person to die in dignity, with loving personal care and without efforts to prolong terminal illnesses merely because the technology is available to do so" [United Methodist Church 1988].

The Views of Evangelical Christians

Evangelical Christians believe that the **sanctity** of life depends only on "being." They define "persons" and the qualities of "personhood" by the essence of their Nature. Life is a gift from God who created man in his image when He breathed life into man. To be human, it is not relevant whether the being has high or low abilities to function, nor does it depend on others in society perceiving remaining value in a person's life. Even unconscious patients are still human and deserve to be treated with dignity as for all humans.

Evangelical Christians fear the developing "Culture of Death," which they define as the attitude that permits the deliberate taking of innocent lives that breaks God's prohibition against murder as codified in His Ten Commandments. They are opposed to weighing the value of human life and its burden on others in society to determine whether or not to continue life-sustaining treatment, as recommended by the outspoken Peter Singer, an ethicist at Princeton University, for example. They reject murdering people merely because there are some people in society who decided that the gift of life from God no longer has value due to a decrease in functional capacity such as not being conscious.

While they recognize that it is prudent to not sustain existence beyond its natural course, Evangelical Christians uphold the belief that providing basic care, including nutrition and hydration, is obligatory. They believe it respects the dignity of all human beings, which does not depend on their functional state. They consider the **Withdrawal of Food & Fluid** to be murder except in the case of patients who have the diagnosis of brain death and whose organs have been temporarily maintained for transplantation. For those patients, when medical treatment is finally withdrawn, the act is not considered murder.

Ruth Graham, the Presbyterian wife of the Reverend Billy Graham (a Southern Baptist), died on June 13, 2007, at age 87. The couple's spokesperson, Larry Ross, said Mrs. Graham had "in recent weeks, asked that a stomach tube used to provide her with food and fluids be removed. When the tube accidentally fell out earlier this week, she again renewed that request." Still, the tube was reinserted. Before she died, Ross said, "In consensus with her family and others who have observed her levels of deterioration, and in consultation with her physician, she has not received foods or fluid for several days." The news report [M. Baker, Associated Press, 6-14-07] was corrected "to show that Ruth Graham's feeding tube is still inserted, but no longer being used to provide nutrients." It explained that Mrs. Graham was "receiving medication through the tube...to help manage her pain and discomfort [and to] allow doctors to treat her at home rather than in a hospital."

Thus the personal end-of-life decision to which the Graham family agreed, like the one Pope John Paul II made for Himself [page 129], permitted natural dying.

The Views of Buddhists

Buddhism prioritizes compassion, which leads to the goal of eliminating, if possible, or at least reducing suffering, and to do no harm. While taking of life is wrong, if a patient's suffering is great, it is natural to eliminate suffering. Under that circumstance, Buddhism honors **Refusing Food & Fluid**, even if that choice is made with the clear intent to shorten the time of suffering by hastening death. Buddhists do not support maintaining life by artificial nutrition and hydration if the treatment exposes the person to further harm and suffering. Buddhists believe that people die when consciousness leaves their bodies. When consciousness has permanently dissociated itself from bodies, there is no reason to continue to nourish the body. This is so because the ability to think is the primary requirement of personhood.

Buddhism recognizes patients' right to determine when they should move on from this existence to the next. What is important is whether their minds remain at peace and in harmony so that they die with an assured state of mind. Survivors are encouraged to respect these choices instead of criticizing them or wishing that those who died had taken another path, or died in another way. Survivors should not harbor negative emotions such as resentment or rejection, or grieve more because they judged the death as untimely. Buddhists also believe that the welfare of all in society should be considered when contemplating spending huge resources on one person where the potential for a good recovery is very small. [Sogyal Rinpoche, 1993; Becker CB, 1990]

The Views of Unitarian Universalists

In 1988, the Unitarian Universalist Association of Congregations passed a national resolution that favored assistance in dying for the terminally ill. They were the first Western religious body to affirm what could be called, "the right to die." They remain outspoken in their support of physician-hastened dying.

The Views of Hinduism

The Hindu religions believe in the high value of human beings since it is so difficult to be reincarnated as a human being. They also believe in non-violence— to not injure other beings. They believe suffering is due to Karma, which generally should be allowed to take its natural course by dealing with it in one's present life. Doing so will increase the chance that the person will have a better life in his or her next reincarnation. Suicide is considered an extraordinarily terrible act that results in many years in hell. Artificial attempts to shorten one's life to reduce suffering are not permitted since it will interfere with Karma and the next life.

Hindus believe that one's present body is like a suit of clothes that one changes for a new life. They hold in highest esteem what they term either "The Great Going Forth" or "Letting Go," which is spiritual fasting at the end of life. When faced with incurable disease and debilitation, individuals are permitted the freedom to leave their old bodies by fasting, by gradually reducing intake of nourishment. The practice is quite distinct from suicide. The person's intent is deliberate and conscious, and the emotions are calm. This highly revered spiritual act is publicly announced and supported by the community. The individual strives to attain the dignified goal of focusing on his or her divine destiny.

In the dying process, deliberate interference from outside is definitely not permitted. Physician-assisted suicide and euthanasia are prohibited. Removing artificial means of sustaining life once such means have been initiated is morally ambiguous and could therefore be the subject of debate.

The Views of Jainism

Jainism considers "voluntary fasting" as the "ideal" death. Other Eastern religions come close to this point of view. Here are some excerpts from Sanjay Mehta's article that Professor Daneshvari R. Solanki sent to me [2005]:

"Adoption of the vow should be spiritual... a religious duty, voluntarily adopted and joyfully observed. There must be full faith in religious and acquired knowledge of the principles... The moment of death should be awaited calmly, with engrossment in deep meditation, complete detachment, and inward concentration. Consequences of death should neither be hurtful nor sorrowful, as all ties have been terminated with common consent. Holy death (that is, without an increase in the build-up of passion) is considered free from desire, anger, or delusion, and hence, is not suicide." There is a stage where one has "attained spiritual purity so as to permit the individual to resort to austerities for release from the physical body. The ultimate decision for whether any particular voluntary death is suicide depends upon the motive, means adopted, and consequences ensuing thereafter."

What About Non-Believers?

The discussion of religion has thus far omitted those who do not believe in God. So atheists have a right to complain.

They might voice these arguments: "Christians have special holidays like Christmas and Easter; Jews celebrate Passover and Yom Kippur; and Muslims have The Holiday of Charity and The Commemoration of Abraham's Sacrifice. It's just not fair. We atheists have no recognized holidays."

Someone, perhaps in poor taste, suggested that atheists could still celebrate April first.

Fasting as a Religious Practice

What religions teach as right and wrong can be influenced by culture. Certain foods and drinks are typically components of traditional religious ceremonies. Yet many religions also practice **fasting** during their holiest of days. Some seekers believe that temporary relief from concerns about the needs of the body can help a person reach higher levels of spirituality, and feel closer to the Supreme Being. For some, it would be a modest leap to consider such **holy day fasts** as "practice" to prepare for the **final fast** that will bring a transition to the highest level of spirituality... complete release from the body... freeing the soul so it can enter the realm of the Supreme Being... or to have the opportunity to be reborn.

The above views could be directed by people of religious faiths (as well as others) to consider **Voluntarily Refusing Food & Fluid** as their **last fast** during which they can intensify reflections, enhance perspectives, and create final, loving connections with family and friends before they make their final spiritual journey. What is paramount for spiritual transcendence, some religions teach, is to maintain a peaceful attitude toward self, toward others, and toward the fasting/dying process itself.

Some people are critical of what they perceive as a recent trend in America "to err on the side of life," which is consistent with the "new Catholic" position that considers **Withholding Food & Fluid** from patients who will never regain consciousness as "euthanasia by omission." With the appointment of the fifth Catholic to the U.S. Supreme Court Justice, Mr. Samuel Alito, Jr., the position taken by this church may be influential. Yet critics of religion point out what they perceive as an inconsistency: some people of faith, who believe in the afterlife so strongly that they glorify it with such terms as Kingdom of Heaven, ardently fight the inevitability of death. Furthermore, some people of faith accept the deontological principle that everyone must follow edicts that come from God through His representatives on Earth. The deontological principle thereby removes these ethical controversies from the domain of what can be argued.

The most critical point about the practice of **materialism** is that it places the highest values in life in the physical area by maintaining biological functioning, as opposed to emphasizing spiritual values. In terms of the four principles of bioethics, critics can argue that **materialism** is wrong if, to prioritize its values:

A) It disregards what patients wanted by superseding ***autonomy***;

B) It causes patients to suffer more and ***does harm***. (Note: Even unconscious individuals can be harmed if materialism violates their previously stated wishes; for example: wanting family members to remember them as they were before they experience further deterioration, dependence, and indignity; and disregarding their wishes on how they wish to spend their financial assets);

C) It is pursued even when there is no hope for return of consciousness, thus failing to provide **benefit**; and

D) It causes huge psychological and economic burdens to both the family and society, thus violating the principle of **social justice**.

The counterargument is that no human being has the right to judge the value of another human being's life. Permitting the right to decide that another's life has no value would lead to a justification to hasten the dying of other human beings, which could begin the slippery slope so that ultimately, the old, the frail, the disabled, and the very sick—the very people who are so dependent on the rest of us to provide care for them—can be disposed of, merely for the convenience of those who are stronger.

To focus this conflict, consider the various meanings of the words "sanctity of life." To some, it means we must preserve any biological functioning until God decides to take the life that He gave. This attitude also requires the belief that God gave us modern medical technology with the intention that we would use it.

Another way to interpret "sanctity of life" is to define those characteristics and behaviors that make a human being a person beyond the potential to donate useful organs for transplantation, or to provide a uterus in which a fetus can develop. Clinically, Susan Torres was "brain dead" by neurological criteria that have been accepted since 1981, when the President's Commission for The Study of Ethical Problems in Medicine and Biomedical and Behavioral Research: She had complete and irreversible brain function. Yet with a ventilator and artificial nutrition and hydration, her organs were kept functioning for nearly three months, at which point, doctors removed a live baby by Caesarean section. Medical technology allowed the organs of Susan Torres to perform an important biological function after she had died.

Newspaper reporters can confuse readers by incorrect writing. For example, the title of Mr. R. Willing's article [USA Today, 2005]: "Brain-Dead Virginia Woman Dies After Giving Birth" has two mistakes: Someone who is dead cannot die a second time; and dead people cannot perform any function of life, including *giving* birth. Still, her organs did perform a very important biological function.

11. Given These Intense Moral Arguments, How Can I be Sure That Others Will Honor My Last Wishes?

In making challenging end-of-life decisions, one person may believe that the administration of Food & Fluid is a medical treatment that every patient has the moral right to refuse, while another may consider the administration of Food & Fluid as ordinary care that every person has the moral right and obligation to receive as long as they exist.

If you want to abide by the late Pope's Allocution, your written **Advance Directive** should state so, clearly and convincingly. Here is one example of specific wording to express this Last Wish:

"I want to maintain life."

"If my doctor or hospital wants to stop tube feeding, I want my Proxy to request my transfer to a Catholic health care facility that is willing to provide artificial nutrition and hydration, and to seek funding for continued treatment since I believe that life is precious and that it is always the right path to maintain life until God decides to take me."

(Then you would list YOUR specific reasons. The answers to subsequent **i-FAQs** provide some examples of possible reasons.)

Such a statement could be critically important because in some institutions, by-laws specifically permit their ethics committees to recommend discontinuing those medical treatments they consider to be **medically futile** (of no further benefit), including medical administration of Food & Fluid. [See W. J. Smith, 2003.] Ethics committees are typically composed of physicians, attorneys, nurses, social workers, ethicists, clergy, and "lay" people from the community. While many of these committees only make recommendations, their opinions could lead to insurance companies' refusal to pay for continuing treatment that the physicians and these committees judge to be "futile." Usually, State laws and institutional by-laws allow a certain amount of time for second opinions and transfer to other institutions and providers who are willing to continue to provide treatment. *Comfort Care* is never discontinued, however, and a reasonable amount of time should always be allowed for families to accept the end.

Clearly stating your wishes in your **Advance Directive** can help your Proxy succeed as your advocate by insisting that you be transferred to another doctor or facility, and to justify searching for alternative financial resources to pay for your extended care—if you want to continue tube feeding (or any other treatment others consider to be providing no benefit). Transferring to another physician is within the standard of medical care since it honors another ethical value—the integrity of health care professionals to "have a right to remain true to their own conscientious moral and religious beliefs." [Hastings Center, 1987.]

Some Catholics have independently decided that God's "gift of life" does not require their unending obligation, just as a gift of an automobile does not require unending replacement of engines and transmissions beyond 300,000 miles. If you want your Proxy to have the authority to exercise the option of **Voluntarily Refusing Food & Fluid** at time in the future when you cannot speak for yourself—then the Proxy you designated in your **Advance Directive** may need to document that you really wanted to **Voluntarily Refuse Food & Fluid**, perhaps over the objections of one of your more observantly religious relatives, and some States require that the evidence your Proxy offers meets the standard of *clear and convincing* evidence. As one suggestion, consider explaining your reasons in words similar to these, either in your Advance Directive or a supporting document:

"I do NOT want to prolong my biologic existence."

"I consider myself Catholic and I am aware of the late Pope John Paul II's Allocution that stated continued administration of Food & Fluid 'should be considered, **in principle**, *ordinary* and *proportionate*.' I construe the words, "in principle," to mean there is still room for interpretation. In deciding my future medical care, I want my doctors to follow the instructions of my Proxy whom I now give the ultimate authority to **Refuse Food & Fluid** on my behalf. I list some reasons below, however they are meant only to support my Proxy's decisions, not to be interpreted by others. I intend this document to be durable so my wishes will transcend my future incompetence. I want to avoid the possibility that my stated reasons will serve as an excuse for further discussion by any ethics committee or court of law:" {Emphasis added.}

(Then you would list YOUR specific reasons. The answers to subsequent **i-FAQs** provide some examples of possible reasons.)

These two Last Wishes are exact opposites. Yet the strategy designed so that others will honor them is similar. You must state your wishes **clearly and convincingly** in your written Advance Directive, anticipate potential obstacles, and empower your Proxy with illustrative reasons. You should also discuss your wishes with your physician and those who care about you.

12. *Was Pope John Paul II Scientifically Correct When He Stated:*

A. "Permanent Vegetative State is frequently misdiagnosed"? ,

B. "Doctors cannot predict which PVS patients will recover"? *and*

C. "Care for these patients is not, in general, particularly costly"?

The short answers are: A) Yes, the **Permanent Vegetative State** can be misdiagnosed, and it is instructive to understand why. B) Yes, doctors cannot predict with certainty which specific patients will recover although many doctors believe they can predict what categories of patients will never recover. The field of medicine has never claimed to be foolproof, and the quality of recovery must also be considered. And C) Yes, the basic cost of liquid nutrients is not significantly higher than the cost of regular food and liquids, but the total cost of care is enormous if we consider the total additional cost of skilled nursing and medical care.

From the scientific and economic points of view, the importance of the three-part premise of the late Pope's Allocution extends beyond the relatively uncommon **Permanent Vegetative State** to the alarmingly increasingly common diseases of **Alzheimer's** and related progressive **dementias**, and the enormous burdens they will impose on individual caregivers and on society as a whole. This topic is discussed at length in the context of the guidelines proposed by the President's Council on Bioethics' report, "Taking Care: Ethical Caregiving In Our Aging Society" [i-FAQ 42, page 329].

SKIP

A. Misdiagnosis of PVS

Some people speculated that the reasons Pope John Paul II changed the 500-year Catholic tradition of weighing ***benefit versus burden*** a year before he died was because he was worried about his own failing health. One of the complications of Parkinson's disease is loss of the ability to swallow. However, at the very end of his life the Pope did not ask to return to the hospital, nor did he ask to replace the NG tube that had been used temporarily, with a more permanent PEG tube implanted surgically. Still, his key point of faith is to consider patients as always retaining their human quality as long as medical technology can maintain their existence.

At England's only unit that specializes in caring for patients in the **Vegetative State**, in two studies widely separated in time, about 40% of referred patients were misdiagnosed. [Andrews and others, 1996; Gill-Thwaites and Munday, 2004.] Researchers in Wisconsin and Texas also found misdiagnosis in 18% and 37% of their **Vegetative State** patients [Tresch and others, 1991; Childs and Mercer, 1993]. Dr. Andrews provided insight on why these patients were misdiagnosed. The referring doctors relied too heavily on visual tracking and voluntary movements in their initial examinations. Misdiagnoses occurred in patients who were blind or could not move. The key to making the diagnosis of Vegetative State requires clinicians to demonstrate whether or not their patient has *behavioral manifestations of awareness.*

The Andrews' group showed that this most critical determination can simply be accomplished by assessing whether the patient can reliably indicate "YES" and

"NO." Yet patients' responses depended greatly on the prevailing conditions when clinicians asked the questions. It was important that evaluating conditions be optimal. To interpret the patients' responses correctly, the clinicians must know enough neurology to distinguish between primitive reflexes and meaningful responses.

Ideally, the patient should be observed by experienced clinicians several times to maximize the chance of observing them when their performance is at its best. Other caregivers should be consulted for relevant clinical and behavioral information; for example, what part of the body can the patient still move? The patient should be maximally alert by sitting up (if possible), and by keeping the dose of sedating medications at a minimum. Sensory input should be simple. The evaluation should be performed after the patient has rested, and rest may be needed during a long evaluation. Often, patients' indication of answers must be augmented: whatever muscle patients can move can be used to activate a buzzer that all can hear; for example, one buzz for "YES," and two buzzes for "NO." It took several years for Andrews and his colleagues to develop their assessment tool. For each patient, it can still take several days for the patient and questioner to "train each other."

Unless this level of thoroughness is applied, misdiagnosis can leave patients lingering in a horrific state of not being able to express themselves even though they are aware of what is happening around them.

If awareness cannot be demonstrated, then the diagnosis is **Vegetative State**. If possible, the clinician should explain what they are observing during the evaluation. Some patients in the **Vegetative State** can laugh, for example, but if they laugh when "talked to in nonsense language or told a very sad tale in high-pitched, rising tones," then it is easier to accept that it is merely a reflex. [Royal Hospital for Neuro-disability web site.] Similarly, some patients grasp a loved one's hand tightly, which could fuel hope that the patient does not want them to leave, yet this may be a primitive reflex, as seen in babies. Educating family members may help them accept that such behaviors are *not* reasons to hope for higher mental functioning if other tests indicate that higher brain function is gone.

Some patients correctly re-assessed by Andrews as *not* being in the **Vegetative State** could communicate their wishes with technology and training. About half could do more than answer "Yes" or No" to the questions of others; they could select one letter at a time by using an alphabet scanner to initiate their own ideas. Some could indicate if they wanted to discontinue life-sustaining treatment.

To permit totally paralyzed patients to communicate, Philip Kennedy and Andreason [2004] put electrodes on their scalps and measured cortical EEG's (brain waves), while the "brain-machine interface" of Hitachi Inc. uses "optical topography" to translate slight changes in the brain's blood flow into electric signals [Tabuchi H, 2007]. The cost of taking futuristic "high tech" tools from the research lab to the bedside is far less than providing years of unwanted care for these patients.

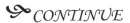CONTINUE

B. Predicting recovery and the essence of personhood

Each person must decide what is essential to his or her definition of the core of personhood, and whether to base it on faith or on science; on existence and history (once a human, always a human); or on function (ability to relate to others). Researchers may be curious to see if patients' EEGs or functional MRIs respond differently to a baby crying versus romantic music; or hearing their own name versus "dog"; or hearing a recording of a loved one's voice versus the same audio tape played backwards [Schiff and others, 2005]. But many consider the essence of personhood as the ability to interact with the environment. Gertrude Stein's "A Rose is a Rose is a Rose" pays homage to the specific qualities that constitute a rose. If personhood is more than the biological functioning of several organs, what qualities must we insist be present? Some people would start with what Descartes said in 1637 ("I think; therefore I am.") and then raise the bar:

"I decide; therefore I am."

Descartes went to a doctor who performed a physical exam and took a medical history. Wondering if he had retrieved all the relevant information, the physician asked, "Is there anything else?"

Descartes answered, "I think not..."

— The words were barely out of Descartes' mouth as he vanished.

The most fundamental way to demonstrate personhood is to consistently give correct Yes/No answers. How consistent? Andrews required his patients to answer correctly, 90% of his simple questions before he would rule-out the diagnosis of **Vegetative State**. The criterion of [Giacino and others, 2002] for Minimally Conscious State requires six correct answers for six simple situations for which the answers are easy and obvious. (Examples of such questions are given in this book's Guideline, "Questions to determine if a brain-damaged person can consistently respond to his or her environment.)

To be clear, Dr. Andrews' research did not indicate that patients could recover from the **Permanent Vegetative State**. Instead, their diligent clinical evaluations showed that over one-third of patients were initially misdiagnosed.

❧ *SKIP*

While many of the misdiagnosed patients learned how to use the alphabet scanner, their limited ability to "recover" was dismally disappointing. In Dr. Andrews' series, "All 17 misdiagnosed patients [out of total of 40 patients referred] were ... totally physically dependent for all care needs. For 15 [of these 17] patients, pressing a buzzer was the only functional movement" [Andrews and others, 1996].

The function of patients who are *correctly* diagnosed as **PVS** was even worse. Jennett [2002] initially described the syndrome; here are examples of their functioning: One patient "uttered single words from a vocabulary of four or five once every two or three days. [There was no mention of any attempt to determine if the words were meaningful or in context]... Another... responded to loud noise or attempts at nursing care by clenched teeth, rigid extremities, and high pitched screaming that abated in response to soothing voices or music."

Neurologists and other medical specialists will continue to work on reaching a consensus and collecting clinical evidence so they can define the differences among brain death, coma, *Persistent* versus *Permanent* Vegetative State, Minimally Conscious State, and the Locked-In State (total paralysis that severely limits or prevents communication by people who can think). Some researchers will invoke high-tech imaging techniques. Yet after 3 to 6 months with no apparent awareness, the most critical way to assess brain function may still be to simply determine if the patient can, or cannot, consistently and meaningfully answer "YES" or "NO."

There have been rare reports of patients with **brain trauma** who can suddenly speak again, after not talking for many years. Wesley Smith [2003] cites Terry Wallis, who "woke up" after 19 years in a "coma." [He was, however, paralyzed; see page 412.] Smith uses such examples to argue for the primacy of "personhood" not based on judging the current perceived **value** of human life. Yet for similar patients for whom clinical data were available, many had been able to indicate what they wanted non-verbally, for years. While they did not talk, they found other ways to indicate "Yes" and "No." Even so, the frequency of such awakenings is extremely rare after brain trauma. In contrast, stable reversals from **progressive dementias** have never been reported to my knowledge. Patients suffering from Alzheimer's or other progressive dementias have never recovered.

❧ *CONTINUE*

If you are wondering why we mentioned these other conditions when the Pope referred specifically only to **PVS**, we will now explain.

Articles in medical journals frequently refer to **PVS** as rare; for example, "The vegetative state is ***extremely uncommon...*** " [Andrews and others, 1996.] Yet it may not be rare at all. Physicians tend to think *inside* the diagnostic box and base the frequency of a "disease" on its ***etiology***; that is, on what caused it. Most **Vegetative States** emerge from comas that were initially caused by physical trauma, by anoxia (lack of oxygen), by vascular injuries (strokes), or by encephalitis (infections). Yet outside this box of etiology, in the all-important domain of behavioral functioning, the **Vegetative State** and its less severe "cousin," the **Minimally Conscious State**, are extremely common—as dementia progresses from the moderately severe stage to the very severe end-stage.

Political scientist James Hoefler reworked information from the work of neurologist Cranford [1991] to compare the similarities between the **Permanent Vegetative State** and **advanced dementia**. He argued that ultimately, advanced dementia mimics the **PVS** in terms of level of consciousness, self-awareness, and even the sensation of pain [Hoefler, 1997, Table 4.3, *Page 96*]. Hoefler was impressed with the magnitude of the problem of dementia. He estimated that for each person in a **Permanent Vegetative State**, there are almost 100 in end-stage dementia. Compared to roughly 25,000 cases of **Permanent Vegetative State**, there are now roughly 2 million cases of severe dementia, according to an Alzheimer's Association Fact Sheet [2005], and this number may triple by mid-century.

Conclusion: While the prognosis for some brain-injured patients is uncertain, these patients constitute a very small proportion of all brain-function impaired individuals. In contrast, those who suffer from end-stage dementia have a far more certain prognosis since their disease is progressive and irreversible. It could be a mistake of huge proportions to apply the uncertainties of the small group to the much larger group. Making end-of-life decisions for patients with end-stage dementia has an extremely low risk of error (perhaps none), while at the same time, the emotional and economic cost of maintaining their biologic existence is enormously greater.

C. The cost of caring for patients with minimal awareness

While the late Pope John Paul II stated that tube feeding is not particularly expensive for people in the **Vegetative State**, the total cost to maintain these patients for years is enormous. Caring for a patient in the **Vegetative State** costs far more than the cost of the fluid. According to the Multi-Society Task Force on PVS [1994]—approximately $150,000 a year (in 1990 dollars). The lowest estimates for some areas of the U.S. are roughly half this amount. The average lifetime cost of care for severe traumatic brain injury is predicted to range between $600,000 to $1,875,000 [Giacino and others, 2002]. Some papers have alarming titles such as "The Six Million Dollar Woman" by Professor Paris, a Jesuit priest [1981]. With Alzheimer's and related diseases affecting 1 in 8 people over the age of 65, and with 5 million cases of severe dementia projected by the year 2040, even Hanrahan's 1995 statement "**epidemiological time bomb**" underestimates the impact of this future problem. (Multiply 5 million by $100,000 to get a glimpse of its magnitude.)

Even now, more than half of personal bankruptcies arise from health-care costs [Jacoby and others, 2001]. Estimates are that between one-quarter and one-third of all medical expenses (depending on who pays for it) are directed towards patients in the last year of their lives. One-third of families with a hospitalized chronically ill patient lost most or all of their savings [Covinsky and others, 1994]. Medical costs near the end of life are disproportionately expensive [Lynn and Adamson, 2003].

If the bar is placed, as Pope John Paul II insisted, on keeping alive indefinitely those who are permanently unconscious, then his edict to continue sustenance would also apply to all patients with higher degrees of functioning. They would include those in the **Minimally Conscious State** who can experience suffering, and all patients who are obviously suffering and have no hope. Clinically, the Pope could not have placed the bar any lower to include more patients without threatening the possibility of organ donation, which depends on accepting the agreed-upon neurological definition of the next most devastating condition called "brain death" (or more properly, "death diagnosed by neurological criteria"). The bottom line is that some people would say that the Pope (or whoever wrote his Allocution) made a colossal and misleading miscalculation. The social context of these issues is so important that this topic is discussed in more detail, along with the President's Council on Bioethics' report, "Taking Care" [starting on page 329].

13. For Physicians, Attorneys, Social Workers, Nurses, and Religious Leaders... Is It Ethically and Morally Right to Inform Their Patients/Clients/Congregants About Voluntarily Refusing Food & Fluid?

Since we wrote these **i-FAQs** and their answers, readers might predict a "Yes" answer; however our two-part response is more complicated: **i**) We do believe it is ethical for professionals to inform lay people about **Voluntary Refusal of Food & Fluid**, but **ii**) We also believe that there are certain ways and circumstances that professionals could present this information that would make the process **immoral**.

Some professionals oppose informing lay people about **Voluntary Refusal of Food & Fluid** and this is our understanding of their reasons: If the person's motivation to **Voluntarily Refuse Food & Fluid** is to hasten his or her death—a goal that some consider as morally wrong—then it is therefore also morally wrong for another person (the professional) to inform them how to perform that wrong act. Some would argue that it is not possible for a professional to discuss this option without subtly recommending it. While proponents may argue that **Voluntary Refusal of Food & Fluid** is merely allowing Nature to take its course, they believe the method is really a deliberate intent to hasten dying (unless the patient cannot absorb the Food & Fluid, or is imminently dying).

Everyone knows **Voluntary Refusal of Food & Fluid** will eventually lead to death, yet one could argue that patients might not consider using this method to hasten the process deliberately unless a trusted authority informed them that...

A. **Voluntary Refusal of Food & Fluid** (**VRFF**) does not lead to death by starvation;

B. **VRFF** is minimally uncomfortable and the process of dying is often described as peaceful;

C. **VRFF** usually takes two weeks or less and for approximately the last half of that time, the patient is asleep or in a coma;

D. **VRFF** is definitely considered morally acceptable in some religious and belief systems, although it is controversial in others; and,

E. **VRFF** is legal since the U. S. Supreme Court ruled that any competent adult can refuse any medical treatment, which includes artificial nutrition and hydration.

Ideally, physicians should also educate patients and families about related decisions. Internists at the Mayo Clinic concluded, "Clinician familiarity with [legal and ethical] concepts" and realize that withdrawal of a cardiac pacemaker is "not the same as physician-assisted suicide or euthanasia" could "lead to *more expeditious withdrawal of unwanted medical support* from terminally ill patients." {Emphasis added to Mueller and others [2003].}

On the other hand, we would be alarmed if professionals offered information about **Voluntary Refusal of Food & Fluid** in improper or **immoral** ways such as *attempting to persuade a patient* to Refuse Food & Fluid immediately...

i. Before the patient is ready to die;

ii. Because continued care of the patient would entail suffering and expense, which reasons are not openly admitted and discussed;

iii. In spite of knowing that the particular patient has deep religious or moral beliefs that **Voluntary Refusal of Food & Fluid** is wrong; or,

iv. If offered as a pre-condition for receiving aggressive *Comfort Care* (which would violate the essence of what it means for the decision to be **Voluntary**).

This last option was dramatized in the 1973 movie, **_Soylent Green_**. In what was *his* final performance, Edward G. Robinson played a character who agreed to undergo euthanasia, in part because the authorities had promised to provide him with the "long version" of a simulated peaceful scene prior to his dying.

❧ *SKIP*

The fine line that professionals must walk is to provide information in a balanced way without trying to influence the patient to opt for **Voluntary Refusal of Food & Fluid** while respecting the patient's autonomous wishes and belief systems. At a practical level, professionals should simultaneously strive to do two things: Support the patient to find meaning in life and neutrally inform the patient of the available end-of-life options. Then the professional should remain non-judgmental as she or he steps back to a posture of being willing to accept *what* the patient decides... and especially, *when*. Knowledge about the common issues can help raise the clinician's index of suspicion. For example, if the patient's decision is motivated by relieving the adult children of the financial and physical burdens of care, then the responsible clinician should also interview those children, perhaps individually and with the patient, to deal with this issue.

Judging whether an act is morally right or wrong is ultimately based on one's belief system. It is presumptuous to judge other people's "intentions" or "motivation" as wrong if that "wrongness" is based on your value system instead of theirs. As we have seen, the moral view about **Voluntary Refusal of Food & Fluid** varies among persons of the same religion, as well as among different religions. Since human behavior is admittedly complex, some reasons may seem right and other reasons may seem wrong for the same behavior, even within the same belief system. For such dilemmas, the principles of bioethics can sometimes help. Below is a simplified version of these principles that considers the theme of this book:

Informing Patients About Voluntary Refusal of Food & Fluid: Applying the Principles of Medical Ethics

1. Patients must be fully informed about **VRFF** in order to prudently exercise their **autonomous** choice;

2. Informing patients about **VRFF** may **benefit** patients who may find this method a peaceful way to avoid prolonged suffering. It may also **benefit** family members who may use the time to say goodbye;

3. Informing patients about **VRFF** does **not cause harm** as long as doctors are careful not to inadvertently encourage **VRFF** by respectfully encouraging patients to continue living and provide the best available *Comfort Care*—so that the patient can make a choice that is independent and voluntary; and

4. If the patient's choice is truly **voluntary**, then **Refusal of Food & Fluid** can help facilitate the **fair allocation** of society's limited medical

and financial **resources** while it reduces the burden on caregiving relatives.

To elaborate on Principle 1 (**autonomy**), recall Dr. Nuland's confession of guilt for what he called the "**worst sort of paternalism**"—withholding information because he was afraid the patient might make the "**wrong decision**" [1994, Emphasis added, *Page 252*]. Given the amount of information required for some patients to seriously consider **VRFF** leads me to disagree with the fine distinction made by Dr. Loewy [2001]: he felt that it is *right* only for physicians to accept patients' spontaneous requests for **VRFF**, and that it is *wrong* for physicians to offer this information if patients did not initiate the inquiry. I believe it is paternalistic for a doctor to judge what the patient should know, and wrong to withhold information necessary for the patient to make his or her decision.

To elaborate on Principles 2 (**benefit**) and 3 (**do no harm**): Providing information about **VRFF** may create good and prevent harm since it may prevent unnecessary and prolonged suffering and further indignity. It also may allow some people to avoid suicide attempts that could be violent, illegal, or unsuccessful. Botched attempts may leave patients worse off. **VRFF** may make it unnecessary for physicians or family members to actively participate to hasten dying, which is illegal and can leave the helpers with guilt. Even if someone else does the helping, loved ones could be in legal jeopardy if they are present during the patient's final hours so they must leave without saying goodbye and violate rule number one about dying: "Do not allow a person to die alone." If the patient's Advance Directive explains the reasons for wanting **VRFF**, those written passages may later provide solace and reduce guilt among the surviving relatives. If the professional explains that **VRFF** allows patients to change their minds and that some alert patients do, then family members who later grieve their loss may find it easier to accept that their loved one maintained his or her resolve to achieve a peaceful transition.

With respect to the fourth Principle of **social justice**, we must again consider the disease that will most challenge the caregiving and economic resources of our society—dementia.

Many sources currently list Alzheimer's disease (which accounts for about 60% of all dementias) as the third most expensive disease after heart disease and cancer. However the $100 billion a year to care for demented Americans is a gross underestimate since another $100 billion should be attributed to unpaid caregiving by family members and the work opportunities they lost. Alzheimer's often wipes out families' life-savings and disrupts the careers of those who assume the task of caregivers. The caregiver burden will affect increasing millions of family members as baby boomers age, since 47% of people over the age of 85 have Alzheimer's. The sandwich generation will especially suffer as they take on the responsibility for both older and younger generations—their sick parents and growing children. And some must also continue their jobs to make ends meet. The cost is also emotional: relatives of Alzheimer's patients have more stress than caregivers of other diseases. Toward the end of the Alzheimer's patient's life, 43% of family caregivers have a clinically significant depression [Schulz and others, 2003]. Caregivers' physical health is also jeopardized and they are at risk for increased mortality. Such is the burden on individuals who care and provide care.

Consider the following example as the tip of the iceberg in creating a burden to society. In 1994, Fleck wrote: "As for medical and economic irrationality, the State of Missouri covers only 40% of people with Medicaid who live below the poverty line. Nevertheless, the State spent more than $900,000 to sustain the life of Nancy Cruzan, who was in a **Persistent Vegetative State** for seven years." There are thousands, perhaps millions, of other examples, where a family's savings was spent on the care of an unconscious person at the expense of college educations that could have increased the productivity and life satisfaction of grandchildren. Similarly, the maintenance of one infant born without a brain, who therefore has no potential for mental development, can drain the health care resources away from thousands of infants and babies who could otherwise have received better preventive medical care including vaccinations. It may be emotionally harder to make decisions for infants than for the elderly who have enjoyed a full life, but what may be critical is an accurate and certain prognosis, combined with a consensus regarding what constitutes the minimal functioning of a human being.

Still, such arguments cause many to worry, including Dr. Hartwig who warned about "slippery slopes" to induce people to feel they have "a duty to die" [1997].

❧ CONTINUE

Our world faces a great crisis. Along with expected increases in Alzheimer's and other dementias, there will be a relative decrease in the number of working and caregiving people to support them in terms of finances and energy. There will soon be a shortage of 400,000 nurses. Unless people's attitudes undergo a major change about the circumstances under which they will no longer want to prolong their existence and the existence of loved ones—society will not be able to meet this inevitable, enormous challenge. I hope this book will encourage policy makers to rethink these critical issues as well as stimulate individuals to be more diligent as they create their Advance Directives.

In practical terms, instead of considering the administration of Food & Fluid as "ordinary care" when there is no hope for improvement in a person with a severe, progressive, irreversible dementia—both the individual's and society's interests could reasonably and ethically be justified by **Voluntarily Refusing Food & Fluid**.

We enjoy religious freedom in America, but implementing our moral beliefs can impact the rest of society. Sometimes Americans distinguish between beliefs and behaviors. For example, America tolerates the *belief* of fundamentalist Mormons that God has mandated polygamy, but America's secular laws do not permit them to *practice* polygamy [Jon Krakauer, 2003]. Similarly, it is fine to *believe* that providing food and water always recognizes the inherent human dignity of the individual every person, but we must also ask, given the expense of keeping so many patients with dementia alive, how many people in our country and others must go with far less than optimal medical treatment, if we permit people to *practice* that belief? In addition, it can be argued that those who insist on providing Food & Fluid to patients in the Permanent Vegetative State or end-stage dementia are not only imposing their belief systems on others; they are also harming those who believe otherwise.

With terribly long waits to receive health care, rumblings have begun to legalize a two-tier system in Canada. Leslie Burke has challenged the British National Health Service in his bid for right-to-life. Obviously, this is a world-wide problem.

The controversy became more intense with the publication of the President's Council on Bioethics' report, "Taking Care," which is discussed in depth, later.

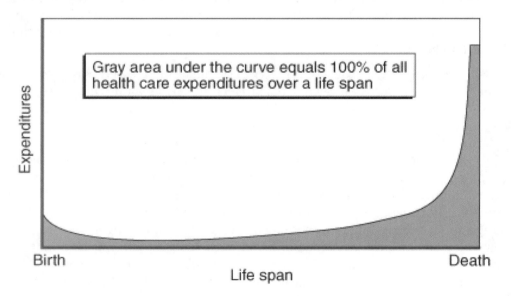

Figure 1. Americans' Current Health Care Expenditures Are Concentrated in the Final Part of the Life Span
J. Lynn, D. Adamson, Living Well at the End of Life, Santa Monica, Calif: RAND, Corporation, 2003.
Reprinted with permission.

The graph above shows the current medical expenditures across the life span in America. The authors estimated that the last one-tenth of one's life uses nearly half the lifetime cost of medical care [Lynn and Adamson, 2003].

The Physician's Ethical Obligation According to the AMA, and, Which Question is "More Moral" to Ask?

The physician has an ethical obligation to help the patient make choices from among the therapeutic alternatives consistent with good medical practice...

The patient's right of self-decision can be effectively exercised only if the patient possesses enough information to enable an intelligent choice.

> —American Medical Association Council on Ethical and Judicial Affairs. *Code of Medical Ethics*, 1998-1999 edition. Chicago, IL: American Medical Association, 1997.

So...

In discussing end of life options with lay people, should professionals provide or withhold the information they have about **Voluntary Refusal of Food & Fluid**?

Or is it "more moral" to ask...

Is it ethical for professionals to withhold the information they have, since individuals can only make an informed choice when they are provided with the information they need, and **Voluntary Refusal of Food & Fluid** is a legal way to avoid prolonged suffering that satisfies the principles of medical ethics.

Chapter 7

QUESTIONS OF LEGALITY, CIVIL RIGHTS, AND SAFETY

Some Wish to Die as They Wish to Have Lived

Some people consider the right to choose how and when to end their lives as one way to express their individual civil rights. This motivation may add passion to their search for a legal peaceful choice at the end of life, but it might also distract them to politics.

---

14. What are the Differences Between Voluntary Refusal of Food & Fluid, and Voluntary Euthanasia?

Voluntary euthanasia is the merciful ending of another's life at the request of a suffering person. Physicians administer a dose of medication that is deliberately set high enough to stop the drive to breathe or to stop the heart from beating. One right-to-die organization distributes buttons with this slogan: "Please let me die like a dog," in appreciation of how peaceful dying seems when a veterinarian administers a high dose of anesthetic medication to pets they have loved, but must finally let go. One problem with legalizing *voluntary euthanasia* is that authorizing physicians to terminate lives gives them power that could be abused in the privacy or secrecy of the intimate doctor-patient relationship.

With *Controlled Sedation for Refractory Suffering*, relief of suffering is the primary therapeutic goal. Although the medication *might* hasten death as an unintended but foreseeable side effect, most medical, legal, and pastoral leaders consider the process as morally correct, and use the term Double Effect to refer to two possible results: relief of suffering without loss of life, or relief of suffering but with the possible but unintended side effect of hastening dying. The positive good is the goal, but the side effect is realistically recognized.

The Catholic Church has embraced the concept of the Double Effect for six centuries, stating that it is "a positive good to relieve a patient's suffering as long as one does not intentionally cause death or interfere with other moral or religious duties." In 1273, when he introduced the concept, Thomas Aquinas referred to the act of self-defense. In contrast, the Catholic Church views "suffering as having special significance in terms of patients' opportunity to share in Christ's redemptive suffering."

The primary goal of **euthanasia** is to end all suffering by immediately ending life. **Euthanasia** is legal only in Holland and Belgium (since 2002). Even before it was legalized, if physicians followed strict guidelines, they were not prosecuted. Euthanasia was legal, briefly, in Australia's Northern Territory. With less publicity, it is permitted in Switzerland. In Colombia a court decision made it legal, based on "human rights."

The U.S. public does distinguish between physician-assisted suicide and euthanasia. Oregon's Death with Dignity Act explicitly forbids euthanasia. The State of Michigan had no law against assisted suicide when Dr. Jack Kevorkian began his "crusade," but even after the legislators passed a law to make assisting suicide illegal, a jury later refused to convict him of that crime. Yet a judge found Kevorkian guilty and sentenced him to serve a minimum of seven years in prison after he performed voluntary euthanasia on national TV. His victim, an ALS patient, was presumably not able to hasten his own death. [Terman, 1999].

Next consider comments about an award-winning film that chronicles the long but unsuccessful attempt to legalize euthanasia in Spain.

Outside "The Sea Inside"—a Deleted Scene

The Academy Award's Best Foreign Film of 2004 portrays the true story of Ramón Sampedro. He lost his long legal battle with the Spanish government to legalize euthanasia. He wanted a doctor to help him end his life peacefully after 28 years of living as a quadriplegic. During that time he was totally dependent on his brother's family, and felt he lived in a state of indignity.

Ramón did not have a "good death." Cyanide caused him to suffer in agony for 20 minutes—alone, in front of a video camera. Why cyanide, instead of a medication that would have provided a more peaceful way to die? As the target of the news media and the police, Ramón feared that using a prescription medication might implicate one of his physician-friends. Why alone? Because Ramón wanted those who helped him die to avoid being charged with a crime. The strategy for having eleven people help was based on the hope that each individual's contribution would be too small a part of the whole process for the authorities to charge any one of them with the illegal act of assisting suicide.

Director Alejandro Amenabar recognized that the story's strong subplot could distract from Ramón's story so he deleted the scene that explained why Ramón's beautiful lawyer, Julia, changed her mind. (The scene is available on the DVD as bonus material.)

Julia suffered from a rare and progressive neurological disease. She had promised Ramón that she would leave her husband and return to Ramón so they could consummate their deep love... by ending their lives together. Her vow gave Ramón much solace since he would not be forced to suffer indefinitely. But Julia insisted waiting to die until after Ramón's book of poems had been published. In the meantime, here is how Julia's husband effectively argued (in the deleted scene): The act of taking care of her—even if her disease progressed to the point where she could no longer recognize him—still constituted an important means *for him* to express his love. As a testament to prove his love, he also bought her a magnificent home that overlooked the sea.

The scene where Ramón died alone in pain, although very sad, is not the one that burns most intensely in my mind. I recall with anguish when Gené, the activist from Spain's right-to-die organization visited Julie, a few years later. At first, Gené was relieved that Julia seemed calm as she gazed out at the sea. Julia was able to greet her with some typical pleasant words, as expected. But when Gené placed Ramón's letter on Julia's lap, she seemed not to understand what to do with the envelope. She just stroked Gené's wrist. When she asked, "Ramón *who?*" Gené turned away from Julia's blank stare and then struggled, but not successfully, to hold back her tears.

While Julia still retained the primitive ability to relate to another human being through gentle touch, her unique personality was devastated by such a profound loss of memory that she could no longer remember or appreciate one of the most loving people she had experienced in her life.

15. What are the Differences Between Voluntary Refusal of Food & Fluid, and Committing "Slow Suicide"?

Ceasing all Food & Fluid can be considered an acceptance of the natural process of dying. For suffering terminal patients who have the capacity to make medical decisions and who clearly do not want to eat or drink, it would be morally wrong—as well as a legal violation of their Constitutional rights—to force them to eat and drink, or to insert tubes or intravenous lines into them, as a way of prolonging their existence and suffering.

In contrast, mentally ill patients rarely **Voluntarily Refuse Food & Fluid** to commit suicide. To make political statements, martyrs like Mahatma Gandhi typically refuse only calories but continue fluid to maintain hydration.

Psychiatric consultation may be necessary to determine that a patient's judgment to make the decision to forgo intake is sound and not the result of a severe mental illness. For patients who suffer from such severe mental illness as *anorexia nervosa* and *severe depressive disorders*, it is clinically, legally, and morally appropriate to insist on inserting an IV or NG tube to save their lives while offering them treatment for their psychiatric illness.

How do clinicians make this critical distinction? Briefly, *Anorexics* have a distorted body image; they falsely perceive that their bodies are too fat. *Depressives* suffer from extreme hopelessness that is not based in reality. When treated, individuals with either disorder often return to a normal life in terms of functioning and duration. There is a gray zone, however, where terminal patients suffer from a moderately severe mental illness but may still retain the capacity to make sound medical decisions and choose **Voluntary Refusal of Food & Fluid** [Terman 2001a, 2001b]. When the ability to make sound medical decisions is in doubt, it is prudent to request a mental health professional to evaluate the patient for decision-making capacity (which is described in general, later).

16. What are the Differences Between Voluntary Refusal of Food & Fluid and "Physician-Assisted Suicide"?

Since words may convey inaccurate or unintended meanings, before we compare **Voluntary Refusal of Food & Fluid** with what is commonly called "Physician-Assisted Suicide" (**PAS**), we first take issue with this term's implications and offer an alternative.

"**Suicide**" most often refers to life-ending acts performed by people who suffer from the most severe consequence of treatable mental disorders, but who are usually not terminally ill. The tragic result is ending a person's life who might have received psychiatric treatment, and then enjoyed many more years of life. Clearly, in practice, "Suicide is a permanent solution to a temporary problem."

"Suicide" also refers to impulsive dramatic acts of manipulation where the person did not intend to die but wished only to make a statement that he or she hoped would have impact on another, but miscalculated. Finally, "suicide" is used to describe the treacherous acts committed by kamikaze pilots and terrorists.

Nevertheless, using the word "suicide" in the context of end-of-life options has one distinct advantage: It makes it clear that the final act *must be performed by the patient*, which clearly distinguishes the act from euthanasia, where the physician administers the lethal dose of medication directly to the patient.

To develop the new term, we first propose that "Physician-Assisted" be replaced by "**Physician-Aided**." Oregon's law does not require physicians to be present **when** (and very importantly, **if**) their patients decide to ingest the medications that the physicians have prescribed; thus, the only way they aid is by writing a prescription. Note: Medical supervision is still available, but the patient or family members must ask for the doctor to be present. Oregon's Death with Dignity Act provides *immunity for all who are present* when a patient ingests a lethal dose of pills, provided they follow the law's strict protocol.

The proposed new term concludes with the words, "**Hastened Dying**" since the present Oregon law and most other proposed bills in the U.S. were limited to terminal patients. These laws clearly intend to hasten only the on-going process for patients who are already dying.

But "Physician-Aided Hastened Dying" could possibly refer to euthanasia so we propose adding the word "patient." The final term is then: **Physician-Aided, Patient-Hastened Dying**, or **PAPHD**. Note: "Physician" was chosen over "Doctor," allowing for the shorter abbreviation **PAD** (or **PHD**) to replace **PAS**.

This new term implies that a **physician aids** the **hastening** of an on-going process of **dying** only if **patients** themselves so decide. Clearly, it takes two separate actions: first, **physicians aid** by writing the prescriptions; second, **terminal patients can then decide** if (as well as when) they want to ingest those pills to hasten their dying.

The Benefits of Physician-Aided, Patient-Hastened Dying

The benefits of **Physician-Aided, Patient-Hastened Dying** can be illustrated by looking at the effects of **Oregon's Death with Dignity Act**.

1. The obvious benefits. Patients who have no hope for recovery from their terminal illness, who feel their current suffering and indignity are unbearable, and/or who no longer want to be totally dependent on others and further drain their emotions and finances—are freed from being forced to endure for an indefinite period of time as their conditions inevitably and progressively decline. **Physician-Aided, Patient-Hastened Dying** provides the option for a peaceful, painless, and relatively rapid method to hasten their dying.

Why is this so important? Because the advances of modern medical technology are like two-sided coins. For example, with surgery and chemotherapy it is now possible to provide several more years of enjoyable life to women who suffer from some types of uterine cancer. A century ago, when the inevitable end came, the patient peacefully drifted into a coma due to obstructive uremia. That is, blockage caused toxic chemicals to build up in the blood, and these chemicals reduced consciousness. Now however, long-term survivors can be subject to unbearable end-stage symptoms, including pain.

2. The psychological benefit of being able to determine if, as well as when. Although 17 days is the minimum time patients must wait after they begin the eligibility process, patients may still have up to six months to live. Relatively few Oregonians actually die by ingesting a fatal dose of medication according to Barbara Coombs Lee, one of the leaders of **Compassion and Choices**. She commented on the work of Dr. Susan Tolle who obtained the following approximate but provocative numbers [2004]:

- 1 out of 6 terminal patients discussed the options legalized by the **Death with Dignity Act** with family members, although more may have considered the option.

- 1 out of 50 terminal patients formally began the 15-day eligibility process.

- 1 out of 800 terminal patients actually took the medication to hasten his or her dying.

Looking at the same data in another way, out of about 1000 terminal patients, approximately 167 discussed the **Death with Dignity Act** with family members, 20 began but did not finish the eligibility process, and only 1 actually took the medication. So... did the 166 or even more patients who considered the option or discussed it with their families, including the 19 who only began the eligibility process, derive any benefit from Oregon's **Death with Dignity Act**?

Barbara Coombs Lee believes, *Yes, definitely*! But her reason may at first seem paradoxical. She explains that the very law that permits people to end their lives before their terminal illness causes death can actually lead many patients to decide to live as long as possible. Why? Because they derive psychological comfort from knowing that the law will permit them to end their lives (and suffering) quickly and peacefully, if and when they decide their existence has become unbearable.

To explain further, once terminal patients qualify to receive a lethal dose of medication, they never again need fear that they will be trapped to exist in a state where they face increasing indignity and unrelenting pain. Knowing they can choose the time to permanently end their suffering provides them an opportunity to change their attitude toward their symptoms. One day at a time, they can decide if their lives still retain sufficient meaning to endure their suffering. If they have ultimate control over ending their lives but choose not to do so, then they have **voluntarily decided to stay alive despite their symptoms**. Thus patients can make an important psychological shift in how they see themselves: *from* "**helpless victims**" *to* "**willing survivors**."

This positive change in self-perception, plus the decrease in anxiety about how intense and long suffering could be, permits patients to direct their energy toward a final search for meaning during the last months or weeks of their lives. A surprisingly high proportion of patients continue living this way, postponing the ingestion of the lethal medication so long that they ultimately die without using the prescription of lethal medication. Thus, legalizing **Physician-Aided, Patient-Hastened Dying** can improve both the quality and quantity of the precious bit of life that remains for many terminal patients. It is ironic that **many live longer when permitted to control when their lives will end.**

The Irony of Legalizing Physician-Aided, Patient-Hastened Dying

The very law that permits people to end their lives sooner, leads many to choose to live longer.

The same can be said for informing people about the option of **Voluntary Refusal of Food & Fluid**. Thus, some of the energy that is now being put into changing the law could be directed towards educating people about other options that are already legal.

3. Arguments against legalizing Physician-Aided, Patient-Hastened Dying. First of all, "Pro-life" opponents prefer to use the term, **Physician-Assisted Suicide**, since this choice of words makes the practice sound horrific. The semantics have already been discussed above, and we believe this term is not appropriate. As a psychiatrist, I am professionally committed to preventing suicide among individuals who suffer from mental illnesses and providing them with treatment so they can enjoy a full healthy life.

The religious argument: Some claim that **Physician-Aided, Patient-Hastened Dying** is morally wrong. Anything anyone does to hasten dying is wrong since each human life belongs to God, not to the person who inhabits the gift of the body. (There are some exceptions that religions have permitted, however, such as virgins committing suicide to avoid being raped by the victors of wars.) Except in such extraordinary circumstances, people are responsible to God beyond and in addition to their personal needs. Attitudes are not quite as opposed to "terminal palliative care" [Burdette, 2005], however.

The secular argument: The legal term, *parens patriae*, refers to that function of government that provides protection to those who are not able to protect themselves; in this case, the State's duty is to prevent its citizens from killing themselves.

The medical role argument: The American Medical Association praises the time-honored concept of physician-as-healer, a role some insist must not be tarnished by any act to hasten dying. Opponents of legalizing **Physician-Aided, Patient-Hastened Dying** fear the process will diminish patients' trust of doctors, especially since much of our current medical system is profit-based, and it is obvious that the least costly "treatment plan" would be to pay for one prescription of lethal medication. Using more highly charged words, the argument is that patients might distrust the medical system because they would worry if managed care included the option of "Managed Death." Yet multiple surveys over the past two decades repeatedly reveal that 65-70% of people consistently want to legalize **PAPHD**. In Oregon, no patient is forced to accept this "treatment plan." Requesting a prescription, and ingesting the pills are both independent acts, each of which must be voluntarily performed by the patient.

Despite the way some politicians, religious leaders, and lawyers characterize it, **Physician-Aided, Patient-Hastened Dying** as practiced in Oregon, has safeguards that ensure it will be voluntary. Seven years of experience in Oregon has not justified any of its opponents' initial warnings. People have not flocked to the State to die. People with disabilities are not being forced to choose an early death. The old and feeble are not being coerced to choose to end their lives early. The number of people who take advantage of the law are small.

Actually, the quality of end-of-life medical care in Oregon is among the finest in America. Almost everyone agrees that hospice offers terminal patients the best care, yet across our nation, only 22% of terminal patients take advantage of hospice. Yet in 2003, of those terminal patients in Oregon who did ingest a lethal dose of pills, 90% died under hospice care. No arguments prove that **Physician-Aided, Patient-Hastened Dying** hurts those who prefer not to choose it.

In 1997, the U.S. Supreme Court explicitly allowed States to experiment with **Physician-Assisted Suicide**. Under Oregon law, physicians and pharmacists are not required to comply with patients' requests if they feel conflict with their personal, moral, or religious values. Some view the standard of care as requiring them to refer these patients to other providers. Still, former Attorney General John Ashcroft and his successor, Alberto Gonzales, wanted to punish doctors by threatening to revoke their licenses to prescribe controlled medications and/or to imprison them, if doctors offered their patients this option. In January, 2006, the U.S. Supreme Court ruled that the 1970 Controlled Substances Act could not serve as the legal basis for restricting physicians by threatening such punishment. While the citizens of Oregon, who voted twice to legalize **Physician-Aided,**

Patient-Hastened Dying, and organizations who favor the ability to choose this option were pleased, in the future there may be reactions at the State level or other attempts made in Congress. Those who feel it is the State's or Federal Government's duty to protect citizens in this way should consider this allegory:

I Just Want to Help

"Oh, let me help you,"
Said the bird to the fish,
As she safely placed him
In the branch of her tree.

The U.S. Supreme Court upheld the ruling of the 2006 judges of the 9th Circuit who considered Ashcroft's threat to prosecute Oregon's physicians as "unlawful and unenforceable," and one judge from the 9th Circuit was quoted as saying, "We note that the attorney general has no specialized expertise in the field of medicine."

The Supreme Court Justices who dissented argued that "assisting in suicide is not a legitimate medical purpose." But the main issue was not a medical but a legal one: whether the Federal government or the States should make that decision. This ruling prevented Federal intrusion by the way States to decide how to regulate the practice of medicine. The ruling will affect people in all states, not just Oregonians, in terms of the way end-of-life medicine is practiced. To understand how, consider how physician-assisted suicide is practiced secretly, how the DEA operates, and how fear can change the behavior of many physicians:

Confidential surveys in San Francisco found that more than half of the surveyed doctors admitted they had helped AIDS patients hasten their dying [Slome and others, 1997]. Several confidential surveys in other States revealed that many physicians are willing to provide assistance to hasten dying.

Experience shows that the behavior of physicians is affected by the possibility that they may be prosecuted through a Drug Enforcement Administration (DEA) action, whose proceedings can revoke their license to prescribe certain medications for anxiety, insomnia, and pain—or worse, put them in jail. Although no exact numbers are available, the impact could be exponential, based on this theory: For every one doctor who was prosecuted for allegedly creating a "drug addict" out of a terminal cancer patient who suffered from pain, or was prosecuted by the DEA for prescribing an opioid for what the doctor believed was a "legitimate medical purpose" (to treat pain) but was duped by an addict and then prosecuted as severely if the doctor committed the crime of trafficking by selling the drug on the street—many dozens of other doctors who learned of their colleagues' misfortune will become afraid to provide adequate pain treatment to dozens of their patients. Thus, many dozens of dozens of patients may suffer unnecessarily. This result may be an example of how little things can make a big difference, as popularized in *The Tipping Point* by Gladwell [2002].

Writing about "what is wrong with the DEA's war against doctors," John Tierney quoted an estimate of Ronald Libby, a professor of political science at the University of North Florida, that the DEA investigated about 1 in 6 pain specialist doctors one year. Including State and local authorities brings the estimate for the annual risk of being investigated, for those doctors who regularly prescribe pain medications, to about one in three. A Pittsburgh doctor was sentenced to over 6 years in prison based on a drug addict's testimony. Now, there is new compelling evidence to charge the *key witness/accused drug addict/presumptive victim* with perjury [Tierney, 2006a, 2006b].

The bottom line: Merely publicizing the Attorney General's attempt to use the DEA to threaten Oregon physicians may still make doctors in other States reluctant to discretely help terminal patients to hasten their dying to end their suffering, since individual States can still decide what constitutes "a legitimate medical purpose," and States may now pass stricter laws that could be applied retroactive, now that the U.S. Supreme Court ruled States must decide.

The reactions and counter-reactions of the U.S. Supreme Court decision may further polarize the issues in the political realm, while individual patients and their families continue to suffer. It is thus imperative to educate people about the alternative—an option that is, and will almost certainly remain, legal: **Voluntary Refusal of Food & Fluid**. Since individual States may create additional obstacles to make it more difficult for legally designated **Proxies to Refuse Food & Fluid** on behalf of incompetent patients via their Advance Directives, the strategies detailed in this book, which are designed to overcome these obstacles, may become even more important in the future.

Comparing Physician-Aided, Patient-Hastened Dying to the Voluntary Refusal of Food & Fluid

1. How active are these methods? **Physician-Aided, Patient-Hastened Dying** is active. Both doctor and patient *do* something. The doctor *prescribes* the medication; the patient may (or may not) *ingest* the pills.

With **Voluntary Refusal of Food & Fluid**, the patient *does not do* something; specifically, does not eat or drink. The doctor is available only to provide additional *Comfort Care*; for example, to prescribe medications to reduce anxiety.

Since **Physician-Aided, Patient-Hastened Dying** is active while **Voluntary Refusal of Food & Fluid** is passive, the latter method may be more morally acceptable to some people.

2. Where are these methods legal? **Physician-Aided, Patient-Hastened Dying** is legal only in the State of Oregon, the South American country of Colombia, and in Europe—Switzerland, Belgium, and the Netherlands. Yet other countries and States quietly do not prosecute doctors if the circumstances of the act are such that juries are likely to be sympathetic and not find them guilty of committing a crime. In April, 2007, Vermont lawmakers voted down an attempt to legalize "Physician-Assisted Suicide" after four hours of debate. Compassion and Choices used the word "paralyzed" to describe the California Assembly on June 6, 2007, as efforts were quietly abandoned for the third time in three years.

Voluntary Refusal of Food & Fluid is legal right now in all U.S. States, Canada, and most other countries. Choosing it should present no legal problem for adults if they are competent when they decline Food & Fluid. Yet many U.S. States present additional hurdles by imposing strict requirements for Proxies when they act on behalf of incompetent patients based on the instructions from their previously created Advance Directives. **Refusing Food & Fluid** on behalf of incompetent patients is far more difficult than refusing other types of treatment.

Note: This book reviews the legal challenges that form the basis for its suggested strategies, whose goal is the success of your Proxy to exercise Substituted Judgment (to make decisions based on knowing your wishes and values), which can include the **Refusal of Food & Fluid** on your behalf. The ultimate success of your Proxy depends on A) how well you word your Advance Directive (others must consider it *clear and convincing*), B) how well you explain and provide examples for why you want this option available under some circumstances, and C) how much you empower your Proxy. This book describes the strategies to accomplish all these tasks.

Briefly, in addition to an empowering Proxy designation, I recommend you create a document I call "**Empowering Statements for My Proxy**."

3. How effective are PAPHD and VRFF? The number of patients who took prescriptions of lethal medication in Oregon from near the end of 1997 through 2004 was 208. In early 2005, one patient woke up after being asleep for 63 hours. His wife reported that her husband claimed God visited him and told him that he was not supposed to die this way. He then suffered for two more weeks before he died of lung cancer. While critics might cite this case as an example that things can go wrong, there are few other medical procedures that have a "batting average" as good as 207/208 (.995; that is 99.5% effective).

Some might find it interesting, however, that many years ago, this 208th patient was convicted of rape and spent seven years in prison. People of religious faith, especially those who believe in redemptive suffering, could cite this case to support the view that God should, and does decide when a person's life is over.

As previously discussed above, **Voluntary Refusal of Food & Fluid** is not the best choice for all people and medical conditions. Two examples are obese patients and those suffering from end-stage liver disease accompanied by ascites. In some of these medical situations, **Physician-Aided, Patient-Hastened Dying** is preferred.

4. What is the time delay to start? In Oregon, **Physician-Aided, Patient-Hastened Dying** cannot begin until the patient waits 15 days to be eligible to obtain the prescription, and another 2 days to receive it. During this time, the patient must request **PAPHD** 3 times, one of which must be in writing. Two physicians must certify that the patient is terminally ill and, if the "patient may be suffering from a psychiatric or psychological disorder, or depression causing impaired judgment, either physician shall refer the patient for counseling" [ORS 127.825]. Once patients receive the prescription, they may fill it any time thereafter, and once filled, they have more time to decide to take it.

Voluntary Refusal of Food & Fluid often requires no additional evaluations or waiting period. The patient can begin to refuse to eat and drink as long as no "interested party" insists on a psychiatric assessment to determine if the patient is mentally competent and his or her decision is voluntary.

5. How long will it take until death? **Physician-Aided, Patient-Hastened Dying** takes an unpredictable number of hours (usually 2 to 24) for death to come. Many proponents of **PAPHD** consider this short time to be an advantage since it reduces how long patients and families must wait for death to occur and makes it easier for them to plan when to say their last "good-byes."

Voluntary Refusal of Food & Fluid takes patients an unpredictable number of days (usually 3 to 17) to die, with 85% dying within 2 weeks. Proponents of **Voluntary Refusal of Food & Fluid** note that the extra days of waiting can benefit patients by providing them time to reflect and to connect with their loved ones and perhaps also to leave their legacy of values. It also provides time for loved ones to gradually accept their impending loss and to begin to support each other in the grieving process.

6. Is it reversible, if I change my mind? **Physician-Aided, Patient-Hastened Dying** is generally irreversible once patients take the lethal dose of pills. A terminal patient could impulsively take the pills in a fleeting moment of despair or a temporary exacerbation of pain and such a decision could lead to the irreversible result of death. Although we know of no reported cases, it is theoretically possible for patients who change their mind to ask the doctor (if present) to initiate temporary ventilator support or to ask a family member to administer Ipecac to induce vomiting; however patients must make such requests before they fall asleep, and treatment must be initiated immediately. The window of opportunity for patients to change their mind is only a few minutes, and will not be effective unless treatment is started immediately.

In contrast, one major advantage of **Voluntary Refusal of Food & Fluid** is that the method allows conscious patients the opportunity to continually reconsider if they want to hasten their dying. There is a relative wide window during which they can ask their physician to supervise their resumption of eating and drinking. [See the **i-FAQ**, "What if I change my mind?" that explains why a physician is needed.]

Of the 126 nurses who each reported on a patient who **Voluntarily Refused Food & Fluid**, 16 patients subsequently resumed eating and drinking [Ganzini and others, 2003]. Not all the reasons were known with certainty but the nurses felt that families may have pressured five of the patients, and that four may have resumed because of feeling hunger or discomfort. One patient may have resumed due to amelioration of depression.

7. How safe are these methods? The availability of a lethal dose of pills is potentially dangerous to others, since another person, for whom the pills were not intended, might find and take the pills to commit suicide due to psychiatric reasons. The pills could also be criminally administered to someone without their knowledge or permission. There is no such thing as a "100% completely safe" medical procedure. (Note: after 7 years of experience with Oregon's **Death with Dignity Act**, these potential problems have NOT been reported.)

8. Is there a difference in esthetics? Dehydration can lead to sunken eyes and dry skin, compared to taking an overdose of sleeping pills, which—unless the patient vomits—begins with a peaceful sleep. (Medications are used to prevent vomiting.) However, when people are near death and suffering greatly from their underlying terminal condition, sunken eyes and dry skin are usually not of critical concern, even though the image evokes an emotional response since we would like to remember our loved ones looking as good as possible.

9. What about the potential for healing relationships? Patients commonly have increased alertness and clarity for their first few conscious days as they **Voluntarily Refuse Food & Fluid**, which provides the opportunity for a healing experience with their loved ones. The improvement in thinking can have several sources: reduced intake of fluid decreases swelling in the brain, increases the ability of the heart and lungs to send oxygen to the brain, and less pressure causes less distracting bodily pain. Also, the mind is free to reflect and reconsider once the patient has made a major decision that embraces "acceptance."

10. Potential pressure on the patient and increased survivors' guilt. If there is a farewell party, family members and close friends may inadvertently exert subtle performance pressure on their loved ones to ingest the pills. After all, some of them may have traveled thousands of miles to say their good-byes, based on the patient's "promise" that these would be his or her final hours of life.

In contrast, the final party is merely to enjoy a last supper, with no other expectation. **Voluntary Refusal of Food & Fluid** can begin, merely by omitting breakfast, the next morning.

The subtle (though inadvertent) pressure of being present during the more active, irreversible, and faster process of **Physician-Aided, Patient-Hastened Dying** is more likely to lead to more guilt than the alternative of witnessing **Voluntary Refusal of Food & Fluid**. In the latter, all are aware that the patient has two to ten days to change his or her mind, based on conversations with others or deep introspective thought. The time and distance between a family member or friend who says goodbye during the last dinner and when the patient finally loses consciousness, can decrease the perceived proximate cause of guilt. In contrast, waiting in the next room, knowing what is happening (ingesting a lethal dose of pills) but not doing something about it right then, can lead to more guilt later on.

Patients' physical ability to function may decline between the time of their evaluation for **Physician-Aided, Patient-Hastened Dying** and when they want to take the medication they received. That situation could put family members in an awkward and perhaps illegal position if they provide assistance so the patient can take the pills. This can happen in progressively debilitating diseases such as Lou Gehrig's disease (ALS), as illustrated in the last story in this book, "She revised her Advance Directives from 16 to 86." If family members do secretly assist, their behavior can increase their potential to feel guilty. It can also increase their anxiety over being accused of performing a criminal act.

11. Insurance, costs, and reducing suffering. There is one class of individuals for which the treatment of emerging symptoms with **Voluntary Refusal of Food & Fluid** is less available or not available at all: those who do not have health insurance. In the U.S., 45 million people do not have insurance. When these people die, not only must they suffer longer because Physician-Aided, Patient-Hastened Dying—an expedient and inexpensive way to die—is not available, but their suffering may be more extreme if they are not currently receiving adequate *Comfort Care*. (Poor people do not have the funds to pay for several home visits by a physician and for nursing care and medications to reduce their suffering. However many hospices have non-profit contributions to help the poor receive the care they deserve.)

While lay caregivers can learn how to provide adequate mouth care, they do not have the skills, training, or license to administer ***Controlled Sedation for Refractory Suffering***, which is sometimes necessary in combination with **Voluntary Refusal of Food & Fluid**.

Since **Physician-Aided, Patient-Hastened Dying** is illegal in 49 States, it is quite unfortunate that some, perhaps many, poor people who have had no access to good medical care while they lived, will also, at the end of their lives, be denied the opportunity to choose an expeditious method to die.

Recently published statistics support the contention that the richer have less pain: People over the age of 70, whose net worth was $70,000 or more, were 30 % less likely than poorer people of the same age, to have experienced pain often during their last year of life. They were also less likely to suffer from shortness of breath and depression. What proportion of patients experienced pain, and how much? More than half had pain, and of those who did, almost 6 out of 10 reported it was severe [Silveira, 2005].

12. Which methods are available for very physically ill patients?

Physician-Aided, Patient-Hastened Dying is generally available only to patients who are not too physically ill. (The novel, **Lethal Choice**, presents a high-tech method to overcome this obstacle.) In order to comply with the law, patients must be well enough to do all of the following:

A. Make three mentally competent requests for **Physician-Aided, Patient-Hastened Dying** to their physician (one must be written);

B. Request the pharmacist to dispense the medication;

C. Put the lethal dose of medication into their mouths, and

D. Swallow the medication without regurgitation.

Many terminal patients cannot perform one or more of these tasks, and if family members risk helping the patient overcome a physical limitation, they may be accused of illegally assisting suicide, of coercion, or of undue influence; for example, if the patient hesitated in making the final decision.

The next story is about an Oregonian who could not use **PAPHD** but could use **VRFF**. It probably took her a bit longer to die because she continued to enjoy her favorite flavor of sorbet.

"She could no longer swallow."

At 84, Francesca Hartman had relentless pain in her chest even though her physician prescribed morphine and cardiac medications. No longer could she enjoy walking, gardening, or playing the piano. A stroke had damaged the nerves that control swallowing. Her cardiologist could not predict how long she might live, so she could not obtain a prescription under Oregon's Death with Dignity Act. Hospice nurse, Teresa Looper, observed her to remain active, alert, communicative, and even gregarious, well into her fast [Colburn, 2005].

It may have been her conscious choice, but others reported that Francesca did sip some water and enjoyed some sorbet daily. That intake of fluids might explain why the process took about a month. Interestingly, she kept a journal that she printed, and those who have read it stated that "her determination, tinged with ambivalence, shines through." Here are a few quotes: At times she felt like a "past-due pregnant woman." At other times, she asked, "What is sustaining me? I can't go on much longer like this—useless days—useless nights.... Strange to be getting ready for bed when I don't know if I'll be getting up in the morning."

᪥ᡠᡠ᪥

13. Are these methods available for incompetent patients? While the patient is the ultimate decision-maker for both methods, with **Physician-Aided, Patient-Hastened Dying**, patients are expected to have the mental capacity to make this ultimate decision *at the very moment* they ingest the lethal dose of medication. Actually, they need to demonstrate decision-making capacity only during the fifteen days when two physicians initially evaluated their request and responded by writing a prescription. Hence, the assessment of decision-making capacity could have been performed a few months before the patient decides to ingest the pills.

In contrast, patients can empower their Proxy to **Voluntarily Refuse Food & Fluid** on their behalf years later, when they are no longer competent. In effect, their Advance Directives provide a method to create a time-shift for patients' competent wishes to be fulfilled via their Proxies.

Proponents of **Physician-Aided, Patient-Hastened Dying** argue that it is an advantage to assure patients that they are in control of the process—from the beginning to the very end—when he or she says, "I am ready. Now is the time."

Yet the requirement that patients be mentally competent to make the decision for **Physician-Aided, Patient-Hastened Dying** leaves no legal peaceful option for those patients who suffer from Alzheimer's or related dementias, or who are in the **Permanent Vegetative State** or **Minimally Conscious State**.

The time-shift potential for **Voluntary Refusal of Food & Fluid**, when combined with an effective Advance Directive allows you to enjoy as much of life as possible. You do not have to die **when you can, but when you want to**. Your Proxies can follow the specific instructions you gave them; for instance, the end-point you describe for when you want them to **Refuse Food & Fluid** on your behalf. (Examples of endpoints are given on pages 397-398 and in FORM II.)

There are many examples of tragedies where it was clear that the person who chose to die, did so prematurely. Below is a well-known example from 1990:

"How much longer might she have enjoyed life?"

Janet Adkins was 54 when she became Dr. Jack Kevorkian's first "patient" to die, although he interviewed her for less than two hours. Other doctors had given her the diagnosis of Alzheimer's disease a year earlier. Three days before she entered Kevorkian's old van and pushed a button that switched the IV from a salt water solution to compounds to make her unconscious and stop her heart, she played a full set of tennis with her son. She won the game, although her mental decline prevented her from keeping score. While she could still be physically active and connect with her son, the former English teacher could no longer read literature or play the piano. These losses could have contributed to her depression.

Tragically, she permitted Dr. Kevorkian to help end her life in an early stage of Alzheimer's while she was still capable of enjoying life. Her stated reason was fear: If she did not end her life while she still had the mental ability to do so, then she might not be able to end it in the future, and then, she would be trapped in a prolonged state of indignity. At trial, one medical expert estimated that Janet Adkins might have lived another three years before her dementia became severe.

She had been a member of the Hemlock Society prior to her diagnosis and she wrote that her decision was made "in a normal state of mind and is fully considered. I have Alzheimer's disease and I do not want to let it progress any further. I do not want to put my family or myself through the agony of this terrible disease."

At that time, Michigan had no law against assisted suicide so Kevorkian was acquitted of committing any crime.

❧

14. How many people could the methods help? Compared to about three-dozen people in Oregon who took the prescription of pills in 2004, there are currently 2 million people in the U.S. who have severe dementia; three decades from now, unless a cure is found, experts estimate there will be 5 million more.

Huge numbers of people who are not competent to make decisions may exist for very long periods of time, and their numbers will increase, unless a cure is found for such diseases as Alzheimer's.

If you have a family history of Alzheimer's disease or if you have recently been diagnosed with possible Alzheimer's, you can plan for **Voluntary Refusal of Food & Fluid** in the future, as explained in this book. That is not possible with **Physician-Aided, Patient-Hastened Dying**.

15. Physician and pharmacist involvement. A physician ***must be involved*** in **Physician-Aided, Patient-Hastened Dying** to prescribe the lethal dose of medication, but may or may not be present as the patient dies.

A physician ***should be involved*** in **Voluntary Refusal of Food & Fluid**— to provide adequate *Comfort Care*, to deal with the anxious family, and to supervise the medical treatment of any patient who changes his or her mind and wants to safely resume eating and drinking.

The Oregon law does not force any physician or pharmacist to participate in the process if they feel it is contrary to their morals, values or religious faith. Similarly, doctors are not required to provide *Comfort Care* to patients who have chosen **Voluntary Refusal of Food & Fluid**. But medical ethics and the community standard of care typically require unwilling doctors to refer the patient to another physician who is willing. While the AMA ethics guidelines generally require such referrals, the argument could be made that if a physician feels that it is morally wrong to hasten dying then it is also morally wrong to refer a patient to another provider who will hasten dying. In that event, patients will have to search for another doctor on their own.

Sometimes it is possible to convince professionals to cooperate, however, as illustrated in the following "case":

But She Had a Prescription

Standing in front of the drug counter, a lady we'll call Mrs. Smith asked her neighborhood pharmacist for some cyanide.

He shook his head and asked, "Why in the world do you need cyanide?"

"I want to poison my husband."

The pharmacist's pupils grew large. "Lord have mercy! I can't give you cyanide to kill your husband! That's against the law! I'll lose my license. They'll throw both of us in jail! Absolutely not. Under no circumstances can you have any cyanide. NO!"

Mrs. Smith then reached into her purse and pulled out a color photograph. It was a picture of a naked man in bed with another woman.

The pharmacist recognized the man as her husband, Mr. Smith.

The woman... it was the pharmacist's wife!

After gazing at the photo—first in disbelief, and then in anger, the pharmacist swallowed hard and looked at the woman waiting on the other side of the counter. He cleared his throat and said, "Well now, Mrs. Smith, why didn't you tell me? I didn't realize that you already had a prescription."

17. What are the Differences Between Voluntary Refusal of Food & Fluid and "Self-Deliverance"?

"Self-deliverance," a term coined by journalist Derek Humphry, describes a method to hasten death that, in theory, can be accomplished without direct assistance from another person (which would be illegal). Popular among members of the organization that Mr. Humphry helped found, the Hemlock Society, the method was hyped as "independent of physicians." Yet members of Hemlock admitted to visiting doctors' offices to obtain prescriptions for sedation and anxiety, which they stored in anticipation of their final event. Such medications may indeed be needed to relieve the source of the greatest anxiety any one can experience—not being able to breathe—since the cause of death is *suffocation*. The recent innovation to use inert gases reduces this anxiety, Mr. Humphry now claims, as the cause of death is *asphyxiation* (replacing oxygen with an inert gas).

(Note: After "Hemlock" changed its name to "End of Life Choices" and merged with "Compassion in Dying" to become part of "Compassion and Choices," some of its former members splintered off to form the "Final Exit Network.")

The term "Self-deliverance" was popularized through Humphry's best-selling book, *Final Exit*. Derek Humphry gave this name to a new organization that launched in September 2004, with this stated mission: "To serve people who are suffering intolerably from an incurable physical condition that has become more than they can bear." The **Final Exit Network** trains non-medical people to offer "counseling, support, and even guidance to self-deliverance." Members must supply "a doctor's medical diagnosis for our Evaluation Committee" and "attest that all relevant family members or caregivers support the member's wishes." If the committee approves the member's request, they "supply information about all methods of self-deliverance that will produce a peaceful, quick and certain death." They can also remove any tanks and hardware used so the death appears natural.

Network President Earl Wettstein said, "We can't postpone our deaths while we wait for the laws to change," and Derek Humphry stated, "Until laws protect the right of every adult to a peaceful, dignified death, **Final Exit Network** will be there to support those who need relief from their suffering today!"

The Network's approach may appeal to those who hate the idea of giving power to physicians to act as stern gate-keepers, and independent types who champion "self-deliverance" as a way of taking their "stand for freedom, independence, and self determination." They do not require members to have a terminal prognosis.

Doctors Stan Terman and Ronald Baker Miller have several concerns about the Final Exit Network's offering, even though they admit they have never observed patients die using the "new technique" of supplying Helium under the plastic bag so that dying, anecdotal reports claim, is *not* associated with great anxiety from accumulating carbon dioxide. We feel the appropriate term for this protocol is: "***Non-Physician-Aided, Patient-Hastened Dying***."   :

1. From the mission statement, we infer that the leaders of Final Exit Network do NOT explicitly inform their members that **laws need not change** in order for the patient to legally opt for **Voluntary Refusal of Food & Fluid**.

2. Since breathing Helium does not cause carbon dioxide to accumulate, proponents of this method claim that dying this way should be peaceful with no **intense anxious fears of suffocation**. Yet we have seen no proof. Inhaling this extremely light gas *might* lead to mass explosions of brain cells and cause a very short painful shock. (Data from EEG's taken during the process might reveal whether dying by Helium is peaceful.) Nitrogen has been considered in capital punishment since at least 1995 [Creque, SA], although it has the obvious disadvantage of being difficult to obtain. While Helium is easy to buy, it can also be "a probably insurmountable drawback," as Wanzer and Glenmullen point out, "if the patient were in a nursing home or other medical facility" [2007, *Page 122*].

3. It is unwise to eliminate doctors from the evaluation process. Doctors can provide much more than a diagnosis and certification that the patient's suffering is incurable and unbearable. They can offer **aggressive palliative care** that might decrease the member's symptoms. They can also assess if a member's clinical depression is greater than that expected for her situation, which would make it reasonable to first offer the member a course of anti-depressant medications, to see if his or her mood responds.

4. Another way to prevent the tragedy of members taking their lives prematurely is to encourage their **enrollment in hospice**. Even physicians encounter resistance to making such recommendations. Such a challenge would be much harder for most non-professionals to overcome, unless they had personal experience of success with hospice. Here is one critical question: how can a committee of non-medical people be certain that a member has had an adequate

trial of *Comfort Care*, if he or she has not enrolled in hospice? Yet the Network's program guide states only, "You will be encouraged to use hospice care, though this is not mandatory."

5. There is a considerable risk to accepting a member at his or her word that "all relevant family members or caregivers support the member's wishes." The motivation of some people who commit suicide is to express anger, which would have greater impact if enhanced by shock. It would be prudent for a social worker or estate attorney to verify the family's consensus.

6. Unfortunately, The Network admits that it has *nothing to offer patients in advanced dementia*. Instead, they advocate premature suicides in cases where the patients' disease will likely render them cognitively impaired in the future. Their web site uses these words: "Because the law requires that the Network must work with a mentally competent adult who is capable of providing the means for self-deliverance and carrying out the act, **a person would have to be in the early stages of dementia**. We appreciate that **there may still be quality of life left at that point** but when competence is lost, the Network would not be able to provide the information and support necessary for the member to carry out self-deliverance. **So it becomes a choice to make in the early stages and not after the disease progresses**." {Emphasis added.} [Policy of the Final Exit Network on Alzheimer's Disease and Dementia, as of 3-4-06: http://www.finalexitnetwork.org/alzheimers.htm.]

The tragically premature death of Janet Adkins, whose story was summarized in the previous **i-FAQ**, is again, the relevant example. Ignorance about **Refusal of Food & Fluid by Proxy** might lead Network members to end their lives prematurely, which would add to the tragedy.

7. It is dangerous to popularize a do-it-yourself method to commit suicide. Non-terminal, mentally ill people might use it. The Lancashire Evening Post (UK) [Nov. 2004] reported the suicide of a 19 year-old girl by the *Final Exit* method. In early 2007, Burt Bacharach and Angie Dickinson's daughter, Nikki, committed suicide at age 40. Mike Feiler of the Ventura County coroner's office was quoted as saying she died of suffocation using a plastic bag and Helium [http://www.cbsnews.com/stories/2007/01/06/ap/entertainment/mainD8MG077O0.shtml].

Dr. Philip Nitschke, who leads Exit Australia, developed a home lab method to manufacture lethal quantities of barbiturates, which he teaches to others. [The Australian, Nov. 29, 2004.] His 2006 book was banned in Australia. Barbiturates were taken off the market or tightly controlled due to the risk of either intentional or accidental suicides by overdose. Yet in a survey, Exit Australia members revealed that 89% preferred the "Peaceful Pill" to other means of "self-deliverance" and about half of the respondents indicated they would be willing to pay $1000 or more for a prescription [Eleanor Limprecht, Australian Doctor, Nov. 19, 2004]. According to *The Australian*, 120 Exit Members had illegally obtained Nembutal from Mexico ["Euthanasia advocates to flout law," June 18, 2007].

18. Could Informing Emotionally Disturbed People About Voluntary Refusal of Food & Fluid Make Their Suicide More Likely?

This possibility is unlikely for the following reasons:

First, everyone knows people can die if they stop eating and drinking so this is not "new" information. The book teaches that the process, especially for terminally ill patients, is not uncomfortable or as prolonged as might have been assumed. For healthy people, however, it can take much longer.

Second, **Voluntarily Refusing Food & Fluid** requires self-determination and persistence. Patients sometimes need support from their physician and family members to help them maintain their resolve. For non-terminally ill people who are emotionally depressed, doctors and loved ones would direct their efforts to convince the person to eat and drink.

Strictly speaking, the term "**Voluntary**" applies only to people whose judgment does not suffer from a mental illness.

Third, most suicide attempts are impulsive [Baca-Garcia and others, 2001], while **Voluntary Refusal of Food & Fluid** is slow. The extra time provides ample opportunity for individuals to change their minds. Unlike other methods of suicide attempts and suicide gestures, beginning **Voluntary Refusal of Food & Fluid** requires only missing a few meals, which—except possibly for diabetics— would cause little or no physical damage.

Fourth, many suicide attempts are done by "claimers," defined as people who want something from someone else; for example, "Don't break up with me, I still love you, and 'this act' proves it." For this purpose, **Voluntary Refusal of Food & Fluid** is too quiet, too slow, and not sufficiently dramatic to make a significant impression on, for example, an unwilling romantic partner. Commenting on prisoner hunger strikes, Brockman pointed out: "Prisoners who refuse food are motivated by the desire to achieve an end rather than killing themselves, and hunger-strike secondary to mental illness is uncommon" [1999].

Lastly, although absence of reports must always be viewed with skepticism in science, we have not heard of any depressed adult or adolescent who **Refused Food & Fluid** to commit suicide unless they also suffered from anorexia nervosa—a psychiatric disorder that must be ruled out and aggressively treated. Anorexia is a serious illness. It possibly caused Terri Schiavo's heart arrest due to dangerously low potassium levels as she was trying to lose weight. Mostly likely, it was the medical reason for how the famous singer Karen Carpenter died.

19. Can I Accomplish Voluntary Refusal of Food & Fluid Without the Help of a Physician?

The Physicians' Role

The physicians' role is to heal if possible; to care, always.

As part of a multi-disciplinary team such as the staff at hospice, physicians can provide *Comfort Care* to the dying person and support to their loved ones. They can help make sure the timing is right. They can rule out depression, be alert to whether the choice is voluntary, and provide potent medications to make the process as comfortable and as peaceful as possible.

To cite Ganzini's 2003 study again, the nurses felt that out of a total of 126 patients, families may have pressured 5 patients to resume eating and drinking, and that 4 other patients may have resumed because they felt hunger or discomfort. Therefore, if you are a patient whose current condition qualifies you to opt for **Voluntary Refusal of Food & Fluid**, select a doctor to be on your team who can deal with the potential anxiety of your family, and who can help reduce any temporary discomfort you might experience. Furthermore, you may need his or her expertise in the event you change your mind. If your choice is for some indefinite time in the future when you want a Proxy to make this choice for you, ask your Proxy to similarly select a willing physician.

People may make mistakes if they try to **Voluntarily Refuse Food & Fluid** without consulting a physician. For example, some over-the-counter pills touted as "sleep aids" cause intense dryness of the mouth and increase discomfort. A low percentage of patients have a paradoxical reaction to such drugs and become what lay people call "hyper." Drinking alcohol causes gastric discomfort and alcohol has a short half-life that often leads to rebound anxiety. Drinking also provides fluid that can lengthen the time it takes to die. Alcohol is just not a useful drug.

Physicians have the expertise to provide *Comfort Care* for a peaceful process. Sometimes specific needs can be anticipated; for example, patients who decide to stop their cardiac pacemakers or intracardiac defibrillators so as not to prolong the process of dying. For patients dependent on insulin, regular doses of insulin without ingesting food could lead to seizures yet stopping insulin abruptly could lead to diabetic ketoacidosis and becoming comatose when they would have wanted to say goodbye to someone who has not arrived. Unexpected events can also occur for which a physician is needed. Consider this analogy: Do women need a physician as a new life begins? If the fetus is in the right position in the uterus and everything goes smoothly, then an allied-professional mid-wife is adequate. But there is always some risk of complications. Similarly, if physicians who know about palliative care are available as patients make their end-of-life transitions, they can deal with both expected and unexpected contingencies.

Finally, if you do change your mind and you want to postpone the process of dying, a physician, by virtue of his or her specific professional training and experience, is best equipped to attempt to handle your request.

20. What Legal Authorities Have Established That Voluntary Refusal of Food & Fluid is Legal?

The Landmark Case of Nancy Cruzan

The first U.S. Supreme Court case to discuss the right to refuse life-sustaining medical treatment, including medically administered Food & Fluid for a patient in a Permanent Vegetative State (**PVS**), was Cruzan v. Director, Missouri Department of Health (1990) 497 US 261.

Nancy Beth Cruzan was 30 years old when her car overturned and her brain was deprived of oxygen for about 13 minutes. Her three-week coma became a vegetative state, which became permanent. She had not completed an Advance Directive. Her parents hoped their daughter would recover, but when it became certain that she never would, and that her implanted gastrostromy feeding tube could sustain her biologic existence for decades, her parents petitioned to remove her feeding tube. Donald Lamkins, the hospital administrator took the Cruzans' official letter to an attorney in the Missouri Department of Health. His answer was "No. Starving someone to death," he said, "was beyond our ability to think, even, at this point, in Missouri."

At the initial trial in conservative Southwest Missouri, Jasper County Probate Court Judge Charles Teel, Jr., determined that Nancy's "best interests" were to remove her feeding tube since it was providing no discernible benefit. The judge granted Nancy's parents permission to withdraw the tube. Nancy's independent Guardian Ad Litem agreed with the decision, but he felt it was his legal duty to ask a higher court to review the case.

The Missouri Supreme Court overturned the lower court's decision and refused to permit Nancy's parents the authority as her guardians to remove the feeding tube. The State of Missouri had a law that prohibited Proxies from making "Quality-of-Life" judgments; its "Living Will" law favored preservation of "life"; and there was no law that specifically permitted rejecting nutrition and hydration on behalf of an incompetent person.

The parents appealed to the U.S. Supreme Court, which accepted the case. (The Court accepts fewer than one in 50 appeals.) By the time her case reached the U.S. Supreme Court, Nancy Beth Cruzan had been unconscious for seven years. Briefly (see more details below), the nation's highest Court ruled that the Cruzans had no Constitutional right to remove their daughter's feeding tube, but that States have the right to insist on whatever level of evidence they decided on, including *clear and convincing*, as proof of what the patient would have wanted (for example, statements the patient made when competent). So the parents' and Nancy's rights were outweighed by the State's interest in the preservation and protection of human life, and the State's duty to guard against potential abuse. But the Court left open the possibility of a retrial based on new evidence since it considered tube feeding to be a medical treatment.

Publicity from the case brought forward three new witnesses whose testimony was considered *clear and convincing*. After six more months of litigation, the Missouri court finally permitted Nancy Beth Cruzan's parents to transfer her to the hospice part of the State hospital. There, the staff was willing to remove her feeding tube. Twelve days later, she died peacefully.

Her father, Joe Cruzan stated that it had been 1206 days since the initial written request to the Missouri Rehabilitation Center. Prior to Nancy's death, a group of protestors announced they wanted to storm the hospice and to chain themselves to Nancy's bed. They made such statements as, "I am Commanded by Scripture to give a friend a cup of water," and "Shake up Satan's kingdom, today, Lord." [WGBH, 1992. See Frontline, 1992, for a contemporaneous view.]

At Nancy's eulogy, attorney William Colby said that after nearly eight "torturous years... of 'winning' the right to allow [his] child to die... [Joe Cruzan] counted the final authorization to set his daughter free from her medical prison as both his greatest and saddest accomplishment in life" [Webb, 1997].

At his daughter's burial service, Joe Cruzan read this tribute:

> "Today, as the protestor's sign says, we give Nancy the gift of death. An unconditional gift of love that sets her free from this twisted body that no longer serves her. A gift I know she will treasure above all others, the gift of freedom. So run free Nan, we will catch up later."

Sadly, the enormous emotional toll of this ordeal did not end with the death of Nancy Beth Cruzan. Critics continued to beat down the family, adding to the stress of their great loss and the intense five-year legal battle that had exhausted their emotions. On August 17, 1996, around 3:00 AM, after he wrote a note indicating how much he loved and still wanted to protect his family, Joe Cruzan "walked out to his carport, set his five-foot wooden stepladder directly under the main support beam and tied a noose to it. He sealed a strip of duct tape tight across his mouth and taped his arms behind his back. Then he stepped up onto the ladder, threaded his head through the noose, and hung himself." [Colby, 2002.]

᎒᎒

Legal Implications of the U.S. Supreme Court's 1990 Decision

In the first right-to-die case ever considered by the U.S. Supreme Court, a 5-4 majority ruled that an *incompetent* person's right to reject life-support was NOT a fundamental Constitutional right, even though *competent* people have this Constitutional right. Since Nancy Cruzan was NOT competent, she had to rely on Proxies whose decision-making, they reasoned, has *potential flaws*: a Proxy's perceptions of the patient and her medical situation can be skewed due to lack of detailed knowledge of the patient's feelings and attitudes toward ending life, misunderstanding of the patient's medical condition and the medical resources for treating it, and by personal prejudice or motives such as expecting an inheritance.

᎒*SKIP*

While none of these potential flaws were considered specifically (that is, if they applied to Nancy Cruzan), the majority of Justices concluded in general that the parents' refusal of life support on behalf of Nancy was only a "Liberty Interest," not a fundamental right, which must therefore be weighed along with the State's right and duty to protect all human life; therefore a State, in this case, Missouri, could require the high standard of proof called *clear and convincing* evidence.

The burden of such a high level of proof would NOT apply to a competent ill person, however. Since the 1914 ruling about unwanted surgery by Judge Benjamin A. Cardozo in Schloendorff v. Society of New York Hospital, it had been established that every human being has an absolute right to determine what shall be done with his body. By accepting this and other earlier State court rulings, the U.S. Supreme Court held, in the Cruzan case, that providing artificially administered Food & Fluid did qualify as "medical treatment."

William Colby, the attorney for the parents of Nancy Cruzan, argued why Nancy should have the same right to reject life support as any competent person. He cited landmark State court decisions affirming the equality of rights between competent and incompetent persons. The U.S. Supreme Court justified its decision for the higher standard for evidence since discontinuation of nutrition and hydration would result in death. This higher standard for evidence would: A) provide a greater margin of safety against error in case some new advance in medical treatment might be discovered; B) if other, more convincing evidence of the patient's true end-of-life wishes might be unearthed; C) if laws on end-of-life decisions changed; or D) if by simply delaying, the patient died.

In addition to considering potential Proxy abuse, the U.S. Supreme Court ruled that States are permitted to prohibit judgments about "Quality-of-Life" when the decision to refuse nutrition and hydration for an incompetent patient is pending.

℘ CONTINUE

Justice Sandra Day O'Connor voted with the majority, however she added her separate written opinion. Referring to competent individuals, Justice O'Connor wrote, "The Liberty guaranteed by the Due Process Clause must protect... an individual's deeply personal decision to reject medical treatment, including the artificial delivery of food and water," which cannot be distinguished from other forms of medical treatment. Furthermore, she cited medical authorities on the degree of intrusion: sometimes "forcible restraint" of a patient's hands is necessary to stop interference with placement of a nasogastric tube.

Comment: This statement of Justice O'Connor's is quite important. There is a continuum of intrusiveness for interventions that provide sustenance. At one extreme is the surgical implantation of a feeding tube, which requires informed consent, is not likely to apply to an incompetent patient.) Next is the degree of forcible intrusion to which Justice O'Connor referred, to place an NG tube. While that procedure *should require* formal consent by a Proxy if the patient is not competent, in practice, patients who are not able to express themselves might have their doctors insert such tubes—despite their behavioral resistance, which is passed off as "not understanding what is in their 'best interest.'" Justice O'Connor's statement is consistent with our clinical experience: Instead of heeding such indications of refusal, health care providers restrain their patients' hands—not only during the placement of the NG tube, but *also* worse thereafter—to prevent them from pulling out these tubes. Next on the continuum would be forced spoon-feeding. (See the description in the story, "Poor Mom had to endure forced feeding" [page 235].) While assisted feeding is generally not as uncomfortable as inserting an NG tube, a patient who is terribly confused may find the procedure extremely intrusive. The significance of Justice O'Connor considering "medical intrusion" as not limited to surgical insertions is this: some day forced feeding by spoon may also be considered a serious intrusion on patients' right to privacy.

By writing that the majority opinion was narrowly focused on one State's laws that affected the burden of proof, rather than on the more general rights of a dying person, Justice O'Connor left the door open to protect such rights in the future: "Today's decision ... does not preclude a future determination that the Constitution requires the States to implement the decisions of a patient's duly appointed [Proxy]. Nor does it prevent States from developing other approaches for protecting an incompetent individual's Liberty Interest in refusing medical treatment."

❧ *SKIP*

Justice Stevens' Dissenting Opinion noted that Nancy Cruzan's parents had no conflicting interests that were adverse to Nancy's. He emphasized the undisputed medical facts: Nancy's cognitive ability was zero, she could not swallow food or water, and she would never recover from her cerebral atrophy. For Stevens, these specific undisputed medical facts were themselves *clear and convincing*, so he concluded that she had the fundamental right to refuse treatment.

Justice Stevens criticized the Rehnquist majority ruling on several levels: A) He saw the ruling as "an effort to define life, rather than protect it… " Missouri's policy "equate[s] [Cruzan's] life with the biological persistence of her bodily functions." He termed this an "aberrant" version of 'life.'" B) Requiring "life" to be continued indefinitely "impose[s] on dying individuals and their families a controversial and objectionable view of life's meaning." C) The ruling was discriminatory since "an innocent person's Constitutional right to be free from unwanted medical treatment is thereby categorically limited to those patients who had the foresight to make an unambiguous statement of their wishes while competent." And D) The ruling implies a permanent "waiver" of all incompetent patients' Constitutional rights. Due to Nancy's lack of "foresight to preserve her Constitutional right in a living will… or… comparable *clear and convincing* alternative, her right is gone forever, and her fate is in the hands of the State legislature instead of… her family, her independent neutral Guardian Ad Litem, and an impartial judge—all of whom agree on the… action that is in her best interests."

Justice Stevens wrote that Missouri's objection to Nancy's choice as expressed by her parents "subordinates Nancy's body, her family, and the lasting significance of her life to the State's own interests," and interferes "with Constitutional interests of the highest order." He clarified the wish to permit dying: "The right to be free from unwanted life-sustaining treatment… presupposes no abandonment of the desire for life… Rather, it expands the freedom of persons and their families to include the unique facts of a persons' history in finding meaning at the end of life."

Justice Stevens also considered how to define the word "life." He admitted that Nancy was "alive in the physiological sense. But… [with] no consciousness and no chance of recovery, there is a serious question… whether the mere persistence of [her body] is 'life' as that word is commonly understood [and]… used in … the Constitution and the Declaration of Independence." He wrote that Missouri's prohibition against defining "Quality-of-Life" has the effect of usurping the definition from all to whom it is meaningful—the dying persons and their loved ones. He noted that Nancy Cruzan's life could be defined by "reference to her own interests, so that her life expired when her biological existence ceased serving any of her own interests."

In terms of accepting the parents' interpretation of what Nancy wanted, Justice Stevens wrote: "... [C]hoices about life and death are profound ones, not susceptible of resolution by recourse to medical or legal rules... . [T]he best we can do is to ensure that these choices are made by those who will care enough about the patient to investigate her interests with particularity and caution."

 CONTINUE

Justice Stevens concluded that the Rehnquist majority went overboard to avoid all possible errors by Proxies, and that, in turn led to an ironic result: "Chronically incompetent persons" have no Constitutionally recognizable interests at all, so they have thus lost the status of being "persons" under the Constitution. Finally, he noted that Missouri spent several hundred thousand dollars on Nancy Cruzan to vindicate this State policy, an expense inconsistent with Cruzan's own interests.

Marcia Angell, M.D., then Editor-in-Chief of the New England Journal of Medicine, wrote: "For the court to... require detailed advance instructions for stopping tube feeding but not for continuing it, is to be out of touch with the widespread recognition that it is cruel and senseless to keep comatose people alive indefinitely. To see the court's decision as erring on the side of life is not to understand fully that for such patients, life in any meaningful sense is already over" [Angell, 1990].

SKIP

What is Meant by "Clear and Convincing" Evidence?

The legal standard of *clear and convincing* is higher than the standard required for most civil disputes, which is "more likely than not," also termed "a preponderance of the evidence," or more than 50%. The highest standard is "beyond a reasonable doubt" in criminal prosecutions, which is required for capital punishment. Lawmakers and judges do not give percentages for *clear and convincing*, so we must rely on the words used by judges, which may vary from court to court.

The ruling in the California Supreme Court case of Robert Wendland provides this rather strict definition of *clear and convincing*:

"The *clear and convincing* evidence standard of proof requires a finding of high probability, based on evidence so clear as to leave **no** substantial doubt and sufficiently strong to command the ***unhesitating*** assent of every reasonable mind." {Emphasis added.}

None of the following critical terms were defined: "high probability," "no substantial doubt," or "sufficiently strong." Although vague, the "high probability" part of this qualitative definition would seem to fit the level of proof as somewhere between "a preponderance of the evidence" and "beyond a reasonable doubt." Yet the phrase "to leave ***no*** substantial doubt" may place the *clear and convincing* standard even higher than "***BEYOND*** a reasonable doubt"—if "**no**" is interpreted as more absolute than "beyond." It is thus difficult to know if the judges intended to make *clear and convincing* the highest standard of all.

In the definition, "sufficiently strong" requires the command of ***unhesitating assent***. The word, "**hesitate**," is also important in the definition of "*reasonable doubt*," which the Merriam Webster Dictionary cited, from Texas penal code, as: "*Often defined judicially as such doubt as would cause a reasonable person to hesitate before acting in a matter of importance.*"

I must ask, shouldn't matters of importance be deliberated for a while? Don't judges give themselves time between hearing the evidence and ruling? Don't juries deliberate for days or weeks on complicated cases? Wouldn't all of us want our future decision-makers to deliberate for a while on matters as important as our life or death? In a word, weighing evidence takes **time**. Hence, the criterion of "unhesitating assent" seems unreasonable as a requirement for a higher standard of evidence.

As a comparison, medical scientists often accept hypotheses as proved when the probability or "p" value is less than 0.05. Roughly, this means that less than one time in twenty would chance alone lead experimenters to the wrong results on which to base their conclusion. Although there is no direct mathematical connection, it is reasonable to assume that when medical scientists testify in court that their opinions are "within a reasonable degree of medical certainty," they intend to state that the event has a probability of being correct of at least 19 out of 20, or 95%.

According to attorney William Colby, who argued before the U.S. Supreme Court, *clear and convincing* evidence "boiled down to the perception of the individual judge. The evidence had to persuade him, to leave a fixed conclusion in his mind." According to attorney Lawrence Nelson, who argued before the California Supreme Court, this Court's definition of *clear and convincing* seemed excessively high.

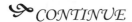 *CONTINUE*

Legal Implications of the U.S. Supreme Court's 1997 Decision

In 1997, the U.S. Supreme Court ruled that there was no Constitutional right to insist on physician-assisted suicide after hearing appeals on these two cases: Vacco v. Quill, 521 U.S. 793, 798, and Washington v. Glucksberg, 521 U.S. 702. The court noted that Terminal Sedation is another way to reduce end-of-life suffering, however it specifically permitted individual States to continue "to experiment" with Physician-Assisted Suicide. The Court did not change its prior position that Food & Fluid artificially administered through tubes is medical "treatment," which all competent adults have the right to refuse.

Legal Implications of the U.S. Supreme Court's 2006 Decision

The ruling focused on one issue: Did the Federal Controlled Substances Act of 1970 explicitly state that prescribing these medications for assistance in "suicide" was *not* a "legitimate medical purpose" or should the issue of how to practice medicine be left to individual States to oversee? The 6 to 3 vote in Gonzales v. Oregon, ruled that the Controlled Substances Act was narrowly designed to prevent the illegal transporting and selling of addictive drugs. Many disappointed conservatives responded by saying they would increase their energy to pass new laws on the State level. Pro-life attorney Tom Marzen told LifeNews.com that Congress should pass "an amendment [to the Controlled Substances Act] that specifically states that assistance in suicide in not a 'legitimate medical purpose.'" This LifeNews.com editorial concluded, "Congress should Constitutionally amend the Federal Controlled Substances Act so that the statute says explicitly what the Bush Administration had believed it said implicitly" [2006]. As discussed later in the context of the President's Council on Bioethics' report, "Taking Care," the National Right to Life Committee proposed "Model Law" insists that every severely demented or barely conscious person has decided by default to receive life-sustaining treatment, even though the more apt term would be *existence-prolonging treatment*—unless there is *clear and convincing* **written** documentation to the contrary. Appealing to the rights of *disabled persons* and the emotionally charged issue of *discrimination*, conservatives may attempt to attack **Physician-Assisted Suicide** and **Refusal of Food & Fluid by Proxy** since it would be harder to attack **Voluntary Refusal of Food & Fluid**.

Current Legal Status of Voluntary Refusal of Food & Fluid

One opponent of **Voluntary Refusal of Food & Fluid**, attorney Wesley J. Smith [2003] wrote, "as a practical matter, all fifty States now permit profoundly cognitively disabled people to be dehydrated to death by withholding or withdrawing tube-supplied nutrition and hydration, as long as their families consent." He argued, "artificial nutrition and hydration [should be] recognized as a unique category of care to be governed by its own rules" [2006]. Neurologists could argue with the gross understatement of the term, "profoundly cognitively disabled," since patients in a Permanent Vegetative State have no awareness.

It is true that individual States have passed laws to impede the right to refuse *Artificial Nutrition and Hydration*. "Twenty States have explicit statutes that require... a higher evidentiary standard, specific preauthorization, or qualifying medical conditions, second medical opinions, or judicial reviews. Some States have laws that do not permit refusal if death would result from 'starvation' or 'dehydration.'" [Sieger and others, 2002] "In eight other States, statutory law contains language that could be misinterpreted, implying, but not rising to, an explicitly higher standard. Four appellate decisions departed from the judicial consensus that *Artificial Nutrition and Hydration* can be refused like other [medical] treatments." As of March 2006, twenty-three states are considering adopting laws similar to the National Right to Life Committee's model proposal.

The effects of these restrictive laws and higher standards for evidence are A) to make it more difficult for Proxies to refuse *Artificial Nutrition and Hydration* on behalf of patients who lack mental capacity, and B) to evoke fear and caution in health care providers when an issue involving **Voluntary Refusal of Food & Fluid** arises. Note the example of Ohio, cited below:

The Restrictive Provisions of Ohio's Proxy Directive

Background: Respecting the dignity of incompetent patients should include granting them the right to refuse medical treatment just as that right is granted to competent patients. What's the difference? Only that they must express this right via a Proxy.

Ohio's Durable Power of Attorney for Health Care Proxy Directive (**Proxy Directive**) is unusual. It states your (Proxy) "attorney in fact NEVER will be authorized to do any of the following: ...(3) Refuse or withdraw informed consent to the provision of artificially or technologically administered sustenance (nutrition) or fluids (hydration) to you, unless: (a) YOU ARE IN A TERMINAL CONDITION OR IN A PERMANENTLY UNCONSCIOUS STATE. (b) YOUR ATTENDING

PHYSICIAN AND AT LEAST ONE OTHER PHYSICIAN WHO HAS EXAMINED YOU DETERMINE, TO A REASONABLE DEGREE OF MEDICAL CERTAINTY AND IN ACCORDANCE WITH REASONABLE MEDICAL STANDARDS, THAT NUTRITION OR HYDRATION WILL NOT OR NO LONGER WILL SERVE TO PROVIDE COMFORT TO YOU OR ALLEVIATE YOUR PAIN…"   {Upper case letters as in the original.}

This restrictive provision effectively changes how you can legally express your wishes about refusing artificially administered Food & Fluid. It transforms a **Proxy Directive** into a **Directive to Physician**.

Refusing oral intake for patients who must be physically restrained as they are force-fed may incite even more opposition than refusing Artificial Nutrition and Hydration by tubes.

Note: Courts of law become involved *only* if there is conflict among members of a family, or if the State decides to become involved (as in the case of Nancy Cruzan, who resided in a State hospital). Family members may find a responsible doctor to discuss these issues in private, consider what they know about the wishes and values of the patient, or base their decision on the "Best Interest" standard, defined as what a reasonable person would want in a similar situation. Decisions to withdraw life-support are made without further review thousands of times every day across the country.

The question remains, should patients who lack decision-making capacity, who have no surrogates, and who left no Advance Directives be kept alive indefinitely? The Southern California Bioethics Committee Consortium [2005] agreed on these guidelines: The physician presents the options to a special committee or a subcommittee of an ethics committee, just as a doctor would provide this same information to a surrogate. Opinions of all concerned about or interested in the case would be aired. In cases of conflict, the entire ethics committee would become involved. If the conflict is still not resolved, then the committee would ask for a judicial review as a last resort.

One must still worry about conflicts that cannot be resolved, where litigation may reach the appellate courts whose decisions have potential to set precedent. Then, highly polarized groups from both sides may join in, to further their political or religious agendas. Meanwhile, the ordeal can last for years as it drains the emotions of the family, sometimes catastrophically. And during this whole time, **To Delay** is **To Deny** the honoring of the patient's Last Wishes.

To avoid the possibility of such prolonged conflicts—for yourself and your family—carefully scrutinize the statutory forms provided by your State with your clinical and legal advisors. As examples illustrate throughout this book, even the exact words codified by your State law in their recommended forms may not be effective to honor your specific wishes. Forms downloaded from the Internet or received by mail may be a good starting point, but they should be considered only an introduction to the underlying complex issues, rather than sufficient to fulfill their primary function: to have others promptly honor your wishes. (Later in this book, the popular **Five Wishes** form is used as a detailed example.)

If you want to be sure that others will honor your Last Wishes, accomplish these three tasks:

Three Tasks to Ensure That Others Will Honor Your Last Wishes

1. Reduce the possibility of your competency becoming an issue by asking a physician, a psychiatrist, or a psychologist, to document that you did possess the mental capacity to make medical decisions near the time you created your **Advance Directive**;

2. Diligently prepare a strategically crafted Advance Directive that states your end-of-life choices in such a way that others must consider them *clear and convincing*, and that authorizes your Proxies maximal power (if you trust them) to advocate your wishes.

3. Select individuals to serve as your Proxies whom you trust to advocate effectively the Last Wishes you discuss with them. Designate them in a sequence so that if one does not serve, the next alternate will, and if you are not sure your Proxies will be available or able, consider designating an end-of-life professional who works with a team to serve as your advocate. (Note: Most States do not allow you to designate your personal physician.)

The case below illustrates how the laws of a State can frustrate the intent of a legally designated and well-intentioned Proxy, and may not serve to honor the actual wishes that the patient expressed when she was competent.

Judge Rules Patient "Not Terminal" Based on Jewish Text

In 1998, Lee Kahan designated her daughter to be her Proxy—but she did not clearly and convincingly state in her Living Will that she wanted her daughter to withhold a feeding tube if she was in end-stage dementia. This is basically all she said:

"I, Lee Kahan hereby appoint Joan Simonson [daughter] as my health care agent to make **any and all health care decisions for me, except to the extent that I state otherwise**.

"I direct my Proxy to make health care decisions in accord with my wishes and limitations as stated below, or as he or she otherwise knows. **If there is any hope of recovery, I want my agent to ask for life sustaining treatment**."

The bold emphasis was added above because Mrs. Kahan did NOT state otherwise; and she had NO HOPE OF RECOVERY.

In many States, these simple sentences would have sufficed to empower her daughter to refuse tube feeding, however the "New York State Health Care Proxy Form" includes this additional paragraph:

"**Unless your agent reasonably knows your wishes about artificial nutrition and hydration (nourishment and water provided by a feeding tube or intravenous line), he or she will not be allowed to refuse or consent to those measures for you.**"

In Borenstein v. Simonson, the 2005 New York court ruled that the agent/daughter "is without authority to make decisions about artificial nutrition and hydration for her mother."

The patient's sister asked the judge to consider what was in the patient's BEST INTEREST given her previous increasing observance of Orthodox Judaism. She argued that, according to Jewish law, neither end-stage dementia nor PVS are terminal illnesses; therefore, life-sustaining treatment is required. Two additional doctors testified that a surgical percutaneous gastric tube (PEG) was necessary to avoid complications that are more common with nasal gastric tubes. The daughter then consented to the PEG.

The patient's sister asked the judge also to remove the patient's daughter as her mother's agent. After a review of the conflicting interpretations of traditional Jewish law, however, the judge denied that request and ruled that the daughter's behavior was NOT in "bad faith."

৵৹৵

Was it appropriate for the judge to rely on a religious document to establish a medical opinion?

The law in New York State requires honoring patient's religious preferences so it was appropriate for the judge to consider Jewish law (*Halakhah*). In terms of separation of church and state, this is not a violation since personal preferences about end-of-life decisions are influenced by one's religious beliefs, and they should be respected. Although the judge spoke to three doctors, it seems that he asked none for their opinion if Ms. Kahan's condition was terminal. Instead, it appears that the judge accepted Jewish law that states end-stage dementia is NOT terminal.

Had the daughter hired a medical expert, a skilled attorney might have argued that Lee Kahan's written intent was to receive life-sustaining treatment ONLY if she had some realistic "hope of recovery," and that she had none with end-stage dementia. Furthermore, many observant orthodox Jews feel that prolonging life beyond what would be natural is not required and according to Jewish law can be considered against God's will.

This case illustrates three points according to attorney Michael Evans: 1) The outcome of a legal case depends on expert testimony and attorney's skill. 2) Citing a person's religious affiliation can be a poor substitute for personal knowledge of her real wishes and can lead to a wrong decision. 3) Judges are reluctant to risk error where "life" is involved and may opt for continued sustenance even when there is no possibility of benefit and there is inevitable further burden and suffering.

In fact, dementia is clinically considered a terminal illness based on the statistical probability that the patient will not be alive in a specific number of months, even though the patient does not strictly die of "dementia." The usual cause of death is an infection; however doctors cannot predict which infected organ system will lead to death [Meier and others, 2001].

This case also is consistent with the usual legal presumption that a person is considered competent unless someone contests it AT THAT TIME. (This is in form, similar to being considered innocent until proven guilty.) Although the patient's sister asked the judge to rule that the patient was already incompetent when she signed the Advance Directive in 1998, the judge ruled that he had to assume she was competent in 1998, since no one questioned the patient's competence at that previous time.

The State of New York could be considered "a leader" in requiring additional specific instructions to empower a **Proxy to Withdraw Food & Fluid**. In that sense, the State seems ahead of implementing the model law proposed by the National Right to Life Committee—the "Starvation and Dehydration of Persons with Disabilities Prevention Act." Yet other States may invoke similar laws retroactively. This possibility brings to mind a story whose moral makes up for its "dry humor":

I Wish He Had Told Me. . .

Lost in the Sahara Desert, a traveler worried whether he could survive as he had run out of water earlier that day. He hoped he'd find water at the next outpost of civilization, but didn't know where that was. He walked on and on, to the point where he felt faint and had to crawl. His hope rose when he eventually noticed a tent.

When he reached the tent he called out dryly, "Water, please—"

A man dressed in a white robe and turban opened the flap of the tent and looked down. "I am so sorry, sir. Here we have no water. But may I ask, would you like to buy a tie? I have a nice selection, starting at only $15 each." He pointed to a display of silk ties, inside.

"You fool! Can't you see I'm desperate for water?"

"I see. There is a tent one mile from here. They have water."

The traveler rested in the shade a while to summon his energy to drag his parched body to the other tent. When he reached it, he practically collapsed in front of its door.

A man came out dressed in a western-style suit.

The traveler asked him, "Please, may I come in? I need water—"

The man shook his head. "I'm sorry, sir. No one is allowed inside without a tie!"

Similarly, when it comes to honoring your end-of-life wishes, it is possible that newly passed laws, especially those pertaining to the highly charged area of **Refusing Food & Fluid by Proxy**, will be applied retroactively. The moral of these stories...

Buy your silk tie now!

Of course, New York State did warn Lee Kahan to grant her Proxy the power to make decisions about **Refusing Food & Fluid**, through the instructions included in the Advance Directive forms that New York State provides. Regardless of your State's current position, however, do not be nonchalant. Instead...

Authorize and Empower Now!

Specifically authorize and fully empower your **Proxy to Voluntarily Refuse Food & Fluid** on your behalf, if that is your wish. If you can trust your Proxies, include the statement that their current decision overrides how others interpret your other writings or statements.

Attach a document that you call "**Empowering Statements for My Proxy**" to your Proxy Directive that expresses your wishes in such a way that others will consider them *clear and convincing*. Include examples in this document that illustrate your preferences.

What you put in writing on paper should reflect your more detailed deeper discussions with those who will share the process of making the ultimate decisions (your Proxy and your physician), and those who will be most affected: the people who love you.

Chapter 8

Questions on Competency, on Brain Function, and on Alzheimer's Disease and Related Dementias

---

The Most Difficult Lines We Will Ever Have to Draw

. . . are the lines that reflect our judgment about whether there is, or there is not, sufficient mental ability:

To create and to revise one's Advance Directives;

To maintain adequate nutritional intake by knowing how to eat and drink without the need for assisted spoon-feeding; and

To retain those human qualities and unique aspects of personality beyond mere biologic existence in a body whose physical characteristics look familiar.

---

21. How are Competency and Decision-Making Capacity Determined?

Competence is a legal ruling—usually by judge, but sometimes by a jury—regarding whether or not a person possesses the mental ability to make certain kinds of decisions. **Decision-making capacity** is a clinical opinion formed by a physician who may be a psychiatrist or forensic psychologist. Such professionals may be asked to provide expert testimony to express their opinions about **decision-making capacity** to help the court rule on **competence**. Courts hear such cases only when an "interested party" raises the question and there is a conflict of opinions. In the absence of a court review, the opinions of clinicians regarding decision-making capacity are usually final.

Decision-making capacity can vary depending the time of day and the length of time since the last administration of certain medications. Of great importance is that decision-making capacity is specific to the complexity of a given subject. Each area of decision-making must be independently evaluated. For example, some people do not possess enough mental ability to complete a Living Will because they do not have the ability to describe the precise level of functioning, prognosis, and suffering at which point they would want specific medical treatment discontinued. Yet these same individuals may still possess sufficient mental ability to sequence the order of whom, among their close relatives and friends, they trust to designate as their Proxies and alternates, to make medical decisions on their behalf.

Typically it is your primary treating physician who will determine when it is necessary to evaluate your decision-making capacity, as this story illustrates:

When Should Doctors Test Mental Ability?

When I was still training to be a psychiatrist, my young colleague asked our professor how to know when we should assess decision-making capacity, especially in patients who appeared normal.

The professor answered, "Start by asking a simple question that everyone should be able to answer without any problem."

My colleague requested an example.

The professor nodded. "Captain Cook made three trips around the world. He died during one of them. Which one?" He stared hard at my colleague as he asked, "Can **you** answer that?"

My colleague hesitated, fidgeted, and then explained, "I must confess that I don't know much about history. Do you have another example?"

You can request a professional to evaluate your decision-making capacity at any time. Your Proxy's decision to **Voluntarily Refuse Food & Fluid** on your behalf, however, could spark the challenge of religious leaders and politicians since it affects life and death. Although in most States the burden of proving mental incompetence is upon the petitioner, a well-documented evaluation of your capacity to make decisions near the time you signed your Advance Directive is prudent. Such a document may completely discourage challenges or reduce their potential impact. If you are in the early stages of a disease that causes progressive dementia, it is important for the interview to determine that your decision is not a result of your being depressed over your recent diagnosis. Ideally, the interview would establish that your current decision is consistent with the life-long values you held prior to your diagnosis, and are consistent over two or three interviews.

The method to evaluate decision-making capacity is applied to **Voluntarily Refusing Food & Fluid**. Some patients may not require such a comprehensive evaluation if it is obvious they are not aware that they have a choice, or if they cannot express any choices consistently. As a safeguard for patients who seem able to make medical decisions, however, a psychiatric evaluation can help rule-out the impact of depression, the presence of anorexia nervosa, and the motivation of not wanting to be a burden to others, if that is inappropriate.

 SKIP

How Clinicians Determine Decision-Making Capacity

The clinician tests mental ability in four ways, to see if you are able to...

Understand the risks and benefits of your choice. In the case of **Voluntary Refusal of Food & Fluid** there are two treatment options: One is <u>to refuse</u> Food & Fluid; the other is <u>to continue to receive</u> Food & Fluid.

Appreciate the probable consequences of each treatment option as it applies to your life and the people close to you. In the case of **Voluntarily Refusing Food & Fluid**, you would die sooner and your loved ones would miss you longer... *however* you might prefer that they remember you as you were before you became sicker, more dependent, or lost control of your bodily functions.

Reason logically, by comparing the probable consequences of each of your options. Your reason to **Refuse Food & Fluid** might be because you prefer to reduce how long you will suffer, how much more dependent you may become, what further indignities you might suffer, and the way you want the assets in your estate to be spent—compared to the value of existing longer.

Express a consistent choice that follows from the above reasoning. Over a period of time, whether you are having a good day or a bad day—when a variety of people ask you in a variety of ways, you consistently state that you want to exercise the option of **Voluntary Refusal of Food & Fluid**.

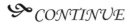 *CONTINUE*

If you have been given a diagnosis that affects the functioning of your mind, it does not necessarily mean you lack decision-making capacity. For example, a person in the early stage of Alzheimer's disease who has also been given the diagnosis of lung cancer might authentically decide not to undergo either surgery or chemotherapy. What is critical is that people can remember the key facts long enough to demonstrate their understanding and appreciation, apply logical reasoning, and then consistently express their choice.

While the woman's choice was consistent in the "example" below, her ability to understand and to appreciate were questionable:

At Least Her Decision Was Consistent

Two elderly people lived in a retirement home. They lived independently. Both had lost their spouses. By now, they had known each other for several years.

One evening, at a community supper, they sat across from one another. When the fruit cup was served, the man glanced at his dinner partner with admiration. While they ate chicken Parmesan he gave her a big grin and said, "You look pretty tonight." And as they finished their chocolate pudding, he took a deep breath, gathered up his courage, leaned over the table, and asked, "Will you marry me?"

Feeling flattered, she smiled. After about ten seconds of silence, she answered, "Yes! Yes, I will."

The meal ended with broad smiles. After they rose from the table, they embraced with a gentle hug. Then they returned to their rooms.

The next morning, however, he felt troubled. "Did she say 'Yes' or did she say 'No'?" He couldn't remember. He tried, but just could not recall. Not even a faint memory. With trepidation, he looked up her name in the telephone directory and pushed the button to dial her phone number. She answered right away.

First, he remarked what a lovely evening they had last night. Then he explained that he didn't remember as well as he used to. Finally, he inquired, "When I asked if you would marry me, did you say 'Yes' or did you say 'No'?"

He was delighted to hear her response. "Why, I said, 'Yes! Yes. I will.' And I meant it with all my heart."

But then she continued, "And I am so glad that you called this morning, because I too have a memory problem. You see, I couldn't remember who had asked me."

So, even if you have a problem with memory or mood, you may still retain decision-making capacity. Your reasoning must be consistent for the decision to be judged sound, however it need not conform to society's majority opinion. You can base the reasons for your choice on values that only a minority of people holds. To take the humorous story above seriously, the gentleman might wonder if the woman's reasoning revealed she was more interested in marriage in general than in him specifically, but he still might want to marry her, if he felt lonely.

22. What Special Considerations Apply to Alzheimer's Disease and Other Irreversible and Progressive Dementias?

Alzheimer's disease and related dementias pose enormous problems—for patients, for family members, and for all of society. The strategies to deal with these diseases are thus important for all to consider. Alzheimer's disease is similar to cancer in one critical way: the issue of *time urgency*. Everyone knows how important it is to diagnose cancer early for the greatest chance of survival. While dementia cannot be cured, the earlier treatment begins, the slower symptoms may progress with treatment. Yet the end-stage of dementia is just emerging from the closet, as the brief descriptions of a series of movies below illustrate. No one wants to face bad news unless there is hope by doing so. Instead, our natural tendency is to invoke the psychological defense mechanism of **denial**. For hopeless situations, denial may be reasonable. Until recently, Alzheimer's was hopeless. Here are two compelling reasons to act now—if you, or a family member, are facing a recent diagnosis of dementia:

Compelling reason number one: The medications that may slow the progression of symptoms may also delay the onset of initial symptoms. Yet in 2003, only one out of ten Alzheimer's patients was being treated with a cholinesterase inhibitor. Details regarding these medications are beyond the scope of this book, but research in this field is advancing rapidly so consult your neurologist or internist. **Remember: the earlier you start treatment with these medications, the more effective they may be**.

Compelling reason number two: Patients in the early stages of the disease must write their **Advance Directives** BEFORE they lose the ability to make medical decisions. The harsh reality is that once their *finite window* of being mentally able to make medical decisions closes, that opportunity will be gone forever. Remember: **don't miss your opportunity to do advance care planning—for both your sake and your family's**.

To prevent future challenges, it is prudent to ask a qualified health professional to assess and to document that you still possessed the capacity to make medical decisions near the time you created your Advance Directive. Discuss your options with your physician. Then discuss what treatment you DO want and do NOT want with the individuals who are candidates for being your designated Proxies. Of course, not all patients progress to the end-stage, but if you do, these discussions can help you decide what you want, will give you the opportunity to inform your doctor what you want, and will let you check out your potential Proxies to see if they will advocate your specific wishes when you no longer can. These discussions may also establish the point at which, as the disease progresses, you will want to refuse certain modalities of treatment, including resuscitation, hospitalization, surgery, antibiotics, and perhaps Food & Fluid.

Recent research has shown that Alzheimer's disease can actually be diagnosed by psychological tests [Tierney and others, 2005] and by special brain scans [Reiman and others, 2004], **five or ten years, or even more, before** clinical symptoms begin. Consider such tests if you have a family history of dementia or if you are worried about the significance of emerging symptoms. Some patients who are eventually diagnosed with dementia exhibit symptoms other than the classic problems with memory. These other symptoms typically include apathy, lack of interest and withdrawal from intellectually demanding work or hobbies, as well as clinical depression that is resistant to treatment.

This excerpt is modified from the newsletter of the Hemlock Society, which changed its name to End of Life Choices, and then merged with Compassion in Dying to become to become Compassion and Choices:

A Daughter's Lament

The cost of my mother's disease was astronomical—both *financially* and *emotionally*. It's easier to cite numbers, but the emotional drain was actually worse. Her disease cost $11,000 per month for the last five years, or $660,000.

My greatest regret was how long it took me to learn how—and how hard it was for me to summon the courage—to support the wishes my mother had expressed: She did not want to be kept alive after the quality of her life was completely gone.

When the diagnosis is first made, it raises the future possibility that the person will exist in the end-stage of Alzheimer's disease for a number of years. It is hard to imagine and talk about what the end stage looks like, and it is natural to avoid thinking about it. For example, Julie Meisner Eagle's acclaimed video, *Alzheimer's: My Mom, Our Journey* [2002], emphasized the high quality of care at a personalized residential facility, and the pleasure that patients derive from art therapy, but her documentary entirely omitted illustrating end-stage disease.

On Alzheimer's Disease—four movies and a book: "The Notebook," "Iris," "A Song for Martin," "Away From Her," and "Losing My Mind"

Art *can* reflect life, but Hollywood's requirement for happy endings often prevails. Three movies provide a continuum of reality. *The Notebook* ends with one last moment of clarity... of recognition... and of being able to express love, after which the couple holds hands and "pass on" peacefully and simultaneously. Neither will be left alone to grieve the loss of the other. While many will cry when they view this movie, the danger in portraying a fairy tale is that the movie may instill false hope in family members whose loved ones have Alzheimer's disease.

Iris portrays the deterioration of a brilliant mind by the tragedy of dementia. Author Iris Murdoch is shown as an innovative leader in contemporary thinking through glimpses of her speeches and her readings from her books. After her disease progresses, she cannot even remember that she wrote books, a profound memory loss that sadly rings true. While the movie did show the burden of caregiving at home, it glosses over the three years of progressive decline in an institution where the details of the huge amounts of care she must have required and her story of deterioration was compressed to only 60 seconds of viewing time in the film.

Only a third film, from Sweden, *A Song for Martin*, had the courage to portray fecal incontinence and the grossly inappropriate behavior of urinating in an indoor potted tree in a public restaurant. My favorite, this movie is not merely about a horrible disease, but a moving story that depicts how a disease can test the endurance of a partner's love.

The 2007 movie starring Julie Christie, *Away From Her*, does not depict clinical validity. Rarely do patients themselves voluntarily decide to be institutionalized, especially after getting lost only once while retaining most other mental functions. It is also rare that facilities resemble five-star resorts that forbid the well spouses from visiting for thirty days. (The "love triangle" story required these contrivances.)

Highly recommended: Thomas DeBaggio's book, *Losing My Mind* [2002]. The audio version offers a rare insight into the feelings arising from being diagnosed.

God's Light Switch

An 87 year-old man returned to his primary care physician after having a normal physical examination the previous week. The plan for today was to discuss the results of his laboratory tests. The results that just came back were all within normal range. Glad to have a well patient, since there was nothing more onerous to disclose, the doctor decided to engage the elderly gentlemen in personal, light conversation. To open him up, he asked, "So how else are you doing, George? Are you at peace with God?

"God and I are tight," George replied. "The all powerful even knows how poorly I see in the dark. So He watches over me. For example, when I get up in the middle of the night to go to the bathroom, poof… the light goes on! And when I'm done, poof again… the light goes off."

"Wow, that's amazing," the doctor said, and patted George on the back. Later that same day, the doctor called George's wife, as he had promised her. "Ethel, George is doing fine. And I must admit that I'm in awe of his relationship with God. Is it true that when he gets up during the night… that the light goes on in the bathroom? And then, when he's done… the light goes off?"

"Oh my God", Ethel exclaimed. "My problem… Doctor, remember I lost my sense of smell a few years ago?"

Confused, the doctor said, "Yes, I remember. But what does that have to do with George and God?"

"It means that he's peeing in the refrigerator again."

It's not easy to laugh at dementia in reality. Consider this personal story.

The Disease That Robs

Leeza Gibbons' Story about Her Mother

Leeza Gibbons shared the tragedy of her mother's Alzheimer's on the July 13, 2004 Oprah show. "It's ugly, it's not just forgetting. This is a disease that kills. It robs not only the person that has it, but the family members' memory of who that person was. All are threatened to be replaced by the stranger that comes to live in that body."

As Leeza shared a video clip of her mother, she commented, "Now she sits, she doesn't respond, she doesn't recognize anyone, she doesn't know who she is. **It's death in slow motion**. As Nancy Reagan said, '**It's the longest goodbye**.' And you can't grieve because they're still there."

Leeza explained the usual reason why families deplete their life savings for residential care: The patient's behavior becomes unmanageably violent or aggressive. As patients lose language, bladder and bowel control, the ability to walk, the ability to bathe and dress, and the ability to feed themselves, they become progressively dependent on caregivers and skilled nurses, up to 24 hours a day. At the end, their muscles have severe contractures without purposeful movement and sometimes they have generalized seizures.

Leeza Gibbons' grandmother also had Alzheimer's, which might have served to motivate Leeza's mother to share some valuable insights. Not long after she was diagnosed, she explained, "When I kick and scream and fight you, know that it's the disease talking, not me."

Leeza remembered, "I watched my mother's face change into a mask. [Now] she looks like she's in some sort of a trance... . It's a desperate feeling to be right there close to her, to hold her hand and to know that she's not there. What's hard is this wanting to reach into her, and to say, 'Where are you?'"

Leeza Gibbons endorsed the importance of early diagnosis, which "gives you the opportunity to participate in your own care... . My mother sat us down and said, 'When I can no longer call you by name... I don't want to live with [any of you]. And you need to help Daddy know that it's time to let me go.' What a gift and a blessing that was, because we didn't fight or struggle. We had our *marching orders*. She even had us visit the kind of place where she would ultimately like to be." (An assisted living facility).

৵৵

What is the answer to the question, "***Where are you***?" Look at the diseased brain. The cerebral cortex *atrophies*, meaning that it shrivels up, leaving huge spaces that fill up with fluid. Under the microscope, millions of nerve cells are damaged by *amyloid deposits*. The arrays of nerves that formerly maintained exquisite interconnections are now *disorganized tangles.*

The cerebral cortex must function normally to retain personality, intellect, and memory. After its cells die and their interconnections are destroyed, what's left? Such devastating brain damage causes the loss of the essence of the person. But family members are often confused. They still see the physical attributes of the person they loved, perhaps only slightly changed. This discrepancy makes it difficult for family members to accept that the essence of the person they have loved is really gone.

The words "***marching orders***" can take on expanded meaning when considering Advance Directives. Do you have the courage that Leeza's mother had, to express the Last Wishes you want your Proxies to carry out, in the event you do reach the end-stage of Alzheimer's disease? Existing with Alzheimer's does not require life-supporting medical technology that can be discontinued. So **Refusing Food & Fluid by Proxy** may be the patient's only option to reduce the duration of suffering and indignity other than to wait until the patient contracts an infection in the lungs, urinary tract, or blood from bedsore-infections. Still, all family members must agree, and one must convince the then-treating doctor not to treat the infection aggressively with antibiotics so that the patient may pass on.

In our clinical experience, all too often, a devoted spouse who really wished for the end, regretfully decides to go along with a doctor's recommendation to treat an infection; and then has to put his or her life on hold again, waiting months or years for the next infection to occur. Sometimes doctors do not even ask, or they ask in such a way that seems to expect the well spouse to consent to treat, as several stories will illustrate.

Nearly half of dementia patients lose the ability to feed themselves within 8 years of diagnosis [Volicer and others, 1987]. The reasons include inability to understand how to eat, inability to move intentionally, or loss of the physical ability to swallow. Some physicians recommend that dementia patients stop oral feeding when the medical risk of choking and aspiration becomes too high [Priefer & Robbins, 1997; McNamara & Kennedy, 2001]. The cited references in this book are only a fraction of those that demonstrate that tube feeding is often of no benefit and may even harm the patient, as it drains emotional and financial resources. These facts lead to what may be for many readers, perhaps for us all, the most difficult question in this book:

The "Most Difficult Question"

Suppose a member of your family had the certain diagnosis of an irreversible progressive dementia, which had progressed to the point where he or she no longer knew how to eat or drink. In terms of observable behavior, if you placed in front of him or her, a bowl of food with a spoon in it and a container of fluid with a straw in it—he or she would just sit there, not knowing what to do with either the spoon or the straw, even if it had been a long time since he or she ate or drank.

Suppose further that he or she had not previously made his or her wishes known by a written Advance Directive.

How would you respond?

Would you **consent** to minor surgery **to insert a PEG tube** to provide Food & Fluid on a relatively permanent basis if the doctor insisted it was obligatory to provide basic care to sustain life for as long as possible?

Would you **refuse to consent** to minor surgery **to insert a PEG tube** because at this stage of this disease, most people would not want to prolong the dying process?

Would you **continue only oral feeding** even if the patient resisted taking nourishment and needed to be tied down and forced to accept it?

Or, would you **not continue oral feeding** if said assistance required force, and instead let Nature takes its course because you believe that it was the disease itself (as it impaired the brain) that was resulting in the patient effectively **Refusing Food & Fluid**?

In our society, it takes courage to **Withhold Food & Fluid** from a loved one, even when the attending physician is willing to provide medications for sedation and comfort.

For such challenges, it may be crucial that everyone in the family agree, given the prevailing political and legal forces that presume that we must err on the side of life, even though surveys reveal that a very high percentage of people would not want to continue to exist in that state.

As you struggle to find an answer, it may help to consider whether Professor Edward Sunshine's description applies in your case. In referring to Terri Schiavo's situation, he wrote in the National Catholic Reporter: "Another moral perspective would see Schiavo's [medical] condition as lethal, because her brain damage was preventing her from eating and drinking" [2005].

Consulting professionals in the fields of medicine, psychiatry, law, and religion can help, but keep in mind that highly publicized court cases usually arise only when a family is divided. Whatever you decide, ensure that everyone in your family who wants to be heard, has an opportunity to participate in the decision. Also keep in mind that 70% of hospital deaths occur as a result of decisions by physicians made with the tacit agreement of the family members [Asch and others, 1995]. Finally, appreciate that the ability of families to make decisions in private with their doctors has been threatened by the actions in Congress over the Terri Schiavo case, and the proposal of a model law by the National Right to Life Committee [May 2005]. If States were to pass a similar laws, they would prohibit family members from **Withdrawing Food & Fluid** based on what most people would consider being in the patient's BEST INTEREST. Such withdrawal would be permitted **only** if the Advance Directive had i) a *clear and convincing* written authorization for the Proxy to withdraw, or ii) a *clear and convincing* written instruction for the doctor to withdraw.

"At what point shall we let Nature take its course?"

I am the oldest child of three. Starting in her early eighties, our widowed mother suffered from severe, progressive dementia. Two years ago, we had to place her in a skilled nursing home. For a year, she was unable to recognize anyone or communicate. At one of my visits, the nurse gave me a note: Her doctor wanted to speak to me. I met with him the next day. He told me that eventually, Mom would **no longer be capable of feeding herself**, and sometime after that, she would **lose the physical ability to swallow**. He asked me if my mother had discussed what level of feeding assistance she would want and if she had given any other indication of how long she wanted her existence to be prolonged.

I explained that my mother had consistently refused to talk about such things, which she called "morbid." The doctor nodded. "Only 1 in 9 patients talk with their doctors about their end-of-life wishes." He suggested that I speak to an elder care attorney before resuming our conversation. Then he gave me three names.

After the lawyer listened to the story, he advised me to speak to my sister and brother. He stated that if all three of us agreed on what was in our mother's **best interest**, we could decide among several options; otherwise, our mother would have to accept society's default treatment plan: Doctors will do everything possible to prolong her life. I called my sister, who lived two hundred miles away, and asked her to drive down the following weekend. My plan was to talk about Mom with my brother and sister.

The next Saturday evening, after dinner, we moved into my living room, and I announced that we had to make a difficult decision. Then I shared my discussions with the doctor and the attorney.

I said, "Of the two treatment decisions we must make, this is the easier one: Should we offer Mom a feeding tube when she can no longer swallow? Most dementia patients do not understand the need for tubes so they require physical restraints to prevent pulling them out. The restraints are uncomfortable, cause further loss of dignity, and increase the risk of lethal infections from bedsores. Even with a feeding tube, Mom might regurgitate and aspirate, which can lead to a lethal bout of pneumonia."

I assured my brother and sister that the doctor could reduce Mom's sensation of thirst as Nature took its course so her life would end peacefully. Both agreed to refuse tube feeding on Mom's behalf when she lost the ability to swallow.

I had carefully planned my presentation for the second and more difficult decision. "Mom is more than confused. To be honest, we must admit she's lost all her personality and humanity. And she's been that way for a year. Furthermore, the doctor says she will only get worse. Recently, I've found it necessary to show her how to use a spoon and straw. So now I must ask the hardest question I've ever had to ask. Why wait? Why wait to **Withdraw Food & Fluid** from Mom until she can no longer swallow?"

My brother and sister just stared at me. Their facial expressions pleaded for further explaining. I responded, "I feel it is both right and kind to **Refuse Food & Fluid** on behalf of Mom when she has **lost the understanding of how to eat and drink**. I've thought deeply about what Mom would want, and what would be best for her." I waited...

As I had expected, my sister asked, "But how can we be sure that Mom **no longer understands how to eat and drink**?"

I repeated what the doctor had suggested. "Either we or the nursing assistants will continue to place food and water on her table, but we will not raise the spoon to her mouth, not put the straw between her lips, and not demonstrate how to use the spoon and straw. We'll just wait and observe. If over a day or so, Mom just sits in front of the food and water without eating or drinking, then we can conclude that either she *no longer* understands how to eat and drink, or she *no longer* wants to eat and drink. The doctor knows some patients who couldn't talk but they still pulled out their feeding tubes. One did so 17 times. So after we observe Mom for a day or so, we can ask the staff to stop offering her further food and water and let her disease of dementia take its natural course."

My brother asked, "Will the nursing home administration let us do that?"

I answered, "The doctor said we might have to bring her home, or enroll her in a sympathetic hospice if someone on the nursing home staff objects. There are a lot of people involved in Mom's care, and all it takes is one to create a fuss, even though the doctor is willing to argue that this would definitely be in her **best interest**."

My sister was sitting like a lid on a pot that had just started to boil. She exploded as stood up. "BEST INTEREST? How can you say that? To starve her to death? How can you even suggest we abandon the very person who brought us into this world?"

"It's not starvation. It's dehydration, and it's—"

"I know it takes four hours every day, for the staff to feed her," my sister interrupted, "but I don't care. As long as Mom is alive, regardless of the condition of her mind and body, she deserves to be treated as a human being with all the ordinary care that every human deserves." I was about to reply as my sister's voice got even louder. "Providing nourishment is a form of care owed to all helpless people. It's how we express our love and concern. I can't stand thinking about your suggestion. Our own mother—" Then she sat down, put her head in her hands, and sobbed.

After she quieted down I gently said, "Think of it this way: We're NOT deliberately hastening Mom's death. We're just letting her die naturally from the consequences of her **mental** disease. A few minutes ago, you agreed to let her die from the consequences of her **physical** disease, when she can no longer swallow. So why won't you let her die when her **mental** disease prevents her from knowing how to use a spoon and a straw? Have you seen what it's like to feed her, recently? She is getting more resistant. I strongly feel we would NOT be respecting Mom's dignity if we decide to force feed her."

As my brother nodded his head, my sister said, "I'm not *convinced*."

So I tried again. "Don't you feel, that if Mom could speak for herself, this is what she would want? Most people would. The doctor gave me an article that summarized an AARP survey showing that almost 9 out of 10 people over 50 felt that total physical dependency would be worse than death. In situations like Mom's, 8 out of 10 felt it would be important to be **off** machines that extend life. Mom's doctor said he thought it would be in her best interest not to force spoon-feeding."

My sister shook her head. "How can you be so sure? Maybe Mom is one of those one or two... out of ten."

Nothing I knew about our mother would ever convince me that she would be in that small minority. But how could I prove that? I thought for a moment and then realized that it was time for me to give up. The next morning,

I called the doctor. "We agreed to withhold tube feeding when she can no longer swallow. But as long as she can swallow, I guess you'll have to continue the spoon-feeding."

For the next eight months, my mother had no vestige of meaningful interaction with any one, including those whom she formerly had loved so much. I tried not to count, but my sister only paid her two visits.

When Mom did lose her ability to swallow, her doctor ordered the staff to stop spoon-feeding. He told me that he wrote in her chart that it would be too great a risk. Two days later, she developed a fever but he administered no antibiotics or hydration. Finally, Nature took its course and Mom died three days later.

I wish I could erase from my memory, the sight of my mother lying in her bed as her muscles became more contracted. She hardly moved from the fetal position except for the many seizures during her last two months. When I recall those eight months, I ask, *What was the point?* My brother agrees. I haven't discussed my feelings with my sister, nor do I plan to.

The huge financial cost was just part of it. Worse was the enormous emotional drain as I was forced to witness the staff fighting with Mom during spoon-feeding, until she was no longer able to swallow.

Two positive things emerged from my mother's awful, prolonged ordeal. It motivated me to try to write my own Advance Directive in a *clear and convincing* way. I designated my brother as my agent and I gave him the authority to **Refuse Food & Fluid** on my behalf. I listed alternates if my brother cannot serve as my agent. I also added two statements to my Advance Directive: I specifically stated that my sister can never serve as my agent, and I waived my right to a court review so that she couldn't challenge my Proxy. My brother knows all this, but my sister does not. She will only discover it if my brother and all alternates are not available. I don't want to hurt her feelings, but if she does find out, she'll know why I made that choice.

৵৶

See the Table on page 219 for 8 possible answers to, "How aggressively should we provide Food & Fluid to patients with severe dementia?"

23. For Patients Who Cannot Communicate, How Can We be Sure They Want to Voluntarily Refuse Food & Fluid?

It is essential that patients' end-of-life choices related to refusing life-sustaining treatments be **voluntary**. If someone suspects "**undue influence**"— that one person is exerting pressure on a vulnerable patient to make the decision that the other person wants—then professionals from the fields of medicine, psychology, social work, family therapy, and the law can, either individually or as a coordinated effort, interview members of the family and caregivers to rule-out this possibility. These professionals look for typical circumstances and behaviors that suggest controlling the patient for malicious or selfish intent. Conflicts can arise when one family member (the loving, well-meaning one) cannot find out what the sick person wants because of the behavior of the other (the mean, selfish person). For example (unlike the story above), the other does not allow the patient to visit or talk on the phone, using the excuse that she is sleeping or not feeling well. Frustrated, the loving person often contacts an elder care attorney, who in turn arranges for professionals to conduct independent examinations. (Beyond this brief statement, this complex subject is beyond the scope of this book.)

One paramount quality of being human is the ability to express a choice. It is an insult of great magnitude to the autonomy and dignity of any sick and vulnerable person to not make every effort, even if it is tedious. We recommend asking the patient crucial questions—even if the patient only has the ability to indicate "Yes" and "No." I consider this point so important that my own Advance Directives includes this statement:

"Please, make every effort to ask me."

As long as I can indicate "Yes" or "No"—even if only by squeezing a hand, or by blinking my eye, I want all concerned to have the patience to ask me what I want. Please "listen" to me, even if I can express myself only one letter at a time. My Proxy may also decide to ask experts to employ enhancement technology to assist my communication, if it seems appropriate.

Sometimes well-meaning relatives think they are being helpful by answering questions that presumably impatient professionals ask, but there is great danger that this process may impose their values and wishes on the patient, who may have different treatment preferences. No decision is more important than refusing or accepting treatments that may prolong life, and for this decision, the patient's preference must prevail.

Beyond "Yes" and "No," technology can expand the ability of patients to interact with their environment. Selecting one letter at a time allows patients to initiate their own statements. Dr. Philip Kennedy [Kennedy and Andreason 2004] developed a *brain communicator system* that can overcome the challenges of even profound paralysis and mutism. Dr. Kennedy and his colleagues measure EEG-like signals from conductive screws placed in patients' skulls. Other neurologists use simple oscilloscopes to help patients indicate "Yes" and "No." The patient either "thinks" the word or letter, or imagines that a part of the body moves in one direction or another, to indicate "Yes" or "No," depending on what mental activity results in a measurable, consistent change in brain-wave pattern.

To make sure the choice is **Voluntary** when a patient suffering from dementia seems to **Refuse Food & Fluid**, it is respectful to continue to offer Food & Fluid since the patient may change his or her mind.

Competent patients who have previously decided to **Refuse Food & Fluid** sometimes "just forget" to forgo intake, perhaps because of their habit to eat and drink, and because their thinking has become clouded. The clinician can then remind the patient of his or her options by stating them neutrally and noting that any choice is acceptable. Trying not to exert influence is important if the patient continues his or her resolve [Terman, 2001].

Although some conscious people may not be upset by the sight or smell of food as they are fasting, which was my experience. If you feel the presence of food would disturb you, however, then direct your Proxy (or add a statement to your Living Will) that you want to be offered NO food or fluid—after you have refused a certain number, perhaps 2 or 4 or 6, meals.

The memoir below, "A Time To Be Sure," demonstrates the extra care and consideration a daughter gave to find out, with high degree of certainty, whether or not her father wanted to **Refuse Food & Fluid**. [Note: The questions she used were further refined for general use, and are listed separately, on page 210.]

A Time To Be Sure

My father had generally been a happy man who enjoyed many aspects of life. Sadly, during his last four years, several strokes caused major deterioration. Once a successful electrical engineer and active in both golf and tennis, now he could only sit in front of the TV in our living room, and open his mouth to eat when someone (usually me) fed him or gave him a drink. I tried to make his life more interesting by sharing the events of my life and by commenting on what I noticed he had watched on TV. I also tried to bring joy to his life by preparing his favorite foods, even though they had to be pureed.

According to his neurologist, Dad had an "expressive aphasia." He could understand language perfectly, but he couldn't talk at all. That's because one of his strokes knocked out the part of his brain that is essential for creating speech. So, to learn what he wanted, I had to guess by asking a series of questions. That was not as frustrating as it might sound. Usually, it didn't take too long to ask him a series of questions and watch whether he shook his head "No," or nodded his head "Yes."

Still, I'm sure he missed our regular conversations as much as I did—No, definitely more, since after all, I could talk with other people.

I could usually guess how Dad was feeling from the expression on his face, whether or not his eyes were keenly focused, and how much enthusiasm he showed as he shook or nodded his head. Sometimes, Dad looked depressed, but I never asked him directly. Why? Because I had no idea how to make him feel better, and the last thing I wanted to do was to even hint that he was a burden to me. There were other times, however, when Dad would brighten up. He seemed to enjoy tossing a volleyball back and forth. I loved to see him smile when I fumbled or threw the ball wild. But his joy didn't last long. When he wanted to stop playing, he would just hold on to the ball. That was his signal that our game was over.

One day, Dad coughed up green phlegm and his temperature rose to 102. I called his doctor and he gave me some advice that shocked me. He said I need not feel morally obligated to treat Dad's pneumonia, and offered this medical fact: "Before the antibiotic era, pneumonia was called the friend of the old and the sick." I don't know what he said next, I felt so stunned that I hung up as soon as I could. Then I realized... Dad's doctor had just given me the clear message that I could let Dad die by not treating him. I gazed at my father, who was so sick now that he could not respond, "Yes" or "No." How could I presume to make a life-or-death decision for him, without knowing for sure what he wanted? After I thought more about it, I called the doctor and asked him to treat Dad aggressively. Dad was treated for five days in the hospital with IVs and antibiotics. He recovered from his pneumonia and returned home.

But then he seemed even more depressed. He refused meals, even when I prepared his favorites. He closed his eyes in front of the TV. Worst of all, he would not look at me as I talked to him. And when I threw him the volleyball, most of the time he held onto it instead of throwing it back—to say he didn't want to play at all. At one point, I had to admit that I was avoiding the harsh reality of what Dad might be trying to tell me—that he no longer wanted to live.

I begged a psychiatrist to make a home visit. He spent more time talking to me than trying to relate to Dad. I guess psychiatrists usually have patients who can talk. He admitted that he had little to offer. He doubted antidepressants would change Dad's perception of his physical state, but he still left two prescriptions—one to help Dad with his anxiety and the other to help him sleep—in case those symptoms got worse. The psychiatrist suggested that I call hospice, which surprised me since Dad's neurologist never said that Dad's strokes were "terminal" and I thought hospice accepted only patients who were expected to die within six months. The psychiatrist suggested that I ask hospice to do their independent evaluation, to mention Dad's high risk for another major stroke, recurrent pneumonia, and major depression.

When the hospice nurse finished evaluating Dad, I asked her how long he might go on living like this. She answered, "He could last many months, even years. Your choices are limited: You can wait until your father has a massive stroke that prevents his breathing. Meanwhile, if he gets pneumonia again, do not treat him with IVs or antibiotics. It could be a year or longer."

That night, I couldn't sleep. Clearly, Dad felt depressed since he had returned from the hospital... Maybe Dad's doctor had been right, to suggest we not treat his pneumonia... Maybe Dad was depending upon me for a way out... Maybe. I was desperate to learn what Dad really wanted... But how could I find out? If I asked him, what would I be suggesting? How could I be sure?

I was in the habit of calling my brother every week. He lived in the Midwest. The next morning, I discussed Dad's situation with him. Always good at logic, my brother had something definite to offer. He referred to the statistics courses he had taken in graduate school and stated, "If Dad answers a number of questions consistently, then we could be certain about what he wanted."

I asked him, how many questions?

"To be 'within a reasonable degree of medical certainty,' scientists and doctors insist on 95%. If Dad can answer five or six questions consistently, we could be sure. Even using only four questions, $0.5 \times 0.5 \times 0.5 \times 0.5 = 0.004$, which means the chances are only 4 in a 1000 (1 in 250) that he would *seem* that consistent. Scientists only required 1 in 20."

I said, "If you say so." (I didn't really understand the math then and I had to call him recently to remind me about the numbers to write this.)

Some days were better than others for my father, so I decided to wait until he had a good day before I posed the series of ultimate questions. Later that week, as we threw the ball back and forth, I tried to rev up his enthusiasm by doing some silly antics. Once, I tossed the ball way over his head. Next, I pretended to strain as I stretched to make a "difficult" catch. It worked! He smiled. That was the moment I was waiting for. I asked, "Dad, aren't we having a lot of fun?" I threw the ball back to him and waited for him to nod... . Actually, I really hoped he would nod.

Instead, he just held on to the ball. I waited for him to throw it back, but he didn't. So I asked a most difficult question: "Doesn't this kind of fun make your life worth living?"

Dad fiercely shook his head to say "No" as he held on tightly to the ball. This was the moment I had prepared for. I had written down a number of questions to ask Dad. Knowing that I would be nervous, I printed them out so I could record his answers. (They are reproduced on the next page.)

A "Yes" / "No" Conversation to Make Sure

1. Dad, do you expect your medical condition will improve?

   He shook his head to indicate "No."

2. So you assume that you must live under these circumstances?

   He nodded to indicate "Yes."

3. Under these circumstances, then, do you want to go on living?

   He shook his head to indicate "No."

4. Can you enjoy enough of life to want to go on living?

   He shook his head to indicate "No."

5. Do you want to hasten your dying by not eating or drinking, as long as you are kept comfortable?

   He nodded to indicate "Yes."

6. Wouldn't you want to continue to eat, as long as I prepare your favorite foods?

   He shook his head to indicate "No."

7. Do you understand that if you decide not to eat or drink, you will die?

   He nodded to indicate "Yes."

8. Are you glad I'm giving you the opportunity to express yourself?

   He nodded to indicate "Yes."

9. Would you like to talk about something else, like this evening's newscast?

   He shook his head to indicate "No."

10. Do you want to go on living under your present circumstances?

    He shook his head to indicate "No."

11. Do you want to continue to eat and drink?

    He shook his head to indicate "No."

12. Do you want to hasten your dying by not eating and not drinking?

    He nodded to indicate "Yes."

Not since before his first stroke, did Dad look at me with such intensity during a conversation. It only took a few minutes even though I asked twice as many questions as my brother recommended. I wanted no doubts later.

To make sure Dad's answers did not reflect a temporary down period in his mood, I ended our conversation by saying, "Dad, I'm willing to honor your wishes, but I must make sure you're not just having one bad day. So, could we repeat this conversation in a day or so?"

In response to my question about repeating the whole series of questions, he nodded his head, to indicate "Yes."

Two days later, every one of Dad's answers was the same. Then I asked him a few more questions—again, several times in several ways to be sure— about what he would want if he seemed uncomfortable when he could no longer nod or shake his head. He indicated that he would prefer medication for anxiety and insomnia rather than resume his intake of Food & Fluid.

As it turned out, he never seemed too uncomfortable.

For the next day and a half, I offered Dad his favorite foods and a variety of fluids, but he consistently shook his head to refuse them. When I asked him if he wanted medication for anxiety or insomnia, he nodded only twice. Every time Dad woke up, I'd offer him the same choice: Food & Fluid, medication, or nothing. He never chose Food & Fluid. As the week progressed, he slept more and was awake less. He always seemed calm and comfortable. After the fifth day, he remained in a very deep sleep. On day eight, he just stopped breathing.

When I reflect on how Dad died, there's *almost* no guilt. (I'll explain the "almost" part in a moment.) Here's why: I asked enough questions to be sure I knew what Dad wanted. I asked the questions when he was in his best mood. And I gave him multiple opportunities in those first few days to change his mind and resume intake of Food & Fluid.

Why "almost"? Because I still feel a little guilty, even though it is only with the benefit of hindsight, about not asking Dad if he wanted to treat his pneumonia before he got sick. My only regret is that I wish I had used the multiple-question technique before Dad got too sick to use nods and shakes to refuse treatment.

When I've told this story to others, some comment that my role sounds like assisting suicide, but I disagree. The two doses of medication that Dad took certainly did not hasten his dying. I always gave Dad the opportunity to change his mind to resume eating and drinking. I only helped him carry out his choice, which the medical doctors and attorneys I've spoken to agree was his right, since there was no reason to doubt whether Dad was mentally competent.

While Dad's choice most likely hastened his dying, my role was limited... I only facilitated *his* choice with great respect.

I found the next point ironic, but it didn't occur to me until three years later. I was telling someone about my experience with Dad, and she in turn was sharing how her mother, in her final days, kept on turning her face away from the food. Whenever the nursing assistant tried to open her mouth, she tightly clenched her teeth.

After I heard her story, I asked myself, why didn't Dad turn his face away and clench his teeth? At first, I was puzzled and had no answer. Then one day, it suddenly occurred to me: All the questions I had asked Dad over and over... they really served a purpose totally different than the one I intended. I assumed the questions would assure *me* that Dad really wanted to **Refuse Food & Fluid**. But in reality, the questions were Dad's way of assuring himself that I, as his daughter, could handle letting him go. I finally came to understand that Dad could have Refused Food & Fluid as soon as he returned from the hospital, but he wanted to wait until he was sure I was emotionally able to let him go. *Dad* got the assurance *he* needed when I asked him all those questions.

One final note: Now that I've seen how peaceful **Refusing Food & Fluid** was for Dad, I will insist that when the time comes for my final transition, the person or organization I've authorized to advocate my Last Wishes will have the courage and patience to discuss this option with me while I have the ability to make medical decisions, and then make sure my wishes are honored.

I also followed the suggestion of my advisor to document my wishes in a document to empower my Proxy. I've prepared a document that states what I want in a *clear and convincing* way, that includes my reasons for wanting my **Proxy to Refuse Food & Fluid** on my behalf in writing, and I had this document witnessed. As one of the examples to illustrate my reasons to support my Proxy's decision against potential challenges, I included a copy of this story about Dad in that document, and attached it to my Advance Directives.

24. How Do We Know if a Brain-Damaged Person Can Consistently Respond to His or Her Environment?

Some loving parents want to remove life support and are forced to fight the States' right to protect life (or existence). This was true in the cases of Karen Ann Quinlan and Nancy Beth Cruzan. Other loving parents litigate intensely for their brain-damaged children to maintain their existence. Examples are the cases of

Robert Wendland who was in the persistent Minimally Conscious State, and Terri Schiavo, who was in the Permanent Vegetative State. Prolonged litigation typically focuses on young adults whose brain damage was caused by trauma or lack of oxygen. This is in contrast to adult children of parents suffering from progressive irreversible dementia. For them, mourning is realistic, and even if there is disagreement, as in the story, "Shall we let Nature take its course," the patient lives months, not years, so litigation cannot be prolonged. It is understandable why some parents of brain-damaged children hold on to remote hopes. No loss is harder than losing a child. But as they cling to the smallest responses from their children, some parents justify continued hope by claiming...

"I can tell! My child still recognizes me."

"When I walk into the room and lean over her bed, I notice a definite flicker in her eyes. Sometimes she even has a slight smile. And she holds on to my hand so tightly.... . That assures me sure that, at least sometimes, she can recognize me."

ভ৶

Professor Lawrence Schneiderman explained that severely brain-damaged people can exhibit confusing reflexes [2005]: "The mere sound of visitors' walking can cause the patient's eyes to flicker." If the cerebral cortex is injured so that only the brain stem survives, the patient can still have "sleep-wake cycles and primitive reflexes such as coughing and blinking [and] a grimace so relatives will say, 'Oh, she is happy to see me.'" Dr. Schneiderman states that, in reality, the patient is "permanently unconsciousness," and the grip reflex is among the most primitive that even undeveloped brains of newborn babies exhibit.

Everyone expects parents will be biased and not objective. However a news release was picked up after Barbara Weller, a new attorney for Terri's parents, spent 45 minutes with her. Her published story had the title "**Very Much Alive and Responsive.**" [See www.LifeSite.net, January 5, 2005.]

The basis for this news article was the account written by attorney Barbara Weller. On the morning of Christmas Eve, 2004, Ms. Weller visited Terri Schiavo at the Woodside Hospice. Also present were Terri's parents, Bob and Mary Schindler, Terri's sister and niece, and Attorney David Gibbs, III. Below is an excerpt from Attorney Weller's published observations of that 45-minute interaction, which I also had the opportunity to discuss with her, on the phone:

"My visit with Terri Schiavo"

by Attorney Barbara Weller

I am a mother and a grandmother, as well as one of the Schindlers' attorneys, and I could understand how parents might imagine behavior and purposeful activity that is not really there. I was prepared to be as objective as I could be...

The thing that surprised me most about Terri as I took my turn to greet her by the side of her chair was how beautiful she is... I saw a very pretty woman with a peaches-and-cream complexion and a lovely smile... She appeared to have an inner light radiating from her face...

When she heard their [the visitors'] voices, and particularly her mother's voice, Terri instantly turned her head towards them and smiled. Terri established eye contact with her family, particularly with her mother, who spent the most time with her during our visit. It was obvious that she recognized the voices in the room with the exception of one... Attorney Gibbs was having a conversation near the door with Terri's sister. His voice is very deep and resonant and Terri obviously picked it up. Her eyes widened as if to say, "What's that new sound I hear?" She scanned the room with her eyes, even turning her head in his direction, until she found Attorney Gibbs and the location of the new voice and her eyes rested momentarily in his direction... .

When her mother was close to her, Terri's whole face lit up. She smiled. She looked directly at her mother and she made all sorts of happy sounds. When her mother talked to her, Terri was quiet and obviously listening. When she stopped, Terri started vocalizing. The vocalizations seemed to be a pattern, not merely random or reflexive at all. There is definitely a pattern of Terri having a conversation with her mother as best she can manage. Initially, she used the vocalization of "uh uh" but without seeming to mean it as a way of saying "no", just as a repeated speech pattern. She then began to make purposeful grunts in response to her mother's conversation. She made the same sorts of sound with her father and sister, but not to the same extent or as delightedly as with her mother. She made no verbal response to her niece or to Attorney Gibbs and myself, but she did appear to pay attention to our words...

Terri definitely has a personality. Her whole demeanor definitely changes when her mother speaks with her. She lights up and appears to be delighted at the interaction. She has an entirely different reaction to her father who jokes with her and has several standing jokes that he uses when he enters and exits her presence. She appears to merely "tolerate" her father, as a child does when she says, "stop," but really means, "this is fun." When her father greets her, he always does the same thing. He says, "here comes the hug" and hugs her. He then says, "You know what's coming next—the kiss." Her father has a scratchy mustache and both times when he went through this little joke routine with her, she laughed in a way she did not do with anyone else. When her father is ready to plant the kiss on her cheek, she immediately makes a face her family calls the "lemon face." She puckers her lips, screws up her whole face, and turns away from him, as if making ready for the scratchy assault on her cheek that she knows is coming. She did the exact same thing both times that her father initiated this little routine joke between the two of them... .

When one of the visitors approached her and started to talk directly to her again, Terri would open her eyes and begin her grunting sounds again in response to their conversations... .

When her sister went to her to say goodbye, Terri's verbalizations changed dramatically. Instead of the happy grunting and "uh uh" sounds she had been making throughout the visit, her verbalizations at these good-byes changed to a very low and different sound that appeared to come from deep in her throat and was almost like a growl. She first made the sound when her sister said goodbye and then, amazingly to me, she made exactly the same sound when her mother said goodbye to her. It seemed Terri was visibly upset that they were leaving. She almost appeared to be trying to cling to them, although this impression came only from her changed facial expression and sounds, since her hands cannot move. It appeared like she did not want to be alone and knew they were leaving. It was definitely apparent in the short time I was there that her emotions changed...it was apparent when she was happy and enjoying herself, when she was amused, when she was resting from her exertion to communicate, and when she was sad at her guests leaving. It was readily apparent and surprising that her mood changed so often in a short 45-minute visit.

Observations of others:

Terri's sister, Suzanne Vitadamo, visited her on March 18, 2005, the day her feeding tube was removed. On March 22, she signed a short Declaration, from which a key paragraph is copied below:

Terri was sitting up in her lounge chair and Mrs. Weller leaned over Terri, took her arms in her hands, and begged Terri to try to say, "I want to live." Terri's eyes opened wide, she looked at Mrs. Weller with great concentration and said, "Ahhhhhhh." Then, with great effort, she screamed, "Waaaaaaaa" so loudly that two people who were standing outside Terri's door could clearly hear her. Terri had a look of anguish on her face and she seemed to be struggling hard, but she could not complete the sentence. Terri began to cry and Mrs. Weller and I began to stroke Terri's face and hair to comfort her.

Terri's mother, Mary Schindler, appeared at a rally outside the hospice, to plead for her daughter's life. Her appearance was taped and televised. She described that she had tried to teach her daughter how to say, "I love you." Mary said, "Terri tried... but she only got the 'I' part."

❦

So... during the Christmas Eve day visit, Terri appeared to be able to vocalize three distinctly different sounds. During the March 18 visit, Terri appeared to be able to vocalize two distinctly different verbal sounds. But in response to her mother's attempts to train her, Terri was only able to vocalize one sound.

What can we make of this? The critical question is whether her two different facial expressions and her one (or two, or three) different sounds are consistent responses that indicate that she is aware, since they reflect her ability to interact meaningfully with others. What is the alternative? According to Dr. Schneiderman, these sounds and expressions might merely be reflexes that do not reflect meaningful communication, even though Attorney Weller concluded, from her observations, that they were consistent reactions to different stimuli.

A critical question thus emerges: Is it possible to tell the difference between "reflex" and "purposeful communication"? I believe there is a way, which is why I proposed, in my declaration that Attorney Weller submitted to Judge Greer, that if Terri could produce two different sounds consistently, as suggested by Ms. Weller's observations in "My Visit With Terri," then Terri might (for example) be able to assign the meaning of "Yes" to the "grunt" and the meaning of "No" to "uh uh." **IF** she could do this, then it might be possible to ask her such simple situational questions as: Is this person your mother? Is your name Joan? Are you standing up? Is it daytime? Are you a man? And so on. If Terri could answer six questions correctly out of six, then according to the clinical criteria of Giacino and colleagues [2002], she could be considered to have emerged from the **Minimally Conscious State** (**MCS**). If she could answer only some of the questions, she would still be in the **MCS**. But if she could not respond by assigning to different sounds or facial expressions, the meanings of "Yes" and "No," then she would be in the **Permanent Vegetative State**.

The next Guideline offers a series of questions to ask patients who have suffered brain damage from trauma or from progressive Alzheimer's disease.

Questions to Help Determine if a Brain-Damaged Person Can Consistently Respond to His or Her Environment

First the evaluator must identify some way for the patient to indicate what will mean "Yes," and what will mean "No." Any sound or behavior can work; for example a grunt and a moan, or a squeeze and a blink. If the patient can produce only one sound or only one behavior, then one squeeze (for example) would mean "Yes," while two would mean "No."

Then the evaluator must see if the patient can consistently respond to the evaluator's request to indicate "Yes" and "No."

For example:

Please indicate "Yes"	(Check if squeezed correctly once: __)
Please indicate "No"	(Check if squeezed correctly twice: __)
Please indicate "No"	(Check if squeezed correctly twice: __)
Please indicate "Yes"	(Check if squeezed correctly once: __)
Please indicate "Yes"	(Check if squeezed correctly once: __)
Please indicate "No"	(Check if squeezed correctly twice: __)
Please indicate "No"	(Check if squeezed correctly twice: __)
Please indicate "Yes"	(Check if squeezed correctly once: __)

If the patient can consistently respond to requests to indicate "Yes" and "No," then see if he or she can correctly respond to these simple situational questions:

Situational Questions:

1. Is it raining outside?	(Check if squeezed correctly: __)
2. Is it sunny outside?	(Check if squeezed correctly: __)
3. Is it daytime?	(Check if squeezed correctly: __)
4. Is it nighttime?	(Check if squeezed correctly: __)
5. Is it sunny outside?	(Check if squeezed correctly: __)
6. Is it nighttime?	(Check if squeezed correctly: __)
7. Is it raining outside?	(Check if squeezed correctly: __)
8. Is it daytime?	(Check if squeezed correctly: __)

9. Are you a man?   (Check if squeezed correctly: __)

10. Are you a woman?   (Check if squeezed correctly: __)

11. Are you a child?   (Check if squeezed correctly: __)

12. Are you an adult?   (Check if squeezed correctly: __)

13. Are you of white race?   (Check if squeezed correctly: __)

14. Are you of black race?   (Check if squeezed correctly: __)

15. Am I a member of your family?   (Check if squeezed correctly: __)

16. Do I work here on the staff?   (Check if squeezed correctly: __)

Recommendations:

If you know someone who has been diagnosed with a progressive dementia, consider administering this protocol soon, even though it may seem somewhat ridiculous. Doing so may help to establish a baseline result that can be compared with his or her subsequent cognitive performance.

If the patient can respond consistently with "Yes" and "No," and if the patient can correctly respond to simple situational questions as above— then proceed to use the 12 questions from "A 'Yes' / 'No' Conversation To Make Sure," to learn if she or he wants to continue to remain alive, or wishes to **Refuse Food & Fluid** in order to end all suffering.

The Question: How Aggressively Should We Provide Food & Fluid To Patients With Severe Dementia?		
Option	**Pros**	**Cons**
1 Provide Food & Fluid by IV, NG or PEG tube to prolong existence indefinitely.	The patient is still a human being so one must continue to provide basic care.	Medical complications; burden to patient & family; financial expense; consumption of finite medical resources; may not be what the patient wants.
2 Forced oral feeding for a patient who did not leave an Advance Directive.	Could be considered "ordinary and usual care" that any human being should expect to receive.	May not really be what the patient wants; could cause medical complications such as aspiration pneumonia; additional suffering if Minimally Conscious.
3 Oral feeding ONLY if the patient voluntarily accepts Food & Fluid; *NO* forced oral feeding. Physician's orders should read: "**As Patient Permits" (APP)**	The disease is taking its Natural course; resistance *probably* indicates patient's Refusal of Food & Fluid.	Gravely disabled patients need the State's protect of their lives; patients who can swallow should be given extra encouragement, as needed.
4 Do *NOT* force-feed but offer Food & Fluid and *DO* demonstrate (role model) how to eat and drink.	Respecting loss of dignity of this human being by not prolonging a meaningless and expensive existence.	To not take extra effort to nurture goes against social custom and what intuitively seems to be compassionate.
5 Do *NOT* force-feed and do *NOT* demonstrate how to eat and drink, but still offer food and drink.	Let Nature take its course; consider the disease as progressing to a "natural" Refusal of Food & Fluid.	To not take extra effort to nurture goes against social custom and what intuitively seems to be compassionate.
6 Voluntarily Refuse Food & Fluid on behalf of the patient; offer *Comfort Care* as needed.	Prevents further suffering and loss of dignity; reduces emotional and financial burden for all.	Some religions view this as morally wrong ("euthanasia by omission") if the intent is to hasten dying.
7 Give the patient sufficient sedatives to cause unconsciousness to relieve uncontrolled suffering.	Certainly ends suffering by *Terminal Sedation* OR by *Respite Palliative Sedation*, if reversed.	Violates the *Double Effect* principle ONLY *IF* dosage exceeds that needed to reduce suffering.
8 Give the patient sufficient sedatives to depress respiration (*Euthanasia*).	Speeds up the process of dying, which is inevitable anyway.	Illegal; potential abuse if motivation not based on patients' best interest.

Chapter 9

QUESTIONS ABOUT CREATING STRATEGIC ADVANCE DIRECTIVES

**To Make Sure Your Last Wishes Will be Honored,
Your Advance Directive Must Include
WHO, WHAT, WHY, and HOW**

Who: Designate **appropriate individuals** to be your Proxies. Also list those you do NOT want to have that authority.

What: Give your Proxies **specific authority** to Refuse Food & Fluid on your behalf (if that is your preference) and also state if this authority includes refusal by the oral route.

Why: Write your **specific reasons** with examples to provide *clear and convincing* testimony to empower your Proxies to Refuse Food & Fluid on your behalf (**Empowering Statements for My Proxy**).

How: State if you want your Proxy's current decision to override your written instructions (really, how others interpret what you wrote), in the event of a conflict, and how much oversight you want for your Proxy's decisions.

A Well Planned Life

Two women met for the first time since they had graduated from high school. The more modestly dressed one asked the other, "I always admired how organized you were in school. Did you continue to live what I always called, a well planned life?"

"Yes, in fact, I have to say I did," said her friend.

"Would you tell me about it?" the first one asked.

"Well, I'll give you a quick overview. My first husband was a millionaire. My second husband was an actor. My third husband was a preacher. And now, I'm married to an undertaker."

Thinking that going through three divorces must have been how terrible, her friend initially did not know what to say. Trying to respond positively, she asked, "So you are the marrying kind. Four times! Wow. Please explain, though, what do your marriages have to do with your well planned life?"

"Honey, you always did need me to draw you a picture. It's simple. You'll get it as soon as you hear it. Here's my four-part strategic plan: One for the money, two for the show, three to get ready, and four to go."

The **i-FAQs** answered below are also a four-part strategy: Who, What, Why, and How. Each answer is more complicated than the four single words used by the female serial monogamist, above.

If you have read this far, you can appreciate the typical motivations and fears of the large cast of characters that includes your relatives, doctors, religious leaders, politicians, administrators, and judges. These people can wield power to prevent the honoring of your Last Wishes.

Attorney Wesley J. Smith is one of the most articulate champions of the "right-to-life" movement. The suggestions he offered were considered important enough to publish twice [2005a, 2005b]; the excerpt below is slightly condensed:

How to Keep People With Devastating Brain Damage "Alive" Indefinitely (modified from Wesley J. Smith, J.D.)

"If Terri's supporters channel their passion into productive democratic reform, we can almost surely prevent future such miscarriages of justice.

1. "The Americans with Disabilities Act['s] ... protections should apply explicitly where they are needed most desperately, in medical situations where discrimination can have lethal consequences."

2. "States need to review their laws of informed consent and refusal of medical treatment to ensure that casual conversations are never again

deemed to be the legal equivalent of a well thought-out, written Advance Directive... . Human lives deserve protection" from "oral statements."

3. "If people don't want feeding tubes... they have the responsibility to make sure that such wishes are put in a legally binding document. Absent that, the law should require the courts in contested cases to give every reasonable benefit of doubt to sustaining life and not causing death by dehydration."

4. "Our laws should... create a distinction between food and water supplied through a tube and other forms of medical care. Withholding a respirator or antibiotics can lead to uncertain results. Take away anyone's food and water and they will die."

5. "We have every right to demand that judges remain acutely sensitive to changes in circumstances that often emerge over time" [to disqualify the durable standing of a court-appointed guardian or the proxy whom the patient previously had designated].

In a related article, Attorney Smith made this explicit recommendation: "If close family members object to dehydrating a cognitively disabled person and are committed enough in their desire to save their loved one's life to take the matter to court, dehydrations can be significantly delayed and sometimes even prevented. If the patient is unquestionably conscious, they may even win" [2003].

If you are among those who want to keep open the option of **Refusing Food & Fluid by Proxy**, you must overcome this formidable opposition. The rest of this chapter presents various strategies to meet this challenge, which are illustrated in the rest of the book.

25. WHO: Should I Base My Selection of Proxies on Their Personal Abilities or Because We Are Closely Related? and Can I Prevent Specific People From Making My Medical Decisions?

We now consider: the ideal qualities of Proxies; the trap of designating someone who **loves you too much** to let go; strategies to **prevent people you know** from imposing their agendas on you; and strategies to **prevent people you don't know** from gaining the authority to make your medical decisions.

The Qualities of "Ideal Proxies"

- They care about you and about honoring your end-of-life wishes;

- They will be **able** and **available** when you cannot speak for yourself;

- They are willing to learn about your end-of-life values and treatment preferences from you and your physician;

- They can be *trusted* to set aside *their* values and preferences as they make decisions based knowing *your* values and preferences;

- They are **assertive**, **articulate**, and **responsive**;

- They have an adequate **knowledge** of the challenges and workings of the health care and legal systems, OR are sufficiently **resourceful** to learn what they need to know; for example, they can ask an ethics committee or an elder-care or estate attorney to consult; and,

- They have sufficient **energy**, **persistence**, and **diplomacy** to vehemently advocate your Last Wishes.

An impressive list, isn't it? By starting with the ideal, at least you will know what to look for, and which possible candidates you might exclude. In our opinion, the most important quality is **trust**. Second is being **resourceful**. Often, that is more important than current knowledge since many challenges are not predictable and your Proxy can learn on an "as needed basis."

Many Advance Directives designate three individuals as Proxies because if the first or second choice is not willing, available, or able, there will still be an alternate. Older, single, and childless people from small families might find it a formidable task to select even one, let alone three Proxies. Many people may therefore need other options, such as a group of peers, or an organization comprised of qualified professionals, who can serve as Proxies.

Although only three States currently require it, we advise you to ask your designated Proxies to sign **written acknowledgments** that they **accept their duties**. Including their signatures in your **Proxy Directive (*Durable Power of Attorney for Health-Care Decision*)** transforms the document into a two-way agreement that can help empower your Proxies by establishing their standing and increase their authority to act on your behalf [see page 409-410], as their signatures attest to your discussing your specific end-of-life preferences.

The challenges of end-of-life decisions are hard enough without adding the "democratic" process. While it is fine for several caring people to discuss your options, and it is a good idea to inform all those who care about the important decisions you must make (to prevent disappointment, or worse, conflict), your **Proxy Directive** should still clearly state that your acting Proxy has complete authority to make health care decisions, and if this Proxy is not willing, or not able, or not available to serve, then your next alternate has complete authority to make those decisions on your behalf.

There are practical and psychological reasons for this recommendation. If your Advance Directive insisted on a majority or a consensus, one person might realize that he or she would be casting the life-determining deciding vote. That might paralyze him or her and cause a delay in decision-making that will prolong your suffering. Personal agendas and sibling rivalries could also cause delays.

Too Much Love?

Carefully consider if you want to designate someone as your Proxy if, from an emotional point of view... this person "cannot live" without you.

Sometimes those who know you best may also love you too much to take on the awesome responsibility to make emotionally wrenching end-of-life decisions. In some cases, you might consider designating a friend or a professional to serve as your Proxy, but then you must spend sufficient time to inform this person of your values and preferences. Lipkin [2006] found that when physicians asked married patients to name a Proxy, they did *not* name their spouses one-third of the time.

Relatives may prolong the dying process by holding onto a romantic or religious view of the caregiver's role. This may apply to "My Mother, My Child. A Caregiving Daughter Shares **Her** Emotional Eight-Year Journey," by Suzie Adams [2007, possibly out of print].

"Did Dad love so much that he could not let go?"

When I was a very little girl, my grandfather went into the hospital for a routine surgical procedure. Everyone expected him to return home in a few days. But something went wrong and he never regained consciousness. It took him five months to die. All that time, my grandmother struggled with some tough decisions. She never knew for sure what her husband of forty-six years would have wanted. Her experience was a lesson for the rest of us in the family on how important it is to discuss such things, ahead of time.

When I was a teenager, our dog, Cody, fell ill. The veterinarian said there was no hope for him to recover and that we should put him to sleep because he was in pain. But my father simply refused to give permission to put Cody to sleep. Dad held the dog in his lap, cleaned up after him, and made sure he had his medications. Emotionally, however, he couldn't bring the poor dog to the veterinarian to put an end to its suffering.

Years later, my mother shared with me that's when she wondered, *If Dad is having this much trouble making difficult choices for a dog, how long might he let me suffer?* Previously, my parents had given each other power of attorney to make medical decisions in the event of incompetence. But after Cody died, my mother contacted her lawyer and changed her designated agent from my dad to her brother. From that, I learned that sometimes even though you know someone loves you, you may not be able to trust him or her to make these most difficult decisions the way you would wish.

ക്കരു

Judges have the power to set aside your designated Proxy's authority to speak for you, if an "interested party" effectively challenges your Proxy as not acting in your "**best interests**." You can proactively avoid such challenges in two ways. You can *waive your legal right for a court review* of your Proxy's behavior by having your attorney add a paragraph to your Advance Directive after you discuss its ramifications. You may wish to re-read this Guideline in Chapter 3, "Waiver of my rights to avoid going to court... **To Delay** is **To Deny** honoring my Last Wishes."

In some States, you can exclude specific individuals or classes of people whom you anticipate might challenge your Last Wishes, for example, relatives who do not share your belief system. Regardless of what you write, however, others still may prevail in a hearing if they can convince the court there is some basis for accusing your Proxy of fraud, conspiracy, malicious intent, or abuse. If such violations are not proved, then the court review may not be prolonged, especially if you have stated you anticipated these people might try to intrude. It is also less likely that the court will appoint them as your guardian or conservator.

The next story is by a well-informed professional person who is justifiably worried. He has reason to exclude a certain relative from being his Proxy. The story explains why this author must remain anonymous. (Compare this story to the one where Vince calls 9-1-1 for Gus, on page 316).

"But they just want to save me."

I am personally and professionally involved with hospice and have read widely on end-of-life issues. I am also passionate about patient autonomy, including my own.

Recently I was told that one of my family members, a Catholic priest, learned that my Advance Directive contained certain specific stipulations that he felt compelled to fight because—in his opinion—I have an "unformed conscience" and thus do not have the capacity to make such decisions. The facts that I haven't been a Catholic in 30 years, only see him every 5 years, and that he has zero medical experience, are no barriers to his perceived right to usurp my autonomy and to impose his "perfectly formed conscience" on me.

It gets worse: He alleges that my suffering benefits other souls in Purgatory, and that makes him feel morally obligated to fight my expressed wishes.

For nearly fifty years, I have made well-informed decisions. I worked hard to put together a team of doctors whom I trust. They respect my wishes and they will HONOR them—at least as long as I have the ability to express myself.

But should I lapse into a state of unconsciousness, then I will suddenly be fair game for a whole host of individuals who want to make a "cottage industry" of my fate. Others are ready to insert their values into my relationship with my doctors and Proxy—to save my soul. The priest I mentioned is just one example of why I am so concerned for my fate.

I am also deeply concerned about other people. The increasing use of "Will to Live" documents that are touted as a better alternative to Living Wills, and the threat of new "Conscience Laws" that allow health care providers to refuse patients' requests, may have significant impact on how hospice can serve the dying, as the opponents' quest for aggressive curative treatment pledges to never stop.

The list of advocacy, religious, and rights organizations that claim they "actually care" about me is growing at an astronomical rate. The fact that they don't know anything about me, even the color of my eyes, is no deterrent to their willingness to speak on my behalf. All it takes is an URL, "charity" status, and a handy PayPal button to solicit donations, and they all get to advocate for what *they believe* is best for me.

But of course, we're not supposed to question their motives or the possible conflicts of interest of these people. "Saviors" are as exempt from such accountability as their institutions are from paying taxes.

◦◦◦

If your advance care planning leaves a door open for "interested parties" to contest the intent of your Proxy in court, honoring your Last Wishes may be delayed for years, especially if the case attracts people unknown to the family, whose motivations are religious and political. Terri Schiavo's fate was litigated for seven years. The fate of Nancy Beth Cruzan hung in balance for almost four years. Let's now consider the case of Robert Wendland, which was litigated for six years.

What Robert Wendland's Case Can Teach Us

The conflict in the case of Robert Wendland concerned which relative had the right to make medical decisions for him—his mother or his wife. Had Robert completed an Advance Directive, it is likely he would designated his wife and excluded his mother since he was estranged from his mother for a decade prior to his automobile accident.

After his mother went to court, advocacy groups representing both sides volunteered their legal experts. As the case dragged on, Robert's previously expressed oral wishes, as heard and reported by his wife, his brother, and his children were never considered *clear and convincing* (even though some experts felt this oral testimony was *clear and convincing*).

The California Supreme Court used the Wendland case to affirm the Constitutional right to life was so fundamental that they would not permit a court-appointed **Proxy to Refuse Food & Fluid** for patients in the Minimally Conscious State, even though the patient might experience suffering and therefore welcome the relief from being allowed to die.

To overcome the Constitutional right to life, the Court insisted on a written document to provide *clear and convincing* evidence even though the relevant law passed by California's legislators did not require this high level standard of evidence. Since Wendland did not have such a written document, his Food & Fluid would have thus continued indefinitely.

At the age of 49, however, one month *before* the Court published its precedent-setting ruling, Robert Wendland died of pneumonia. Obviously, the California Supreme Court was strongly motivated to establish this precedent.

The potential to reduce family conflict by creating Advance Directives is illustrated in the next story, a piece of fiction based on the known facts.

Several weeks after Robert Wendland died, his
wife Rose "received" this letter (fiction*):

"Why didn't you listen? Why didn't you ask?"
by Robert Wendland from the Other Side

Dear Rose:

It's rare to get a chance to write a letter after you've died, but in my case, it's not so much a privilege as a duty. It's because I made such a terrible mess of things. Here's my deal: if you send this letter to others who can learn from my mistakes, Rose, then I can rest in peace.

I know it's not enough to write it, but I'm really sorry I caused you and others so much suffering for so long. I apologize for what I did, and also for what I did not do. Time is different here so I've had an opportunity to think about all that happened, and it all seems so much clearer now...

Back in 1993, I should not have driven my car after I drank alcohol, but everyone already knows that.

I appreciate that you, my family, and my doctors had the patience to wait two years to see if I would come out of my coma. I also needed to see for myself what kind of mental and physical state I would be in. The truth is that after I woke up, I clearly realized that my life stunk. Even after lots of frustrating physical therapy, I could not walk, talk, drink or feed myself without help. It was embarrassing to be cleaned up and changed like a baby. As far as recognizing people: For a time, sometimes I could; but mostly I couldn't. As I now look back, it was horrible to see how much that hurt you and our children.

What made me most miserable? Not being able to express myself. I wanted to die, but the only ways I could express myself were to be agitated, irritable, and uncooperative. I'm sorry, but when I bit that nurse who was trying to treat me, inside I was really screaming, "Let me go. Let me die."

Finally, after I pulled out that damn feeding tube for the <u>fourth time</u>, people got my message. I was really happy when you refused to sign the consent for surgery to replace that feeding tube, Rose. Enough is enough!

I was also glad that the hospital's ethics committee unanimously voted in favor of your decision. Well done! But the committee members made a terrible mistake. They failed to ask if any other members of my family might object. Of course they didn't know my mother was visiting me secretly. They had only been told we'd been on the outs for ten years. Still, they should have tried to contact her.

I know that woman. She was furious that no one told her about my condition. She felt ignored, like she didn't count at all in my life. That's why she dug in her heels. She probably also wanted to try to make up for all our lost years and to prove she really was a good mother. Then things got more complicated when she went to court and all those lawyers with their own private crusades got involved.

If only the ethics committee had contacted my mother early on... It might have avoided this conflict.

Moving ahead to August 2001, I was shocked that the California Supreme Court did not accept your knowledge of my wishes. For God's sake, my brother and our daughters and son all backed you up. Of course I said, "I would not want to live like a vegetable." I said that several times.

So my first lament is aimed at the court: <u>Why didn't you listen?</u>

I can understand why the judges were worried. Removing my feeding tube would lead to an irreversible result. But I did not want to live like a vegetable. I heard the court's strict definition of <u>clear and convincing</u>— "so clear as to leave no substantial doubt [and] sufficiently strong to command the unhesitating assent of every reasonable mind." Yet I thought you were <u>clear and convincing</u> in expressing my wishes!

I regret not completing a <u>Proxy Directive</u> to make sure that you could make my medical decisions, or a <u>Living Will</u> to indicate my Last Wishes. But I was healthy and only 41. How could I know what would happen? Yet if I had completed an Advance Directive, my case would probably not have gone to court. Even if it did go to court, it would have been decided quickly. But since the court had to appoint you as my conservator, the judges felt they were obligated to consider my "best interests."

My second lament is that my doctors did not give me enough opportunity to express my wishes. Back in 1995, I could still understand questions... But it was not until 1997 that Dr. Leon Kass asked me the most important question: "Do you want to die?" But he only asked me once. Just once! The California Supreme Court made a big point that I did not answer. Believe me, I wasn't thinking deeply about the alternatives. I was just out of it! Simply and totally out of it.

You know what I wish? That back in 1995, when I could still understand such questions, that Dr. Kass, or another doctor would have asked me several times in several ways to be sure if I wanted to die. At that point, I could have indicated, "Yes," every time!

So my second lament is aimed at my doctors: <u>Why didn't you ask?</u>

I realize it would have been tedious to ask me questions that I could answer "Yes" or "No." But if a doctor did have the patience, he could have saved me six years of suffering, six years of feeling *indignity and frustration as I lived like a vegetable, and for you, six horrible years of terrible legal battles. Doctors should not have assumed I could not answer consistently in 1995. They should have tried. A few minutes for six years? I so wish they had.*

My duty to write you ends with these two requests, Rose. First, tell everyone to complete an Advance Directive; otherwise, the courts may not listen. Second, for people like me who end up without an Advance Directive, tell their doctors to make every attempt to ask them what they want—several times and in a variety of ways—to see if their responses are consistent. There is no question more important than, "Do you want to live or to die?"

So, Rose dear, please: Send this letter to people who can learn from my mistakes. Then I'll be able to rest in peace.

Your husband,

Robert

*No one knows what actually went through Robert Wendland's mind, of course, but this fictional interpretation is one possibility. It was based on the following: the "Conservatorship of the Person of ROBERT WENDLAND, S087265," filed August 9, 2001; on conversations with attorney Jon B. Eisenberg, of Eisenberg & Hancock, Encino, CA, who wrote the amicus appeal brief for a group of ethicists; on discussions with Lawrence Nelson, the attorney who represented Robert Wendland's wife, Rose; and on the video, "Who Speaks for Robert: The Importance of Having an Advance Health Care Directive," Center for Humane and Ethical Medical Care, UCLA Medical Center, Santa Monica.

❧ *SKIP*

Would a Proxy Directive have been sufficient to avoid the Wendlands' six years of litigation?

On the video mentioned above, Attorney Lawrence Nelson stated that the family could have avoided six years of litigation if, before the accident that rendered him incompetent, Robert Wendland had signed a **Proxy Directive** to designate his wife Rose as his Proxy.

—Possible, but not certain. While Attorney Nelson stated his opinion prior to the final acts of the Terri Schiavo saga, he still [as of September 2005] stands by his claim that the California Supreme Court would have honored Rose's decision to refuse to consent to the reinsertion of the feeding tube if she had been authorized to speak for her husband via a legally valid, durable power of attorney for health care. Consider this possibility, however:

Those who generally oppose removing feeding tubes from patients who have not clearly and convincingly stated that is their wish (for example, attorney Wesley J. Smith), could have argued along these lines:

1. Our neurology expert thinks Robert can function at a level higher than the Minimally Conscious State if we offer him the opportunity to benefit from _____ , a new treatment program;

2. Rose is dating another man so it is obvious that she would benefit both financially and emotionally if Robert were dead. Even though Robert designated her as his Proxy, Rose now has a highly questionable conflict of interest so the court should consider if her decisions are really in Robert's Best Interest; and,

3. How could it ever be in the Best Interest of someone who is conscious to endure the cruel and barbaric ordeal of starving to death?

This was Attorney Nelson's reply: "Yes, they could have used those tactics for delay, even though they were not consistent with the facts. MediCal stopped paying for further treatment for Robert's rehabilitation since it was obvious that it was not providing Robert any benefit since he was not improving. I don't know if Rose had another person in her life, but that's irrelevant: She would not have had to 'bump off' her husband to have a [new] relationship. Moreover, Robert would not have suffered after discontinuance of the feeding tube; he would have been sedated as all patients should be when they might suffer if treatment is stopped." Attorney Nelson shared that when Robert developed signs of pneumonia, he was given a broad spectrum antibiotic for one week, but never deprived of hydration, and the judge did not permit petitions to force doctors to treat Robert with IV antibiotics. However Attorney Nelson did agree that the opposing attorneys' tactic **To Delay** is tantamount **To Deny** since they consider it "winning" to prolong the biologic existence.

Would a Living Will (**Directive to Physician**) have sufficed? Only if the description of his diagnosis or functional status was worded so precisely that all physicians agreed that he had reached the state described. Even if written, the words, "I do not want to live like a vegetable," might not have sufficed. At the time Robert was still able to create his Living Will, neurologists had not yet reached a consensus on how to diagnosis the Minimally Conscious State.

What would it take for Wendland's Last Wishes to be honored? In our opinion, a **Proxy Directive** worded to give Rose maximum power, supplemented by a document called **Empowering Statements for My Proxy** that explained and provided reasons for his choices. This is all discussed below.

&❧ *CONTINUE*

26. WHAT Specific Wording Will Empower My Proxies to Have the Authority to Refuse Food & Fluid on My Behalf?

It is prudent to **specifically empower** your designated Proxies to exercise **Voluntary Refusal of Food & Fluid** on your behalf in written documents that have been signed by qualified witnesses.

&❧ *SKIP*

Some States will accept your Proxy's decisions to discontinue other life-sustaining treatments but will not accept your **Proxy's decision to Refuse Food & Fluid** on your behalf unless you specifically authorize this power in writing. Other States permit individuals whom you have specifically designated in writing to serve as your Proxies, but deny the same powers to your next of kin if you have not used a witnessed written document to designate them. Some States also deny court-appointed guardians to have the power to **Refuse Food & Fluid**. A few states require second opinions from doctors to determine that you are terminal or in a Permanent Vegetative State before your **Proxy can Refuse Food & Fluid** on your behalf. Many States restrict **Refusing Food & Fluid** for patients in the Minimally Conscious State, even though it is likely that these patients may experience more suffering than patients in the Permanent Vegetative State [Sieger and others, 2002]. As previously noted on page 184, Ohio converts Proxy Directives into Living Wills for this option.

&❧ *CONTINUE*

Even if a diligent review of the relevant laws in your State reveals no current restrictions, do not be complacent. Legislators may pass new laws and judges may interpret existing laws in a restrictive manner. "Interested parties" may argue that providing Food & Fluid is basic, ordinary, usual, customary, humane care that is always required to honor the dignity of all human beings whose quality of life and potential for recovery is inappropriate for other human beings to judge, even if their doctors provide a nearly certain prognosis that the state of unconsciousness or minimal consciousness will be permanent.

The potential for vehement challenges to **Refusal of Food & Fluid** increased after the legal battle over Terri Schiavo's fate in 2005, and the U.S. Supreme Court decision in Gonzales v. Oregon [2006]. In May 2005, the National Right to Life Committee published a "Model Starvation And Dehydration Of Persons With

Disabilities **Prevention** Act." The model law's purpose: Unless *clear and convincing* written documents state otherwise, doctors must presume you want artificial administration of Food & Fluid to continue indefinitely. Discussed in detail later, the law has problems such as not defining the group of people to whom it would apply, or who would pay for the additional cost of medical care. Yet as of March 2006, twenty-three States were considering it or similar laws.

The situation may change in 35 years however, according to Peter Singer, who wrote that in cases where "some living, breathing human beings have suffered such severe brain damage that they will never regain consciousness... with the hope of recovery gone, families and loved ones will usually understand that even if the human organism is still alive, the person they loved has ceased to exist. Hence, a decision to remove the feeding tube will be less controversial, for it will be a decision to end the life of a human body, but not of a person" [2005]. Perhaps this jargon will become as familiar as **DNR**: "Permit Natural Dying" (**PND**) for patients in Devastating Irreversible Brain States (**DIBS**). Some bylaws of hospitals and State statutes (including Texas, as previously mentioned) now permit doctors to refuse to treat patients if they feel such treatment is futile.

The bottom line is, if you want to empower your **Proxy to Refuse Food & Fluid** on your behalf, you should state so, specifically. On a procedural level, State laws can require a statement that...

A. You wish to **empower your Proxy** to make decisions about nutrition and hydration;

B. **Your Proxy knows** what your wishes are (without specifying what they are);

C. Your Proxy can carry out only exactly **what you specify**; for example, most boilerplate and State-provided forms use the words "**artificially** administered," but you may wish to authorize your Proxy also to refuse forced feeding by another's hand where Food & Fluid is placed in your mouth to swallow.

If you trust your Proxy and want to authorize the broadest possible powers, consider using words similar to these in your Advance Directive:

It is frequently important to add the word "**oral**" to your Advance Directive, to overcome the bias of culture that has become imbedded in the law. For terminal patients, Winter stated, "the evidence suggests that unrequested nutritional support provided by either the enteral [by mouth] or parenteral [not by mouth] route to a terminally ill patient may be both medically and ethically indefensible because it may increase suffering without improving outcome" [2000].

Consider again, in more detail, the law of the State of New York:

The wording of the "New York Health Care Proxy" form has these clear instructions: "**Unless your agent reasonably knows your wishes about *artificial* nutrition and hydration (nourishment and water provided**

by a feeding tube or intravenous line), he or she will not be allowed to refuse or consent to those measures for you." The form's instructions even suggest sample wording for your consideration: "If you want to give your agent broad authority, you may do so right on the form. Simply write: *I have discussed my wishes with my health care agent and alternate and they know my wishes including those about* **artificial** *nutrition and hydration*." {Original emphasis in Italics; bolding the word "artificial" added [New York, 2005].}

Note: The instructions state "broad," not "broadest," authority. The "broadest" would be to include both **oral** (assisted by another's hand) as well as what is called *artificial* nutrition and hydration. So residents of New York State who want their agent to have the legal option to **Refuse ORAL Food & Fluid** under some circumstances, must add the word, "**oral**," to their additional statement on the form. This is how the final statement might look: "*I have discussed my wishes with my health care agent and alternate and they know my wishes including those about both* **oral** *(manually assisted) and* **artificial** *(that is, artificially administered) nutrition and hydration*."

Readers who may be wondering if the detailed consideration of the above wording belabors a minor point can re-read the case of Lee Kahan, and then imagine how many times this demented woman may have been force-fed in a way similar to the woman who is described next:

"Poor Mom must endure forced oral feeding."

As I observed the staff interacting with my mother at meal times, it looked like assault, but the attorneys I consulted told me that "battery" is the correct legal term. Three times a day, my mother suffered from an ordeal that the nurses called "assisted feeding." I would instead call this procedure, "forced-feeding against her wishes."

One person held her down and squeezed her cheeks to open her mouth while the other placed some puree deeply in her mouth. After she swallowed, the process was repeated, again and again.

One day, after they finished feeding her, I stood in front of the door and insisted that they explain to me, exactly what they were doing.

They said my mother's higher brain function was gone, so she did not understand that she needed to open her mouth. I cannot imagine that she derived any pleasure from the taste or feel of the food since the staff was trained to place the food at the back of the tongue to stimulate her primitive swallowing reflex. Her intact lower brain helped prevent anything but air from entering her windpipe. This primitive reflex is what prevents food being aspirated that can cause a fatal pneumonia. But that leaves no enjoyment from the taste or the feel of eating food.

This additional understanding motivated me to take the necessary steps so that I will never have to endure this ordeal. I empowered my **Proxy to Refuse manually assisted ORAL Food & Fluid** on my behalf.

A listener called me during a radio interview [KPBS, *These Days*, Dec. 4, 2006] to relate discovering her mother's broken tooth. Unfortunately, this is not rare. Doctors write orders for nurses and nursing assistants to carry out, but they rarely stand at the bedside to see how those orders are carried out. Family members may have to insist that the attending doctor add specific words to their orders. Instead of merely writing, "Full liquid diet," or "Soft diet," doctors should add, "**As Patient Permits**," to respect patients who wish to decline food nonverbally. Perhaps someday, the acronym "**APP**" will be commonly recognized. The Table on page 219 puts this doctor's order into perspective for patients who suffer from severe dementia.

27. WHY Must My Reasons be "Clear and Convincing" to Support My Proxy's Future Refusal of Food & Fluid?

[BASIC FORM: I Authorize My Proxy to Refuse Food & Fluid on My Behalf]

You must **clearly and convincingly** write specific reasons why under some circumstances, you want your Proxy to have the option to **Refuse Food & Fluid** on your behalf, as the *BEST* option at some point in the last chapter of your life. Without an adequate explanation, others may challenge your wishes and they may not be honored. A relative, a doctor, an administrator, a religious leader, or a politician could argue that your Proxy's decision is not in your BEST INTEREST. Even if your wishes eventually prevail in court, **To Delay** is **To Deny** and the process of litigation itself could effectively deny your wishes for a very long time.

Even if you reside in a State that has not (yet) adopted the legal standard of evidence that certain end-of-life wishes must be *clear and convincing*, if your case were litigated or if the legal standard for evidence were changed, you might be held to the new standard. That is what occurred in the case of Robert Wendland: The judges of the California Supreme Court legislated from the bench by invoking a requirement for the higher standard of evidence. Although it was not part of the law when legislators passed it, or when Mr. Wendland had his accident, it still applied to him. Now, their ruling that requires *clear and convincing evidence* for certain types of patients has set a precedent for others, in California.

Authorization for My Proxy to Refuse Food & Fluid

I. General Considerations:

I may reach a point in the progression of a serious illness when I would no longer want nutrition and hydration by any route—whether its administration is considered "medical" or "artificial" because it enters my circulatory system or gastrointestinal system via tubes; or considered "non-medical" and "natural" because the route is oral; that is, even though I still could swallow what another puts into my mouth.

I have discussed my values and preferences with my designated Proxies and informed them about MY criteria for when I want them to refuse nutrition and hydration on my behalf since at that time I would no longer possess decision-making capacity. My criteria are NOT diagnosis-dependent although I clearly would **NOT want to continue Food & Fluid** in the Minimally Conscious State, the Permanent Vegetative State, end-stage dementia, or if I were suffering as I was dying.

I expect my Proxy (and alternates) to consult with my future treating physicians about my condition and any advances in medicine. Then I want my Proxies to advocate my Last Wishes, as they understand them. I authorize my Proxy's decision to override (other people's interpretation of) what I wrote in my Proxy Directive. (If I used only a Living Will, the statements below may help my physician learn what I want.)

II. Empowering Statements for My Proxy to Refuse Food & Fluid on My Behalf: "Let My Proxy Decide"

I empower My Proxy to **Refuse Food & Fluid** on my behalf based on any of the following reasons:

With adequate *Comfort Care*, **Refusal of Food & Fluid** would provide a compassionate, humane method for me to avoid prolonged physical, spiritual, and existential suffering;

Refusal of Food & Fluid would reduce the time of emotional suffering by my family members and close friends as they wait for me to pass on from a disease from which I have no, or a very unlikely chance of recovering;

Refusal of Food & Fluid would limit the bad memories my family members (especially younger ones) might have of me in a state of indignity, when most of my energy was devoted to medical care, or when I was totally dependent on others for basic care, or when I lacked control over my body functions, or when I could no longer interact with other human beings in a positive and meaningful way;

Refusal of Food & Fluid would reduce the consumption of financial resources of my personal estate and/or of society so that these resources can be put to better use than to merely prolong my biologic existence;

Refusal of Food.& Fluid is NOT a "cruel sentence to die by starvation and dehydration," but rather MY preferred way to Permit Natural Dying.

My mental state as I write this statement:

I *understand* the choice to forgo nutrition and hydration compared to its alternatives. I *appreciate* the consequences of this choice for myself and others. I have used *reasoning* to authorize my Proxy to let my future physician know when I want him or her to **Withhold Food & Fluid** on my behalf. I have considered this decision long enough to *express consistently* my preference for this way to hasten the process of my dying. This choice, which I fully discussed with my Proxies, is consistent with my life-long values, made voluntarily without undue influence, and without my feeling I am currently a burden on others, or the result of an acute depression.

To those who visit me in the future, "Let My Proxy Decide":

Human behavior in severely brain damaged people can be confusing for those not trained in Neurology. Primitive *reflexes* from the still functioning lower brain may appear similar to the *purposeful movements* from higher brain functions that are meant to communicate intent. To help reduce confusion, I provide some examples below but the actual circumstance may be different so let me be clear: I trust my Proxy so **"Let My Proxy Decide."** (These four words will be my poetic refrain.)

> A. If I moan and "an interested party" argues that I appear to be suffering, **Let My Proxy Decide** if I should receive only *Comfort Care* (including medications for thirst, pain, insomnia, agitation,shortness of breath, nausea, itching) instead of resuming administration of Food & Fluid.

> B. If I seem to enjoy ice chips or if I move my head toward a spray of water, and "an interested party" argues that I appear to be thirsty, **Let My Proxy Decide** if I should receive only *Comfort Care* (especially mouth care) rather than administration of fluid.

The words I am writing now express the wishes I wish to be **durable** as I currently possess the mental capacity to make medical decisions. If in the future, I no longer can communicate a choice, I do not want an "interested party" to argue that my reflexive behavior indicates that I have changed my mind. Instead, **Let My Proxy Decide**. I also do not want an "interested party" to argue that my wishes would change based on a subsequent edict by a political or religious leader. Instead, **Let My Proxy Decide**. If I have made a mistake in granting this durable authority to my Proxy, I will accept the consequences. I prefer this alternative to granting other individuals the opportunity to challenge my Proxy's authority since **To Delay is To Deny**.

You must TRUST YOUR PROXY and alternates for this decision to be prudent. Consider designating a professional as your Proxy, or modifying the FORM to: Empowering Statements for *My Living Will Advocate* to attach to a Living Will. (See the on-line version at www.caringadvocates.org/articles.php.)

Specific examples from your personal experience, or from your reactions to movies, books, plays, or newspaper or magazine articles, can support your decision to **Refuse Food & Fluid** by Proxy. Perhaps you knew someone who remained unconscious for a very long time before they died, or you had definite feelings about the highly publicized cases of Karen Ann Quinlan, Nancy Beth Cruzan, Robert Wendland, or Terri Schiavo. You may also have had feelings about movies where end-of-life choices were important themes (see below).

Caveat: When writing your Advance Directive, use general words to describe the medical condition exemplified in movies, such as, "If my condition became *similar* to hers." This will reduce the possibility that a court of law will interpret your comments in an overly restrictive way. Also, provide several different examples. Consider the differences in the three movies below. (They were chosen in part because they also illustrate other important points.)

"Million Dollar Baby"

" I saw the movie, 'Million Dollar Baby,' and realized that I would agree with Maggie's decision not to live. She was the boxer who became quadriplegic, as played by actor Hilary Swank. The fighter's conviction to die was so strong that she purposefully bit her tongue and almost bled to death.

"If I were trapped in a paralyzed body and dependent on others because of such severe limitations in functioning or in a similar medical condition (as determined by my Proxy after consulting my physician), and I could no longer speak for myself, then I would want my Proxy to have the power to refuse on my behalf, all nutrition and hydration, mechanical ventilation, and other life-sustaining treatment since I would not want to be kept alive indefinitely, dependent on machines."

❦

Writing clear examples like this one may help your Proxy argue effectively with those in power, including resistant doctors and administrators at nursing homes or hospitals, who might otherwise fear a lawsuit based on a theory of neglect if your Proxy requested **Refusal of Food & Fluid** on your behalf.

Comments on how "well" Maggie died:

Maggie's life ends on an exquisitely loving note as Frankie, her trainer and her only friend in the world, kisses her cheek after he finally reveals the meaning of the words she had heard the crowds chant at her boxing fights: "Mo Cuishle." Frankie's translation from Gaelic will be the last words Maggie will ever hear: "My darling, my blood."

This scene is tender and touching, however we strongly disagree with the medical way Maggie dies. Frankie injects a huge overdose of adrenaline into her IV line. That would cause the muscles of her heart to increase the speed and strength at which they contract to the point where her heart becomes totally disorganized and fails to pump at all. When the resulting painful sensations in her chest are added to the direct anxiety-producing effect of adrenaline on her brain, it is clear why dying from an overdose of adrenaline is definitely NOT peaceful. What is? Doctors would **first** sedate her sufficiently to eliminate all anxiety with an anesthetic type of medicine, and **then** turn off her ventilator.

Maggie's decision to die came in the immediate shadow of two great losses. Previously, she regained some of her fighting personality, and Frankie suggested that she enroll at City College. But after a visit from her critical and derogatory mother, Maggie has no doubt that her mother is only interested in getting her money. The other loss: Maggie's leg was amputated. Losses can lead to depression; however it is possible to overcome them. Yet no psychiatrist ever sees her, despite her suicide attempt of biting her tongue.

After he is asked to help, Frankie consults with his priest and explains, "But now she wants to die. And I just want to keep her with me. And I swear to God, Father, it's... it's committing a sin by doing it. But keeping her alive is killing her. You know what I mean? How do I get around that?"

"You don't. You step aside, Frankie. You leave her with God," the priest answers.

"She's not asking for God's help. She's asking for mine," Frankie says.

After the priest notes Frankie is the kind of person who cannot forgive himself, he says, "Forget God, or Heaven and Hell. If you do this thing, you'll be lost... You'll never find yourself again." The dramatic point was well made: Despite the moral toll of great guilt, Frankie did what he thought was right for his friend.

However, "In the real world she would not make such a request of her friend," wrote Dr. Arthur Caplan. "Instead, she would ask her doctor and nurses to shut off her ventilator. She would ask to be allowed to die, not be killed... Every competent American has the right to stop any and all medical care that they do not want. 'Million Dollar Baby' makes us think we are more powerless than we really are." Dr. Caplan concluded that film audiences were grossly misinformed about end-of-life options by the movie's "one glaring flaw" that "made too much of assisted suicide." [MSNBC, 2-17-05.]

This movie reflects an unfortunate trend for patients to leave doctors out of planning for, and the facing of, end-of-life challenges. A research study by Dr. Kolarik and his colleagues [2002] asked whether patients would prefer to indicate specific treatment instructions or general statements about values and goals in their advance planning, but an unexpected result had even greater significance. The researchers initially approached 206 eligible patients but the majority refused to participate; of those who were interested enough to spend a third of an hour thinking about end-of-life choices, only 2 initiated a discussion about Advance Directives with their personal physicians. The study thus demonstrates a huge reluctance to involve physicians in advance care planning.

My harshest criticism of "Million Dollar Baby" is that it did not portray a good way to say goodbye. While it won four Academy Awards—for best picture, best director, best actress, and best supporting actor in February 2005—and while it made sense for a trainer to have access to the drug, adrenaline, the film does not get our votes for illustrating how to maximize peacefulness for the patient. Nor does it show how to minimize guilt for the caring survivor.

Let's now consider another example, a British play by Brian Clark [1978]. It was made into a movie nine years before the U.S. Supreme Court decision on Nancy Cruzan that asserted the right of every competent patient to refuse any medical treatment.

"Whose Life Is It, Anyway?"

After I saw the movie, "Whose life is it, anyway?," I realized how much I identified with the philosophy of Ken, the quadriplegic character who was played by Richard Dreyfuss. He described what his life had become, to answer the judge's question of why his choice to decide to die was reasonable: "It is a question of dignity. Look at me here. I can do nothing, not even the basic primitive functions [of] urination [or moving my] bowels [or] turn over [or] act on any conclusions... I find the hospital's persistent effort to maintain this shadow of a life an indignity that is inhumane... If I choose to live, it would be appalling if society killed me... If I choose to die, it is equally appalling if society keeps me alive… Dignity starts with choice. Without it, it is degrading because technology has taken over from human will."

While Ken could argue for himself, if my medical condition was similar but I could not speak for myself, then I would want my Proxy to have the power to decide to Refuse Nutrition and Hydration on my behalf. I would also want an impartial psychiatrist to evaluate my mental status, to determine if I was suffering from a depressive disorder severe enough to affect my judgment, that was not based on the reality of my current situation or could be treated.

In the play and movie, an expedited hearing was held on a *writ of habeas corpus*, which is the legal procedure to release a person from **unlawful restraint**. Ken's doctor knew that discharging Ken would give him the opportunity to allow his life to end. Although Ken's doctor wanted to restrain him and argued that Ken's judgment was impaired from a depressive disorder, the judge agreed with Ken and allowed him to leave the hospital.

The end of the play has an interesting twist, one that underscores a major advantage of **Voluntary Refusal of Food & Fluid**. The doctor asks Ken, "Where will you go?"

Ken answers, "I'll get a room somewhere."

The doctor responds, "There's no need. We'll stop treatment, remove the drips. Stop feeding you if you like. You'll be unconscious in three days, dead in six at most."

Skeptical about the doctor's sudden change in attitude, Ken asks, "There'll be no last minute resuscitation?"

The doctor answers, "Only with your permission."

Ken says, "That's very kind; why are you doing it?"

The doctor explains, "Simple. **You might change your mind**."

A recent movie has a similar beginning, yet warrants a different set of remarks:

"Just Like Heaven"

A successful young female physician has a horrible automobile accident. The only person who can see her, and save her life, is her roommate, with whom she has fallen in love. The character played by Mark Ruffalo tries to steal her body from the hospital, but fails. But when he gives Reese Witherspoon a loving kiss, she awakens from her three-month coma—just seconds before the competitive, opportunistic doctor would have "pulled the plug." After she regains her memory, the two live happily ever after.

You might write: "Based on my viewing the movie, 'Just Like Heaven,' and other information I have learned, if I were in a coma for three months, I would NOT want my life to depend on a single signature and one physician's opinion about my prognosis. One physician could be wrong or even biased, as in this movie. For the most important decision of my life—to end it—I would want at least one other, independent physician to examine me and provide his or her opinion on my prognosis. I would also want to wait at least six months.

Comment: This remake of "Snow White" fulfills Hollywood's goal to entertain at the expense of deliberate and gross misinformation. To provide conflict and give the hero an opportunity to save the girl in distress while supporting the theory that "love conquers all," this modern-day fairly tale would have its viewers believe all of the following: a) doctors cannot be trusted; b) their personal ambitions can lead them to not give patients the chance they deserve to live; c) doctors can be "dead wrong" that a prognosis is hopeless and ignore well-established neurological criteria that hope is quite appropriate at three months in cases of mechanical head injury; and d) hospitals have no mechanism for reviews and appeals such as ethics committees whose members would deliberate at length before discontinuing life-support.

No comment about this movie could be more pithy than the original title of Marc Levy's book from which it was adapted: "If It Were Only True."

28. HOW Can I Empower My Proxies so Their Decisions Will Override What I Have Written in Other Documents if There is a Perceived Conflict? Should I?

If a controversy arises between what you wrote in your Living Will (in practice, how others interpret what you meant by what you wrote) and your Proxy's current decision about an end-of-life medical treatment, unless you have clearly stated otherwise, your words in the Living Will (depending on the State) will, or may, override your Proxy's decision. However you can change this order of priority by stating in your Advance Directive that you want your Proxy's decision to override what you have written in your other advance care planning documents.

Caveat: Do not designate others to serve as your Proxy unless you trust them to advocate *your*, not *their*, end-of-life choices, based on *your* values and preferences, not *theirs*.

Consider one legal battle that resolved near the end of 2004:

Wife (Proxy) Tried to Override Her Husband's Living Will

The Case of Hanford Pinette

In 1998, Hanford Pinette signed two documents. In his Living Will, he stated that in the event of a terminal illness with no probability of recovery, he wanted "to die naturally" and to receive medication only to "alleviate pain." But his Durable Power of Attorney for Health Care designated his wife Alice as his surrogate. So she would make medical decisions for him if he ever became incompetent.

In February 2004, 73 year-old Mr. Pinette was admitted to a hospital in Orlando, Florida. His diagnosis was severe congestive heart failure. After trying to improve his functioning, his doctors agreed that further treatment was futile so they wanted to remove him from life-prolonging machines, in accordance with the instructions of his Living Will. But his wife Alice, functioning as his Proxy, refused and said, "No."

While **To Delay** can be **To Deny**, Mr. Pinette was fortunate since his case was expeditiously litigated. The local trial court promptly responded in favor of the doctors' consensus of opinion that was consistent with his Living Will. His wife did NOT file an appeal. Perhaps by then, Alice had spent enough time grieving so she felt she could let her husband go. Thus it took "only" a few months rather than several years for the court to authorize his doctors to follow his written instructions to discontinue life-support.

໔໐

If Hanford Pinette's Advance Directive had given top priority to his Proxy's decisions over the written instructions in his Living Will (which this book recommends only when you do trust your Proxy), then his real wishes, at least as his doctors and the court interpreted them, might NOT have been honored. So his story is an **instructive warning**: Granting your Proxy such power is recommended only if you can trust him or her, and all the people you name as alternate Proxies.

While you are still capable of advance planning, it is *your responsibility* to make sure your Proxy understands your wishes and that you can trust your Proxy to advocate them. To reduce the risk that your Proxy will make decisions based on "loving you too much" instead of what you really want, and the risk of a conflict between your Proxy's decisions and your Living Will, consider these five suggestions as you create or revise your Advance Directive:

1. Be diligent about the wording in your Living Will by completing it in the context of discussions with your physician who knows your specific medical situation;

2. Direct your Proxy to consult with your doctor when making critical decisions;

3. Give your Proxy the option of consulting independent professionals in the field, and to consider their second opinions;

4. Consider naming a professional in the field to serve as your Proxy to spare your relative, or as an alternate Proxy to whom your relative can pass the torch; and,

5. Include guilt-reducing statements in your Advance Directive; for example: "Serving as a Proxy is not easy. I would understand if you were too emotional to make tough decisions and you allowed the alternate Proxy to assume these awesome responsibilities. If you do serve as my Proxy, I realize that many decisions would be close calls even if I could still make them myself, and that there is no way even I could be certain that I had made the right decision. So, all you can do is to try to make the best decision you can with the information you have available at the time. Don't be upset, for example, if a cure is found a few months later..."

It might help to put the challenge in perspective to consider an example of what many would consider selfish behavior by a relative:

"But we still watch football games together."

A husband kept his wife alive for many years even though she was in a Permanent Vegetative State. She was maintained on artificial feeding and sometimes required mechanical ventilation to breathe. On Sundays, he wheeled her into the nursing home's common room to sit beside her. Both wore jerseys of their favorite quarterback of their local team as they watched the Cleveland Browns play football.

About this story, Dr. Post wrote [1995], "The concept of quality of life might be the quality of lives, including family members." Dr. Koch wrote [1998], "Many would argue that personhood ends with the onset of a persistent vegetative state, that life in a permanent coma is 'no life at all.' Even that is rejected, however, by those who live with and care for such patients." Attorney Lois Shepherd [2006a] argued that "PVS patients have absolutely no interest in living"; therefore "continued tube feeding…cannot be justified as an action taken in their interest" but "in the interests of others, whether they be politicians or loved ones... even, at times an exploitation."

Comment: Again, do NOT empower your Proxy if you do not trust him or her. In this particular case, an interested third party could actually have requested a consultation from an ethics committee and challenged the husband's maintaining his wife's existence on the basis of her continued existence that was NOT in her best interest. However on a practical level, this would probably not happen unless a second relative also agreed.

In some States, including California, your Proxy can make medical decisions with you as soon as you sign the Advance Directive form—if you so choose—rather than wait until a health professional determines that you no longer have the mental ability to make medical decisions. As long as you have decision-making capacity, you can still override medical decisions your Proxy makes. In practice, you need not have decision-making capacity to prolong life; only to hasten dying. Collaborating with your Proxy may expedite routine medical care long before there is any need to make life-or-death decisions. The process may help you learn if your Proxy would likely make the same decisions that you would, if someday, you no longer have the mental ability to make your own medical decisions. Listening to physicians when you are ill is an emotional experience, and sometimes, you may not hear or remember everything that your physician tells you. These are many good reasons to have your Proxy collaborate immediately.

If you discover that you and your Proxy have divergent points of view, as long as you have decision-making capacity, you can eliminate this person and designate another to serve as your Proxy.

Some ethnic traditions do not accept the mainstream standard of individualized "informed consent." Instead, patients may leave decisions to the family head, or sometimes to a group, for consensus. In such subcultures, the immediate empowerment of Proxies may be particularly appropriate.

If the laws of your State do not specifically allow Proxies to have instant authority, ask your attending physicians if they would agree to such an arrangement; if so, ask your lawyer to create a power-of-attorney document that will accomplish this. Also consider carefully whether or not you want this power of attorney to be "durable" if you are not yet sure you want this person to be your Proxy. (An alternative could be to require you to renew the power-of-attorney every couple of years, but to continue indefinitely if you became incompetent.)

29. WHY is it Risky to Rely Solely on a Living Will?

I prefer the term, **"Directive to Physician"** to **"Living Will"** since some authors and some laws use the term "Living Will" to mean "Advance Directive" or vice versa, which creates confusion. In this book, an **Advance Directive** consists of either or both: a **Proxy Directive** and a **Directive to Physician**. (See also, the **Glossary** beginning on page 457, and the **Table** of *New* and Recommended Terms about Advance Care Planning.)

Experience has shown a variety of reasons for why it is risky to rely on a **Directive to Physician**. Here are some:

1. It is difficult to predict your future condition accurately. Unless your doctor has given you a specific diagnosis, you may find it difficult to accurately predict your future condition. For example, Michael Martin and Robert Wendland used the imprecise word "vegetable," which judges in Michigan and California ruled did NOT include the Minimally Conscious State.

If the words you use to describe your future medical condition are *too specific*, they may exclude your future state. But if your words are *too vague*, others may argue whether or not your treatment preferences should be applied. Any word can become the focus of controversy; for example does the word "persistent" when modifying "severe brain damage" imply that the condition is irreversible? Whenever something can be argued, **To Deny** is **To Delay** your Last Wishes.

Example of a Vaguely Worded Living Will

After living together a long time and sharing many experiences, spouses can learn each other's values so they can **usually** make correct end-of-life decisions. Usually, not always... Misunderstandings can occur, as illustrated below:

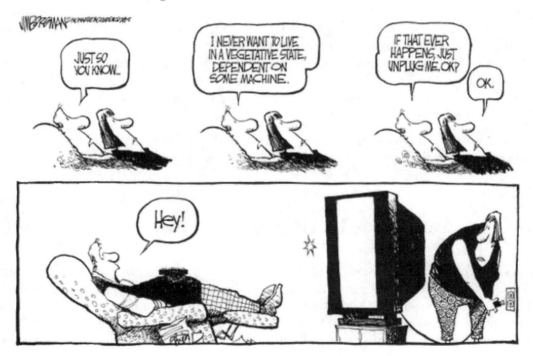

2. The typical format of a Living Will or **Directive to Physician** consists of a number of statements in the "IF" / "THEN" format:

Typical Format of a Living Will (Directive to Physician):

To my future doctor, who may be the last physician to treat me:

"**IF** I am in this particular medical (or mental) condition, _____,

THEN these are the medical interventions I DO want: _____,

and these are the medical interventions I do NOT want: _____."

Most bioethicists and the AMA make no moral distinction between withholding treatment and withdrawing treatment, yet some religions do. You may further clarify that your wishes are not to initiate these interventions, but if they are presently being provided, they should be (or should *not* be) withdrawn.

3. Have Living Wills been widely accepted? Although many professionals had high hopes for **Living Wills** to improve the responsiveness of physicians to patients' Last Wishes, the experience of the last fifteen years has been disappointing. Many reasons have been suggested. In 1991, the Federal government began promoting Advance Directives through the Patient Self-Determination Act where certain medical institutions and facilities that received federal funds were required to **inform patients** as they were being admitted, that Advance Directives were available and that they had the right to complete them. However there was **no requirement to discuss**, let alone complete, Advance Directives. Only about 40% of adults over 40 have Living Wills, according to a 2003 AARP survey, and those people that have Living Wills rarely revise them, even when they experience major changes in diagnosis, prognosis, or personal and family circumstances.

4. Are Living Wills available when needed to make a difference? One study showed that 3 out of 4 times, doctors were not aware that a patient's Advance Directive even existed when they had to make critical decisions [Monmaney, 1995]. Even if the document is known to exist, sometimes it cannot be located when it is needed to make a decision in a crisis. People need to be educated that it is inappropriate to lock up Advance Directives, since safekeeping is less important than availability.

The landmark study called SUPPORT (Study to Understand Prognoses and Preferences for Outcomes and Risks of Treatments) involved over 9000 patients [Teno and others, 1997]. Even when a specifically trained nurse was provided to communicate the patient's preferences to the physician, the intervention resulted in little difference in satisfying patient preferences or in reducing end-of-life cost of medical care.

5. Will your doctor know how to interpret what you wanted? Even if your Living Will is delivered directly to your doctor, he might be confused as to how to apply your written instructions. In Scotland, where failure to comply with written directives can be prosecuted, Thompson and others [2003] did a study that examined how several health professionals responded to a written Living Will when presented with one hypothetical clinical situation. There was a wide variety of professional interpretations: The interviewed doctors and nurses offered **11 (eleven)** different reasons **TO OFFER** treatment and **8 (eight)** different reasons **NOT TO OFFER** treatment. These published reasons provoked another **6 (six)** readers of the British Medical Journal to send in letters to offer additional interpretations. The study's results do not justify peace of mind that one's Last Wishes can be consistently interpreted and thereby honored.

6. Is your doctor required to abide by your Living Will? You might hope that the instructions in your Living Will would require your doctor to follow them, but a survey of American internists indicated that about **two-thirds of the time**, they would let other factors trump written instructions. The doctors who were surveyed stated that they would instead heed their own estimate of the **patients' prognosis** and **perceived quality of life**, and/or the **expressed wishes** of the family or friends [Hardin and Yusufaly, 2004].

The laws of many States include "conscience clauses" that allow physicians to refuse to provide legal treatment if it conflicts with their personal values, morals, or religious beliefs. A survey by Dr. Curlin & others [2007] revealed about 1 in 6 would physicians surveyed would object to **terminal sedation**—an alarming figure since their "conscience" would **unnecessarily prolong intractable unbearable suffering** for what others have estimated as **5% to 15%** of terminal patients. Objectors were less than half as likely to feel obligated to disclose all legal treatment options and about half as likely to refer these patients to another doctor (who might provide this most aggressive form of *Comfort Care*) as non-objecting physicians. This is one reason why the Living Will on page 259 recommends that you appoint an individual to be your **Living Will Advocate**. A document of several pages, no matter how clearly written, cannot vehemently advocate your wishes. Unlike the cartoon on page 251, Living Wills are NOT self-enforcing. Unfortunately, rulings by some courts will not encourage doctors to have more respect for Living Wills since they sided with doctors whose defense was to "err" on the side of prolonging life, as in the following story:

Is it Elder Abuse to Ignore a Patient's Living Will?
The Case of Margaret Furlong

In February 2001, Margaret Furlong, then 81, told her primary physician that she did not want cardiopulmonary resuscitation (CPR), so her doctor filled out a "Preferred Intensity of Treatment" form. In July 2001, Mrs. Furlong signed a "Consent to Withhold CPR," which she renewed monthly with one of her nursing home physicians who signed it. She also signed an "Emergency Medical Services Pre-Hospital DNR" (Do Not Attempt to Resuscitate) form. These last two documents were in her medical records at Glenwood Care Center in Oxnard, California and Margaret Furlong's step-daughter brought these two documents to the staff at the Emergency Department of St. John's Regional Medical Center on March 2, 2002, along with the list of her current medication orders. The treatment plan for her severe pain was aggressive: Vicodin, at least one every four hours, or two, if needed; plus Vioxx.

It is alleged that no one asked Mrs. Furlong what her wishes were when she was first admitted, even though she was lucid at that time. Her admission paper work (mistakenly) indicated she did NOT have an Advance Directive.

Nine hours after admission, Mrs. Furlong had a **cardiac arrest**. She was **resuscitated!** Subsequently, she was **not provided adequate pain medication** (perhaps because she could no longer communicate how much she was suffering). She died ten days later after life-support was withdrawn.

While under the care of her doctor at the hospital, she evidently received pain medications only on an "as needed basis" (based on the nurses' or doctors' perception or guess). Yet the Critical Care Flow Sheet, which regulations require filling out every 12 hours, was blank for 17 of the last 19 twelve-hour shifts. For three shifts, the nursing staff documented only that Margaret's pain was "difficult to assess," "unable to assess verbally," or "unable to assess completely." By this time, Mrs. Furlong was unable to communicate verbally if she had intense pain, and the pieces of paper of her Living Will were NOT Self-Enforcing to end her suffering. See the cartoon on the next page.

According to the appeal brief written by family's attorney Jody C. Moore, Margaret Furlong "thought long and hard about the kind of medical care she wanted at the end of her life. Margaret took every possible step to ensure that her profoundly personal wishes on this momentous, final matter would be known and respected. Defendants allegedly violated their duty to ascertain Margaret's clear wishes, and consequently defendants did not honor those wishes. As a direct result, **Margaret died the lingering death she had sought to avoid, a death filled with invasive, painful, undignified treatments**."

Her family sued on the basis of elder abuse [Ventura County Star, 2004; Case number B172067, Furlong v. Catholic Healthcare West, plead by attorney Jody C. Moore, March 18, 2004].

The judge ruled for a Summary Dismissal after "Respondents argued that the amended complaint pleaded facts showing only professional negligence, not culpable, reckless conduct as required by the Elder Abuse Act" [2004 Cal.

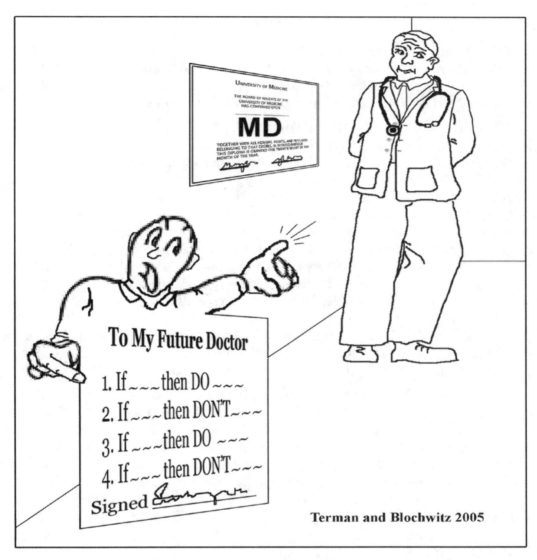

A "Self--Enforcing" **DIRECTIVE TO PHYSICIAN** (Living Will) .

App. Unpub. LEXIS 11667]. The possible reasoning: The Elder Abuse Act provides a list of examples of acts that fall into the category of *failure to provide necessary required treatment,* **but the law does not list providing unwanted treatment.**

Legal professionals at Compassion and Choices are now focusing their efforts on changing the law. I wonder if designating a "Living Will Advocate," as described on pages 258 to 262, could have prevented this sad outcome.

The Furlong case shows that sometimes, pieces of paper can be ineffective, including the document that contained the instructions to doctors about precisely what medical care the patient did, or did not want. Furthermore, the outcome of this lawsuit did little to warn other doctors that they should be more responsive.

7. Could I use the additional form called the POLST? Informed consent is not the only standard for providing treatment. When physicians and their agents (including emergency medical technicians) act in good faith to save a life (or limb) under emergency conditions, they are not expected to wait to confirm whether or not there are documents that refuse such treatment. Still, if a relative provides a document when the patient is admitted, it should become part of the chart so that the patient's wishes are honored. While Advance Directives may serve this purpose, they are complicated documents with many parts that are not relevant. The **Physicians' Order for Life-Sustaining Treatments (POLST)** form was designed to communicate patients' wishes about emergency life-sustaining treatments as effective medical orders. A national initiative spread the use of the **POLST** from Oregon to West Virginia, Washington, Pennsylvania, New York, Utah, New Mexico, Michigan, Georgia, Minnesota, and to parts of Wisconsin, as of August, 2005. The importance of using such a document to prevent unwanted resuscitations is illustrated and discussed on page 316.

8. Why is making decisions for future conditions so difficult? The task of creating a Living Will requires that you anticipate a variety of unpleasant future medical and/or mental states, and then describe exactly what treatment you would, or would not want. Yet research shows that people are reluctant to make specific decisions; that their decisions are not as durable as previously assumed; that their decisions can change based on a variety of factors such as mood and current health status. Having children made adults' decisions more stable. Declines in physical or psychological functioning correlated with less interest in life-sustaining treatment. So did being male. [See the works of Peter Ditto, 2003; Hawkins and Ditto, 2005.]

9. Making life-determining decisions even in real time can be complex. Elderly people often have several diagnoses, which makes even current decisions more complicated. One diagnosis may eventually be terminal, while another diagnosis may be life-threatening but reversible. It can be difficult for ill patients to sort out the complex possibilities and come to a decision, and then argue vehemently what treatment they want. This is one reason why it is prudent to authorize your Proxy to collaborate with you, even though you can still make your own medical decisions. The next story illustrates these points. In this case, it was fortunate that the blood relative surrogate was a physician. Here, useful life was prolonged.

"Please, treat my grandmother's pneumonia!"

If I hadn't been a physician myself, I doubt the daytime secretary and the evening answering service of my grandmother's physician would have put through all my phone calls—all five. To overcome the doctor's resistance, I needed to plead repeatedly as well as delicately:

"... Yes, you're right. Her lung cancer **is** terminal. And yes again, you're right. Eventually she will die from it." (I started with the strategy: First, agree.) "But otherwise, she's in pretty good health for a 76 year-old, don't you think? And her mind is still clear, don't you agree?" (I thus laid the foundation for my next argument.) "So Doctor, if you did decide to order antibiotics to treat her pneumonia, isn't it *possible* she could return to her previous level of functioning and thus enjoy a bit more of what remains in her life?" (Ending strategy: State an outcome as a possibility so it will be difficult to argue against.)

So my strategy worked; I changed the physician's behavior. Time is critical in the war between bacteria and the human body, but my grandmother's doctor promptly started high-powered antibiotics administered through her veins. She recovered.

Four months later, my grandmother was well enough to join her husband and the rest of our family at church for the baptism of their first male grandchild. I will always cherish the memories of this happy occasion, just as I will never forget that evening when it seemed doubtful that she would live to that day.

❧

10. Have Living Wills failed? A few years after the introduction of Living Wills, Dr. Joanne Lynn delineated the flaws and disappointments of these documents, from both her personal and professional perspectives. She wrote these three statements in her 1991 article:

- "I do not have a Living Will because I fear that the effects of having one would be worse, in my situation, than not having one... A Living Will of the standard format attends to priorities that are not my own, addresses procedures rather than outcomes, and requires substantial interpretation without guaranteeing a reliable interpreter.";

- "When people feel that having signed a Living Will serve to ensure that they will avoid medical torment of all sorts, they are misconstruing the document"; and

- "Thus, the Living Will can also lead to errors of under treatment [and] is thoroughly disappointing as a legal document."

Slow-forward one-and-a-half decades. For many people, subsequent experience has only validated Dr. Lynn's brilliantly perceptive vision. One example is

"ENOUGH. The Failure of the Living Will"—the emphatic title of a strongly worded article by Fagerlin and Schneider [2004]. Its conclusion is "Living Wills were praised and peddled before they were fully developed, much less studied. They have now failed repeated tests of practice. It is time to say, 'Enough'" [*Page 39*]. When the authors addressed public policy, they were adamant: "If Living Wills have failed, we must say so. We must say so to patients... [and] frankly warn patients how faint is the chance that Living Wills can have their intended effect."

Yet their condemnation was not absolute. Fagerlin and Schneider did "not propose the elimination of Living Wills [for] patients whose medical situation is plain, whose crisis is imminent, whose preferences are specific, strong, and delineable, and who have special reasons to prescribe their care." Dr. Lynn similarly stated "a good use for Living Wills" is "to document unusually specific preferences or unusual preferences." We would add to this set of requirements, identifying a specific physician who is willing to respond to the terms in the Living Will. That is one reason we prefer the term, **"Directive to Physician."**

One preference that could be considered "unusual" is the **Refusal of Food & Fluid**—not because YOU as a patient, or because we as authors, feel that this request is unusual, but because others do and their opposition can be vehement and sometimes effective since they have the strong cultural bias on their side. There is much controversy over this specific preference. To avoid conflict with two sets of directions (Living Will and Proxy Directive), however, I recommend adding the reasons you want this option to your Proxy Directive and call the document, **"Empowering Statements for My Proxy."** Yet Living Wills might also work if there is no identified Proxy. Fagerlin and Schneider acknowledged that Living Wills could satisfy the States requirement for *clear and convincing evidence* in the Wendland case (in a footnote), and they quoted the Michigan Court *in re Martin*: "[A] written directive would provide the most concrete evidence of the patient's decisions, and we strongly urge all persons to create such a directive."

A closer look at Fagerlin and Schneider's argument reveals their underlying assumption, which they stated twice: "Patients **sign Living Wills without adequate reflection, lack necessary information**, and **have fluctuating preferences** anyway... " and "People who sign Living Wills have generally not thought through its instructions in a way we should want for life-and-death decisions. **Nor can we expect people** to make thoughtful and stable decisions about **so complex a question so far in the future**." {Emphasis added, as this sentence was quoted by The President's Council on Bioethics, and their report will be the subject of much discussion, later in the book.}

Although provocative, the authors' assumption could be considered arrogant and ironic. The words, "Nor can we expect people," most likely refers to more than the "we" of Fagerlin and Schneider. If my inference is correct, this "we" includes, in their words (from other sections of their paper): "bioethicists, doctors, nurses, social workers, and patients [who are] loyal advocates" of Living Wills. Yet the past performance of lay people may not predict what they will do in the future.

Here is the ironic part: The words, "Nor can we expect," constitute a forward-looking statement based on the authors' prediction on what lay people will NOT be able to do in future, the reason for which is, according to the authors, the "question" (problem) is "so complex... [and] so far in the future." Yet the authors' prediction is itself based on the assumption that Living Wills cannot work [in the future] because their problems are too complex. Hence, the authors grant themselves the right to predict what is, or is not, possible in the future, as they simultaneously assume that patients cannot exercise the same right.

As authors of this book, however, we do have hope in the future ability of patients to create more effective end-of-life documents. We support efforts to improve such documents in the future. That is precisely why we wrote this book.

Why We Can Expect More People to be More Motivated to Create More Effective Advance Directives Soon

They will learn from tragic cases such as that of Terri Schiavo;

An increasing proportion of our population will be elderly; and

Awareness is growing about the impending economic and people-power burden of long-term care compared to available resources.

> —In the near future, such reasons will stimulate people to actively seek informational and advice.

Fagerlin and Schneider's generalization is overly sweeping: There has always been and there will always be **some individuals** who are diligent and who will make thoughtful and stable decisions. There are even some who will make thoughtful decisions and then revise these decisions at appropriate times. One positive outcome of the Schiavo tragedy is that more people will diligently pursue advance care planning.

Yes, Fagerlin and Schneider are correct when considering the **past** on a statistical basis: A minority of people completed Living Wills, and most completed documents were inadequate. However, there exists another solution to the underlying problem. Instead of completely discarding Living Wills, why not educate people on how they can diligently craft better documents? The prospect of success will add to the motivations listed above.

Living Wills (Directives to Physician) are highly recommended and can be expected to be effective provided they are used by patients whose doctors have given them a diagnosis whose trajectory is terminal and their physicians promise to treat them to the end, and sufficiently discuss the options so they can develop a plan. If these conditions are met, they can collaborate on creating effective Living Wills, place them in patients' charts and distribute them to close relatives.

I suggest, for people who are medically well, that they consider NOT completing Living Wills. Instead, they could provide their Proxy ENOUGH information to effectively discourage legal challenges from third parties (first choice), or to prevail quickly in court (second choice). To accomplish this goal, people should attach to their **Proxy Directive**, a document called "**Empowering Statements for My Proxy**" (**ESMP**).

The **Empowering Statements for My Proxy** explains *what you want* and *why you want it*—**clearly and convincingly**. While this document may sound similar to a Living Will, its purpose is different. It is designed to arm your Proxy with effective arguments rather than to request direct responses from your physicians. Rather than trying to predict the kind of conditions for which you want your proxy to **Refuse Food & Fluid** on your behalf, **Empowering Statements for My Proxy** includes such statements as: "I have discussed the general guidelines for when my Proxy should decide to honor my request to **Voluntarily Refuse Food & Fluid**, but my Proxy knows much more than what I have briefly indicated below... " Then your **ESMP** would list *some* general reasons and illustrative examples. Putting less directive information in the document reduces the risk that part of the document will become grist for the mill of a prolonged litigious controversy.

If you want your Proxies to know even more about you than what you state in your **Empowering Statements for My Proxy**, you can express your values and preferences in another document that you could call, "**Private Values and Treatment Preferences**." The **PVTP** can include your completed values questionnaires, discussion notes, and narrative summaries of interviews about your end-of-life wishes. Since you know this document will be kept private, you can express yourself freely without worrying about apparent internal contradictions that a litigating attorney might pick at. The document could be useful to an alternate Proxy, including a professional end-of-life advocate, to quickly learn enough to make medical decisions for you based on the Substituted Judgment standard. Your **Private Values and Treatment Preferences** document can also include another kind of statement—something you would be willing to submit in support of *clear and convincing* evidence—but only if necessary, since you would prefer not to reveal this material. Consider this example based on the case of Terri Schiavo:

Terri's parents, the Schindlers, tried to attack the DURABLE aspect of Terri's (orally expressed) Living Will and her Proxy's current decision to remove her feeding tube. They stated that she was an observant Catholic, so that the 2004 Allocution of the Pope would lead her to change her mind about removing her feeding tube. Her hypothetical **PVTP** could have stated that she had not been to Confession or taken Communion for the last 18 months of her conscious life (as some observers stated). This is a personal piece of information that shy Terri would not have wanted to reveal publicly, unless necessary.

One possible reason why few people have Living Wills is that creating them can be a grim process that requires considering unpleasant options for awful medical conditions, which healthy people would rather not think about. If they were only asked to complete a **Proxy Directive**, perhaps they would be more willing, along the lines of the allegory below. (See also, the last story in this book, "She Revised Her Advance Directives From 16 to 86.")

A Strategy for Success

Tibetan monk in training: "What possible value could there be, to teach people how to meditate for only five minutes?"

Sogyal Rinpoche: "It is better to be successful in teaching people how to meditate for five minutes... than NOT to be successful in teaching them how to meditate for a whole hour."

Michael Lipkin [2006] added this strategy: ease into the subject. He first asked patients, "In case you had a medical emergency, who is the person you would want your doctor to notify?" and then asked, "In case you were unconscious or too sick to make decisions about your medical care, who is the person you would want your doctor to talk with... to make health care decisions for you?" Asking to name a "contact person" first led 96% to name their Proxy. About 9 out of 10 interviewed thought that doctors should routinely ask patients to designate a Proxy and would name a Proxy if asked. Only 5% of their charts had advance directives.

11. Is there hope for Living Wills? Yes, we believe there is, and always has been. Yet designated Proxies (frequently family members) often are guided by what they would choose for themselves, or by their urgent desire to keep their loved ones alive [Fagerlin and others, 2001]. Often, they ask for more treatment than patients really want. In contrast, physicians often offer less treatment than patients really want. Yet "with a therapy-specific advance directive supported by a Proxy and prior patient-physician discussion, 100% of physicians were willing to withhold cardiopulmonary resuscitation." While only 82% of physicians were willing to withhold intravenous fluids [Mower and Baraff, 1993], perhaps this percentage would increase if Living Wills included specific, convincing reasons.

30. If My Future Doctors Must Rely on My Living Will, What Criteria Should Trigger Withholding Food & Fluid from Me? and Should I Name Someone as My "Living Will Advocate"?

If you trust your Proxy to make the decisions that you would make, then the **Living Will** (**Directive to Physician**) part of the Advance Directive is NOT required. (Note: If you are worried about giving your Proxy too much power, remember that this individual must still consult with your future physician about your prognosis for recovering an acceptable degree of functioning and the benefits versus burdens of continued aggressive treatment compared to the alternative of *Comfort Care*.) If you live in a State or in a Country that does not recognize **Proxy Directives**, or if you have more confidence in your physician than in any individuals who might serve as your Proxy, and if your doctor has given you a serious or life-threatening diagnosis and discussed possible trajectories and promises to be there when "that time" comes (when you are close to dying), then a **Directive to Physician** may serve well as your Advance Directive, if legal. You may use a document similar to **Empowering Statements for My Proxy** to help your physician learn about your wishes, however, and you may still want **Private Statements about Values and Treatment** for the reasons stated above.

If you cannot identify a friend or relative to be your Proxy whom you can trust to be able, available, willing, and effective, consider designating an end-of-life professional to serve as your advocate, as an alternative to depending solely on a **Directive to Physician** (**Living Will**). If you decide you prefer to rely solely on a Living Will, consider the detailed form that appears at the end of this chapter.

If you decide to rely solely on a **Directive to Physician** (**Living Will**), consider designating an individual or an end-of-life professional to serve as your **Living Will Advocate**. Even though this person would have *no* authority to make medical decisions, he or she could help make sure your last treating physician receives and considers the written document that contains your Last Wishes. This person could be the solution to the problem illustrated in the cartoon on page 251. Your **Living Will Advocate** can also request a second doctor's opinion or a consultation from the local ethics committee, if he or she feels your physician is not responsive to your written directives.

As you compose your own document, keep your audience in mind: You are actually writing to a future physician or group of physicians who will be your health care providers when the criteria you prefer require action. These are the professionals who must interpret what you have written, and who must decide based on what you wrote, what medical treatment to administer or to withhold or to withdraw.

31. How Can I Create an Effective Living Will, if My State or My Country Does Not Recognize Proxy Directives?

[FORM I: Doctor, Please Honor My Living Will]

In the Preface, I admitted how many times I had "finished" this book. One of the "last" times was when Rev. Mettanando Bhikkhu, Ph.D., M.D., visited me and asked me to write a Living Will for him. He explained, "Thailand does not recognize Proxy Directives." As many as ten U.S. States have *no* laws that fully recognize Proxy Directives. In his book, *Power of Attorney Handbook* [2006], Attorney Edward Haman still recommended Proxy Directives "on the chance that one would be honored, it would still be better for you to have one. You can also ask your doctor or local hospital administrator whether they accept and honor health care powers of attorney" [*Page 35*]. Mr. Haman does *not* point out the hurdles, however: Physicians may know they will not be immune from prosecution if they follow instructions on forms that their State has not approved. Haman's book noted Alaska, Arkansas, Kentucky, Louisiana, Massachusetts, Missouri, New Jersey, and South Dakota as States that either do *not* authorize Proxy Directives or that *confuse* Proxy Directives with forms that merely allow naming an advocate to facilitate wishes expressed in your Living Wills. Always check for updates: Michigan's legislature deleted a previously authorized form that Haman noted. Ohio law requires *certain* decisions by Proxies be approved by physicians. Haman suggested expanding State-recognized generic or financial power of attorney forms, and/or using his book's generic medical Proxy Directive on *Pages 95-96 [of his book]*. Yet even completing State-approved forms may result in documents that are inadequate to accomplish certain end-of-life goals. Here is a hint about potential bias that readers of Haman's book might find interesting. **Attorney** Haman wrote this **clinical comment**: "Withholding of food and water for a certain period of time can cause great pain and discomfort" [*Page 39*]. We disagree.

In accepting Rev. Mettanando's request I asked myself, What would it take to make Living Wills as effective as possible? That stimulated the idea of a "Living Will Advocate." I also consulted an expert on why Living Wills fail, Dr. Peter H. Ditto. My concerns resulted in the form below. This form would permit the physician to choose choosing the legal peaceful choice of **Withholding or Withdrawing Food & Fluid**, if the creator of the document desired to keep this option available.

The Living Will presented next explains most choices in context (*in Italics*), but the issue of whether or not you can trust your doctor is so important that it is covered in a separate section following the FORM.

Living Will (Directive to Physician): Withhold Food & Fluid *and* Aggressive Medical Treatment Under Certain Conditions

<u>These are my two greatest end-of-life fears:</u>

• If my brain is so devastated by dementia or trauma that I am not aware of my environment and I cannot respond to the people I love, but others force me to exist in a prolonged state of total dependence and indignity; and

• If my brain is intact, but there is no reasonable hope that my body will ever function normally, AND others force me to endure unbearable pain and/or suffering for an unnecessarily prolonged amount of time. (In this case, if I can express my Last Wishes, I may **Voluntarily Refuse Food & Fluid NOW**.)

The goal of this Living Will (Directive to Physician) is to inform my future doctors what treatment I would want and what I would NOT want, based on my striving to write *clear and convincing* descriptions of those medical and mental conditions I consider unbearable or intolerable.

Because Living Wills are NOT self-enforcing; that is, pieces of paper cannot "get tough" with a treating doctor to vehemently advocate your wishes, as the cartoon on page 251 illustrates, we recommend designating one or more "Living Will Advocates." Unlike a Proxy or Agent, this individual has NO legal authority to make medical decisions on my behalf but clearly has a moral responsibility to advocate on my behalf.

|__| I have appointed a "Living Will Advocate," whose role is TO FACILITATE my stated wishes. If he or she is not available, not willing, or not able to serve in this role, then I wish the next person listed below to serve, in this order of preference:

1. _____

2. _____

3. _____

|__| I have NOT designated any individuals as "Living Will Advocates." I hope my physician or his or her colleagues will be informed, available, able, willing, responsive, and accurate as they interpret and honor my Last Wishes.

Note: *If you do not know anyone you can trust to serve in the role of "Living Will Advocate," consider naming an end-of-life professional or a member of an end-of-life professional organization that provides this service.*

The two functions of my "Living Will Advocate":

1. Logistic problems related to getting the document to my physician:

I want my "Living Will Advocate" to deliver this document to my physician whenever the document may be needed. Although I signed this "Directive to Physician," had it witnessed or notarized, and asked my personal physician to place a copy in my medical chart, it is still possible that, at the very moment when a critical life-or-death treatment decision must be made…

- My chart may be temporarily missing or unavailable;
- My personal doctor may be temporarily unavailable;
- A copy of this document may be unavailable (use your refrigerator instead of a safe deposit box), but I am too sick to retrieve it; or,
- I may have reached the medical condition or mental state described below while I was traveling in another State or country.

In these and similar situations, I want my "Living Will Advocate" to make sure that a copy of my Directive to Physician is given to my current doctor(s) and encourage him or her, as my clinical decision-maker, to read it carefully.

> **Suggestion**: *An "alert" bracelet or necklace or wallet card can provide names and contact information of your "Living Will Advocates." A mini-CD or flash drive can provide a copy of your completed Living Will. You can also register the document (see Further Resources, page 469).*

2. To make sure my future physician interprets and follows my Last Wishes:

Although I have discussed my Last Wishes with my current physician, I realize that, when a critical life-or-death treatment decision must be made, my future physician may not be the same doctor with whom I have discussed my Last Wishes, or may interpret my Last Wishes differently. For example…

> A "new" doctor, with whom I have *not* discussed my Last Wishes, may disagree with my specific Last Wishes based on clinical judgment; or on personal, moral, or religious values (conscience); or,

> Any doctor may not agree that my future mental or medical condition (the "IF" part of my Directive to Physician) has been reached so that the time has indeed come to write orders to withhold aggressive treatment or to **Withhold Food & Fluid** (the "THEN" part of my Directive to Physician).

...In these or similar cases, I authorize my "Living Will Advocate" to request a second medical opinion, and if necessary, also to request I be transferred to the care of another physician, and/or to request a consultation by the local ethics committee. I realize this inherent limitation of Living Wills: The ultimate authority for medical decision-making remains in the province of the physician. So after all these attempts if my "Living Will Advocate" is still not successful in convincing my doctors to follow his or her interpretation of my Last Wishes, I understand and hope that my "Living Will Advocate" will not feel guilty. (It is also possible that my future physician is correct in interpreting my wishes.)

I also recognize three problems about "Directives to Physicians" that are my current responsibility as I create this document, knowing that once I am not competent there will be no way for me to change what I have written: 1) There might be a discrepancy between what I now assume I would want in the future, compared to what I do actually want then. 2) What I wrote might not be considered *clear and convincing*, or be sufficiently specific or encompassing to prevent challenges that *deny* as they *delay* the honoring of my Last Wishes. 3) New treatment modalities may become available that are not available now. In these situations, after my Living Will Advocate consults with my doctor:

|__| I authorize complete LEEWAY for my physician to interpret my Last Wishes.

|__| I want my physician to follow STRICTLY my Last Wishes as written.

The "IF part" of my Directive to Physician:

With respect to the specific medical conditions in which I would want not to continue to exist, I realize that neurologists and other physicians may use a variety of diagnostic terms such as "permanent coma," "persistent vegetative state," "severe or advanced or end-stage dementia," and "minimally conscious state." In contrast, I consider it more relevant to describe limitations of behavior than to list the names of specific diagnoses. Below is a partial but representative list of the kinds of limitations or problems in behavior for which, if my behavior reaches such or similar states, I want my physician to withhold life-sustaining treatment and to **Withhold Food & Fluid**. But first, I state one safeguard for withholding Food & Fluid and medical treatment:

|__| I DO want another physician, if possible a specialist in the relevant area, to render an independent opinion. If both physicians cannot agree that the probability of my improving to overcome the limitations listed below is less than __ percent after __ months of observation and therapeutic trials before

they embark on the "no aggressive medical treatment" and "**Withhold Food & Fluid**" option, they should request an ethics committee consultation.

|__| I do NOT want other physicians to render opinions. I trust my physician to decide when to embark on the "no aggressive medical treatment" or "**Withholding of Food & Fluid**" option for any of the reasons below:

> 1. I cannot recognize the people I used to love;
>
> 2. I cannot recall the essence of the person who I was, or the life that I led, in terms of its fundamental values or significant events;
>
> 3. I cannot communicate my wishes by words, gestures, or sounds;
>
> 4. I cannot indicate "Yes" or "No" by any means, even after a trial of technological assistance (if such a trial seems appropriate [p 141]);
>
> 5. I am not aware of my environment through my senses so I cannot respond;
>
> 6. I cannot make meaningful plans to change my environment;
>
> 7. I am totally **dependent** on others or machines for nurturance since I do not have the physical ability to eat or drink, OR I do not have the mental ability to know how to eat or drink, OR I actively resist people as they try to spoon-feed me by fighting them or by turning my face away from them or by clenching my teeth;
>
> 8. I seem extremely confused or scared, or to be living in horror;
>
> 9. I seem to harbor delusions that lead to behavior so dangerous that I could hurt myself or others unless I am physically restrained;
>
> 10. I seem extremely withdrawn, apathetic, despondent, irritable, or angry—even after I have received treatment attempts including medications to improve my mood (if appropriate);
>
> 11. I am incontinent of urine or feces or so totally dependent that prolonging my biologic existence merely increases the chance that my loved ones, especially younger relatives, will remember me only in such a state of **indignity**;
>
> 12. I have such intense pain or unbearable suffering that relief can be achieved only by medications that sedate me so much that I can hardly be aroused (**Palliative Sedation**);
>
> 13. The burdens of treatment to maintain my existence have become my, and/or my caregivers' overwhelming concern, despite there being almost no potential for benefit (**Futile Treatment**); or,

14. I seem unaware or unable to appreciate being alive and being cared for, yet my caregivers are making huge sacrifices on my behalf—by ignoring other enjoyable activities or responsibilities in their lives, by physical exhaustion, by mental depression, or by draining their financial resources to the extent that my continued existence has become a hardship, and/or is preempting the economic opportunities of my children and/or grandchildren, and/or precluding the use of my assets to benefit the poor and hungry of the world, as I would wish to be done (**principle of Social Justice**).

The "THEN part" of my Directive to Physician:

If my physician considers that enough of the reasons described above apply to my medical or mental condition, or my social situation, then I want my physician to **Withhold Food & Fluid**, regardless of whether Food & Fluid are administered directly into a vein or into my gastrointestinal system, or by another's assistance into my mouth. I DO NOT want any potentially life-sustaining aggressive treatments, including but not limited to: attempts to resuscitate the functioning of my heart and lungs, antibiotics, renal dialysis, surgery, or to have mechanical ventilators breathe for me.

If I am not in a hospital, I do not want to be transferred to a hospital. *Attach to this document a Physicians' Order for Life-Sustaining Treatment (POLST) and a DNH (Do Not Hospitalize) request signed by your physician, or a similar document if you reside in a State that has not yet authorized specific forms for these purposes. (More details on* **FORM III** *are on* page 316.*)*

A further explanation of why I have asked **my physician to Withhold Food & Fluid** on my behalf under these or similar conditions can be found in an attachment that includes general and specific reasons why I may, at some point in the last chapter of my life, want Food & Fluid withheld. (*The* **Basic Form** *on* pages 237-239 *can be* modified from authorizing your Proxy to instructions for your physician, if you are using a Living Will.)

If I have made a mistake in granting this durable authority to my future physician, I will accept the consequences. I prefer this alternative to granting other individuals the opportunity to challenge my future physician's authority to follow the instructions in this "Directive to Physician." I thus embrace the arguments of Professor Ronald Dworkin on **"precedent autonomy,"** psychological continuity, and a single life narrative. Dr. Dworkin wrote, "A competent person's right to autonomy requires that past decisions about how he is to be treated if he becomes demented be respected, even if they do not represent [any longer], and even if they contradict, the desires he has [now] when we respect them, provided he did not change his mind while he was still in charge of his own life" [that is, when competent]. For example, if my dementia progresses to the point where I have become a danger to myself or others, keep me in a skilled nursing facility even if I consistently and repeatedly make *clear and convincing* requests to go home.

Have this document signed by legally qualified witnesses or notarized and bring it to your physician, with whom you should have had previous discussions. Ask your doctor to place a copy of these documents in your chart, in addition to other forms (from your State, "Five Wishes," or other sources) that indicate your preferences for non-medical end-of-life care, whether you authorize an autopsy, your willingness to donate your organs, and your preferences about ceremonies as you are dying, funerals, and memorial services.

In case your last treating physician does not receive, does not read, or does not wish to follow your written instructions—give your Living Will Advocate(s) copies of: 1) Living Will; 2) modified Basic Form; and 3) FORM III, and discuss how active a role you wish your Living Will Advocate to take.

The Key to Success with Living Wills: Can You Trust Your Doctor?

We prefer the term "Directive to Physician" to "Living Will" because it reflects its intended audience: your future (and often last) physician. While your loved ones will have great interest in your Living Will, the ultimate decision-maker will be your physician. Since refusing treatment can hasten dying, decisions are best shared with loved ones when patients cannot speak for themselves. Such discussions should strive to achieve four goals. Your physician should: gather more information about you from your family, interpret what you have written in light of your current medical prognosis, accommodate your family members in terms of their readiness to let go, and then make the final medical decision about continuing or withdrawing your treatment. Unfortunately, conflict may arise if your family members disagree with each other or with your doctor.

In some States, your personal physician is prohibited from being designated as your Proxy and is disqualified from being a witness to signing your Living Will. While the American Medical Association's policy states [E-10.01], "The patient has the right to receive information from physicians and to discuss the benefits, risks, and costs of appropriate treatment alternatives," there are disturbing trends. The previously cited surveys of Hardin and Yusufaly [2004] and of Curlin and others [2007] cast serious doubt that all physicians will honor your written wishes in your Living Will. Focusing on **terminal sedation**, a procedure many consider the last resort for terminally ill patients who have unbearable suffering, Curlin's survey concluded, "Many physicians do not consider themselves obligated to disclose information about or refer patients for legal but morally controversial medical procedures. Patients who want information about and access to such procedures may need to inquire proactively to determine whether their physicians would accommodate such requests." To this, Dr. L. Ross responded [2007], "To impose the philosophy of *caveat emptor* is morally inadequate." And I agree: Terminally ill patients are vulnerable and weak and may not know what specific questions to ask so it is unreasonable and unfair to expect them to proactively determine the moral convictions of their physicians if they will need **palliative sedation**. (Note the use of the less morally charged term, "palliative sedation," which means to relieve the symptoms of disease by sedation).

Jerome Groopman's *How Doctors Think* [2007] could have been entitled, *How Patients Can Help Doctors to Think Better*. He shifts some of the burden of making a correct diagnosis to patients by suggesting they ask their doctors if anything else could be going on in the symptomatic area of their bodies, and to reveal possibly relevant medical or personal history about which the physician had failed to inquire. Furthermore he stated, "Informed choice means, in part, learning how different doctors think about a particular medical problem and how science, tradition, financial incentives, and personal bias mold that thinking. There is no single source for all this information about each disorder..." [*Page 233*] There is unfortunately no source of information about physicians' moral and religious biases that heralds doctors' unwillingness to offer all available and legal modalities of palliative care.

"In unpacking the problem of [refusing] hand feeding" as an end-of-life option, Attorney Lois Shepherd [2006b] noted the "growing vitalist movement in the country." She considered if our Constitutional right to refuse unwanted treatment "really furthers a person's right to die" then "the right to refuse looks like it is grounded as much or more in **autonomy** than bodily integrity." Yet as will be explored in Chapter 12, The President's Council on Bioethics undermines the principle of autonomy by endorsing instead as a higher priority, the moral judgment of physician and caregiving decision-makers. It is likely that more physicians would morally object to Voluntary Refusal of Food & Fluid than to Palliative Sedation. So... if you decide to use a Living Will, your greatest challenges will be to have your doctor agree to reduce your pain and suffering and to Withhold Food & Fluid. While you are competent, try to identify your "last" doctor and discuss your Last Wishes with him. Also appoint a Living Will Advocate who will have the energy to actively seek the most aggressive *Comfort Care*, to question your physician's decisions, and if necessary to ask for a second physician's opinion, a change of physicians, an ethics committee consultation, or even a judicial review.

Chapter 10

QUESTIONS REGARDING THE FAMILY

Some *BEST WAYS* Family Members Can Help

They can show they care by broaching the subject of end-of-life decisions with a loved one;

They can use a discussion with a loved one as the basis to create a legally effective document;

They can realize that they need to deal with their grief separately so that their loved one can independently make his or her decision;

They can try to accept their loved one's decision;

They can still "do something" by shifting the acts of *caregiving* from providing Food & Fluid to providing *Comfort Care* to the mouth;

They can ask the right question during the dying process: "**Is your mouth dry?**" instead of: "**Do you want something to drink?**"; and

Sometimes, they may be called upon to make a decision for a loved one who did not previously indicate his or her end-of-life wishes.

---

32. How Can Family Members Handle My Request for Voluntary Refusal of Food & Fluid if I am Competent?

If you wish to **Voluntarily Refuse Food & Fluid**, discuss your decision with your family members and close friends. Express your right to choose the *least worst death*. State your preference to die from dehydration as a far more peaceful way than to die than, for instance, pneumonia. You don't want to cough, be short of breath and run a high fever. Today, "Pneumonia is the old man's friend" is an outdated myth. This old saw was really only true in the pre-antibiotic era (before 1950) when *Comfort Care* was rudimentary.

Loved ones may initially resist deviating from society's deeply rooted cultural norm of "nurturance" by providing Food & Fluid so ask them to participate by actively providing *Comfort Care* to your mouth. Since you may become confused during the process, request them to ask the most appropriate questions. "Is your mouth dry?" is best. "Are your thirsty?" is fine if they have agreed to treat *thirst as a symptom*. They should *not ask*, "Would you like something to eat or drink?"

Remind them that dying is an inevitable part of life over which they have no ultimate control, but there is still much they *can do* to make it peaceful for you and meaningful for them. Some family members may find comfort in conceptualizing your final *fast* as a religious experience. (See page 136)

Ask for professional help from hospice, palliative care specialists, family and pastoral counselors. End-of-life organizations like *Compassion and Choices* and *Caring Advocates,* and certain disease-related organizations may have volunteers in your area to provide advice and support to you and your family. (See the "Further Resources" section that begins on page 469.)

Sometimes, deep psychological forces must be dealt with and respected, as illustrated in the next story:

"Whose Choice Is It, Anyhow?"

At twenty-four, Stuart was entering the prime of life. He had finished college, obtained his MBA, and had begun a promising career with a position in a leading international business. Then it happened. The car accident that almost killed him. Lucky? Perhaps. He was left quadriplegic. After six months of rehabilitation, he asked his physical therapist how much more improvement he could realistically expect. He found the answer so disappointing that the next time his doctor visited, he asked if there was a way he could hasten his dying. Without any discussion, the doctor replied, "Sorry, that's not legal in this State, and even if it were, I would not offer it to you."

Then Stuart read about **Voluntary Refusal of Food & Fluid**. He asked his doctor what he would do if he just stopped eating and drinking. Would he force-feed him? Insert a tube down his nose or into his stomach? Or just let him be?

His doctor stated he could not answer this question until he had discussed it fully with his colleagues. He promised to return with an answer in a day or two. Although he did consult his colleagues during that time frame, the first people whom the doctor contacted were Stuart's parents.

Did the doctor break the normal rules of patient confidentiality? No. A patients' well being—especially his life—has higher priority.

Years ago, the doctor had a similar patient. After a swimming pool accident the local newspaper had a feature article that included a photo of the young patient and his girlfriend, and described how the community was rallying—with prayer, with hope, and with generous contributions—to help pay for his medical bills.

Then, without warning, news arrived: The young man had found a way to take his own life. Every one was shocked; especially his mother. To this day, she has not recovered.

The doctor was very concerned for the parents: Stuart was their only child.

Stuart's mother burst out crying when the doctor told her of Stuart's inquiry. "I can't stand the thought of losing my son." His father remained silent but bit his lip so hard that he drew a small amount of blood. After a while he said, "Thank you for coming to us and telling us what Stuart intends to do. Doctor, you can see how very upset my wife is. Please doctor, do everything, absolutely everything you can, to change our son's mind."

When the doctor returned to Stuart's hospital room, he brought with him a social worker and a psychiatrist. They often worked as a team to counsel patients who suffered from catastrophic injuries. They explained that each person's life affects many others, which for some people, is reason enough to stay alive. Also, one's attitude can change from one decade to the next, and from one state of sickness or wellness to another.

The psychiatrist then interviewed Stuart alone. Together, they delved into the meaning of Stuart's life, now that he was paralyzed. He also assessed whether Stuart was depressed and if his depression was influencing his judgment. Then he left and the social worker interviewed Stuart about his family of origin and his circle of friends, and what activities in life might still retain pleasure for him. After the two professionals conferred about their separate clinical assessments, they both admitted they could not persuade Stuart to remain alive. They shared this information with Stuart's doctor, emphasizing that his patient did not suffer from a clinical condition that impaired his judgment even though he stated he wanted to **Refuse Food & Fluid**. The three then discussed other ideas to try to persuade Stuart to change his mind. They decided to ask a spiritual or religious counselor and an occupational therapist to visit with him.

The occupational therapist brought along a forty-five-year old man who had been quadriplegic for eleven years. He had formerly been a very active man. After spending the first few years after his accident in relative inactivity, he started writing. Now he has two books out, and he gives lectures on how to overcome severe disabilities. The disabled man explained to Stuart that he discovered that helping others had become the main purpose of his life and had given his life deep meaning. Despite presenting such a positive example, Stuart remained steadfast in his desire to hasten his death.

The religious counselor referred to suicide as the ultimate sin, but this line of persuasion did not seem to impress Stuart, so the counselor moved on to more hopeful themes. He said it was possible that further advancements in medicine could improve Stuart's functioning, using the words, "a scientific miracle." He tried to inspire hope by saying, "You're young and otherwise healthy. Sure, your loss is devastating. I can only imagine it, not having gone through it myself. The change in your life has been huge. But give yourself more time to try to find a reason to live as you give science a chance to advance in the next few years. Have hope, or faith, or whatever you want to call it… "

Neither the occupational therapist nor the religious counselor had good news to report to Stuart's doctor about changing his mind. The doctor knew only one other profession to ask for help—a family psychologist.

First the psychologist interviewed Stuart alone, then he interviewed his parents, and then he interviewed all three, together. During the family session, some deep emotions emerged. Old issues over control, expectations and disappointments, the burden of being the only child, the issue of trying to please his parents, and now the great loss they were experiencing were all touched on. While there was not enough time to go into detail, it was obvious that Stuart's condition and his attitude had touched some old psychological raw nerves.

At one point during the family session, Stuart's mother stopped sobbing and blurted out something she had thought, but planned NOT to say: "Maybe you don't want to stay alive for yourself, at least not right now… But would you consider staying alive for us? I just can't stand the thought of losing you." As she heard what she had said, she put her hand over her mouth and stopped abruptly. Silence filled the room for what seemed a long time. No one knew who would speak next.

Finally, the psychologist said, "I think there is a middle ground." The others all turned to him, in partial disbelief. How could there be? "A compromise, I mean." What? Miffed, they waited for him to continue.

"Stuart, you've seen a doctor, a psychiatrist, a social worker, a religious counselor, and an occupational therapist, and a disabled person, right?" he asked.

"Yeah, right. Six people. Now, seven, with you. Enough, don't you think?"

The psychologist turned to the parents. "Do you think it's enough?"

They shook their heads.

"Well then, who else would you like your son to visit with?"

The father said, "Well, maybe another specialist in neurosurgery, and… " As he hesitated, the mother said, "More visits from his cousins and aunts and uncles. They had no idea, when they visited last month, that Stuart was contemplating—" She sobbed and her voice got so soft that the psychologist could hardly hear her say, "I can't even say it."

"What?" asked the psychologist.

The mother took a deep breath. "Stuart's always been close to Sally. His cousin is like a sister. Maybe—" She did not know how to finish the sentence.

The psychologist turned to Stuart. "Would you consider a proposal? It's the compromise I mentioned before. So, let me ask... Stuart, would you postpone starting your fast for one month so you can visit with members of your extended family and other specialists?" The psychologist did not wait long for his reply, and then turned to the parents, "If after one month of visiting with everyone you asked him to, Stuart still does not change his mind, would you be willing to respect his decision?" No reply from the parents, either.

As silence again filled the room, the psychologist broke it with a smile and said, in a surprisingly bright tone, "Since I hear no objections, the motion carries!" He then walked out of the room, leaving Stuart and his parents staring at each other, still at a loss for words.

Ten days later, the doctor called the psychologist to drop by his office. He was not yet seated as doctor asked, "Do you hear? Stuart's parents have accepted his decision to start his fast. This morning, he refused breakfast. How come? Didn't they all agree to wait a month? What happened? Did you see them again?"

"No, I didn't see them again. This is the first I've heard—" He paused and then asked, "Would you like me to speculate?" Without waiting for an answer, the psychologist continued, "His parents probably realized that additional meetings, consultations, interviews, and visits with family members would not change their son's mind. Perhaps they realized, more than anything, that it is Stuart's choice, not theirs—Just like it is Stuart's life, not theirs."

"But why wouldn't they insist on waiting another twenty days?"

The psychologist glanced at the ceiling, as if reflecting quietly. After a moment, he said, "Every life affects many others, but the closer and more loving, the greater those other lives are affected. Nothing has more impact than dying, and nothing can make someone feel as helpless. Often, the last chapter of one's life is an opportunity to accomplish much important work. It's possible that the effort to have so many people talk with Stuart helped decrease his parents' guilt and move them towards acceptance. Perhaps Stuart also worked on his feelings of obligation toward his parents. It's also possible that they are still working on these very issues."

The doctor related the story of his other patient whose surprise suicide was a total shock to his parents. The psychologist responded, "The greatest loss is when your child dies. But it is much worse if the parents feel they had not participated in the decision-making process. Still worse, if they were not given the opportunity to try as hard as they could to change their son's mind. If they were denied this, it would add so much to their loss... It would begin with shock and last forever from not being given the chance to make an impact. That's why some people never recover from their grief. I'm glad Stuart gave his parents that opportunity. It doesn't matter whether it was for ten days or thirty. Perhaps at this point, it would be harder to prolong the process."

He glanced at the ceiling again. "You know, starting a fast is not the same as going through with it. Stuart can postpone his dying just by asking for something to eat or drink. When I interviewed the family, I noted a great mixture of emotions and complex conflicts in their relationships. This could be a time for much healing in their relationships. I planted some seeds for them to think about. I expect Stuart will be alert for five to seven days—"

At this point, the psychologist seemed to drift off...

Impatient for him to finish his sentence, the doctor said, "And—?"

"Oh, sorry, I was just recalling something that Harriet Beecher Stowe wrote. It just popped into my head. Perhaps you know it?

"'The bitterest tears shed over graves
are for words left unsaid
and deeds left undone.'"

The psychologist stood up. "I can't guess whether Stuart will go through with this, but I'm sure he will feel compelled to think deeply about whether or not he wants to end his life as his parents sit at his bedside. It is a great opportunity for deep discussions. If Stuart does maintain his resolve, they will have enough time to complete their best good-byes."

The psychologist focused on the doctor's eyes. "Call me and let me know what Stuart decides, okay?"

ৡৡ

33. How Can I Discuss "A Legal Peaceful Choice" With a Person Who has Some Mental or Physical Impairment? and How Can I Make Our Discussion Legally Binding?

These questions were designed to broach this difficult-to-discuss subject for patients with mild to severe impairments. If the problem is mental, they may not be able to make detailed medical decisions in advance, as required for creating a Living Will. Yet they may still be capable of convincingly designating whom they wish to serve as their first choice and alternate Proxies. Important: Some States require specific additional authorization for Proxies to make decisions about Food & Fluid so patients' answers must demonstrate that their judgment is sound when they authorize their Proxies to make decisions on their behalf about artificial nutrition and hydration, and about **Refusing ORAL Food & Fluid**.

For patients with physical problems, an audio or video recording can create a legal document. If time is urgent, begin with the last two questions to obtain recording permission, and then proceed in the presence of a notary public or qualified witnesses. If possible, I highly recommend *discussing* first and *recording* second. Many patients need time to discuss the implications of their answers, especially if they are hearing them for the first time. They should not feel pressure to answer *clearly, convincingly,* and *consistently.* Instead, they should be encouraged to *think out loud* and *explore* any feelings of *ambivalence* about their range of choices. The interviewer may also feel more relaxed not having to worry that an attorney might, in the future, argue that the patient was *uncertain* based on a recording that is full of (thoughtful) *hesitations.* The second time, patients are likely to answer *quickly with conviction* because they have made up their minds, having heard all the questions even in the presence of unrelated people who are serving as witnesses and/or a notary. Asking twice is also a good way to confirm that their answers are consistent. The recording might even be done on a different day. So, unless there is a great time urgency, divide this important task into two parts that maximize the purpose of each. First: Explore. Second: Establish legal effect.

Note: Not every patient need answer every question. Consult an attorney in your State about witnessing requirements.

A Guide for a Difficult Discussion

1. Is this a good time for us to talk about a difficult subject? (Y/N)

2. You don't expect to live forever, do you? (Y/N)

3. Do you know that many people lose their mental ability to make their own medical decisions at some point—sometimes years before their lives end? (Y/N)

4. Do you know there are ways you can make sure your Last Wishes will be honored if you no longer can make medical decisions? (Y/N)

5. Do you know you can designate a person as your first choice, and others as alternate **Proxies**? (Y/N)

6. Have you decided on a first choice? (Y/N) Who? _____

7. If your first choice is unwilling, unavailable, or unable, do you have alternate Proxies? (Y/N) Who? _____ & _____

8. Are there any individuals you do NOT want to have any power to influence your medical decisions? (Y/N) Who? _____

9. Are you aware that you can also specify what treatment you DO want and what treatment you do NOT want your doctors to provide, based on your possible future medical or functional condition? (Y/N)

10. Do you want to discuss these options with your physician? (Y/N); OR: Do you want to discuss these options with your Proxies? (Y/N); OR: Do you want to discuss these issues further, now? (Y/N)

11. If, near the end of your life, you are in unbearable pain, do you want your Proxy to ask for enough pain medication to relieve your suffering, even if this request might *unintentionally* hasten your dying? (Y/N)

12. Do you want your Proxy to have the authority to decide about your receiving artificially administered Nutrition & Hydration (**AANH**)? (Y/N)

13. Do you want your Proxy to have the authority to decide about your receiving oral Food & Fluid with another's manual assistance? (Y/N)

14. Would you like to hear read, or to read, the behavioral criteria for severe dementia? (Y/N)

15. If you had severe and irreversible dementia and were not happy, what kind of treatment would you want for "A" through "E" below:

  A) Would you want aggressive treatment for cancer? (Y/N)

  B) Would you want aggressive treatment for pneumonia? (Y/N)

  C) Would you want other kinds of infections to be treated? (Y/N)

  D) If you could not swallow, would you want tube feeding? (Y/N)

  E) If you fought caregivers as they tried to feed you by clenching your teeth, turning your face away, or spitting out your food, would you want your caregivers to try harder to force-feed you? (Y/N); OR, would you want to instead be given Food & Fluid by tube feeding? (Y/N) OR, would you want to receive only *Comfort Care*? (Y/N)

16. Are you aware that currently only Oregon and a few European countries allow doctors to prescribe medication to intentionally permanently end your suffering by Physician-Hastened Dying? (Y/N)

17. Are you aware that **Refusing Food & Fluid** is, for most people, a legal and comfortable way to let Nature take its course, and that dying usually occurs in two weeks from dehydration? (Y/N)

18. Are you aware that **Refusing Food & Fluid** can permit you to avoid prolonged suffering, or indignity and dependency? (Y/N)

19. Do you want your Proxy to have the authority to **Refuse Food & Fluid** on your behalf, by removing your feeding tube? (Y/N)

20. Do you want your Proxy to have the authority to **Refuse Food & Fluid** on your behalf, even if you are able to swallow and doing so will hasten your dying? (Y/N)

21. (For Catholics): Are you aware that in March 2004, Pope John Paul II called **Refusal of Food & Fluid**, when performed with the direct intent to hasten dying, immoral and "euthanasia by omission"? (Y/N)

22. Are you aware that, for five centuries, Catholic bioethicists advised patients and families to weigh the relative burdens and benefits of treatment to decide whether or not to continue treatment? (Y/N)

23. Would you like to learn more about **Refusal of Food & Fluid**—from the religious, ethical, or clinical point of views—by reading or listening to relevant portions of *The BEST WAY to Say Goodbye*? (Y/N)

24. Have you had an adequate chance to consider and ask additional questions about **Refusal of Food & Fluid by Proxy**? (Y/N)

25. Do you want to empower your Proxy with the authority to request **Refusal of Food & Fluid** on your behalf if your Proxy feels that your medical or functional condition reaches the point where it meets certain criteria that you have discussed with him or her? (Y/N)

26. If none of your agents and alternates is available, would you like your professional caregivers to **Refuse Food & Fluid** on your behalf if your medical or functional condition declines to the point where it meets the criteria you discussed or wrote, or if family members or close friends or appointed guardians feel that it would be in your best interest? (Y/N)

27. Are you aware that, if a self-designated "interested party" disagrees with what your Proxy decides on your behalf, that party could go to court and thwart your preferences for end-of-life treatment? (Y/N)

28. Are you aware that States can insist on *clear and convincing* evidence that you want your Proxy to discontinue nutrition and hydration before they will recognize your Proxy as having authority to honor your wishes to **Refuse Food & Fluid**? (Y/N)

29. Can you cite some specific reasons and examples why you would want your Proxy to **Refuse Food & Fluid** on your behalf? (Y/N)

30. Would you be willing to make a permanent audio or video recording of what we just discussed and ADD MORE SPECIFICS, so that if anyone were to raise a question about what you wanted, you will have documented your specific wishes in a *clear and convincing* way? (Y/N)

31. To make sure your communication is legally valid, would you be willing to have present, two witnesses who satisfy your State's requirements for eligibility, during this audio or video recording, or would you permit a notary to witness your signature on this document and/or have an independent person indicate how you answered these questions about your wishes for your future end-of-life care? (Y/N)

For ill patients, someone can read these questions to him or her, marking Y or N as the conversation proceeds. If the patient cannot read the relevant material in this book or elsewhere, a person they trust could summarize this material. Two qualified witnesses could record their copies of Yeses and Nos to the questions as the patient answers, and then sign the appropriate State-approved document or have their personal documents notarized. Consult your legal advisor for specifics.

34. What Steps Should I Take Before I Begin to Voluntarily Refuse Food & Fluid?

I'll Have to Put Him Down

A man takes his Rottweiler to the vet. Once inside the office, he says, "My dog is cross-eyed. Is there anything you can do for him?"

"Well," says the vet, "let's have a real close look at him."

So the vet picks the dog up and looks at him, straight on, directly in the dog's eyes.

Meanwhile, the pet owner anxiously awaits the doctor's final diagnosis.

After a few moments, the vet finally says, "I think I'm going to have to put him down."

"What?" yelled the man. "Just because he's cross-eyed?"

"No, that's not the reason. It's because he's so heavy!"

The moral of this story is that you want to take a careful look at your decision, and make sure you are doing it for the right reasons.

First, enroll in a **hospice** program. Not only will you benefit, but so will your loved ones, who will be entitled to a year of bereavement care after your death, at no further cost (under Medicare).

Many hospices have extensive experience with **Voluntary Refusal of Food & Fluid**, although condoning it publicly varies from hospice to hospice. Similarly, many doctors will not recommend **Voluntary Refusal of Food & Fluid** but will facilitate it, if you directly request it. Even in Oregon, twice as many nurses in hospice had cared for patients who chose **Voluntary Refusal of Food & Fluid** as had cared for patients who chose **Physician-Aided, Patient-Hastened Dying** [Ganzini, 2003; Harvath, 2004]. The criteria for admission to hospice with Medicare payment includes a prognosis that with usual treatment, the end is expected within six months. This definition is harder to apply to patients who suffer from dementia, since most of them die from an infection and doctors cannot predict which infected organ will lead to death, or when. But there are statistics that include most people, and the most common sites for infections are the lungs, urinary tract, and blood stream, sometimes starting with a bedsore. Yet if a patient is choosing **Voluntary Refusal of Food & Fluid**, death would be expected in about two weeks.

As the option of **Voluntary Refusal of Food & Fluid** becomes better known and is chosen more often, I hope hospices will accept this legal peaceful choice as satisfying their criteria for admission and their patients' Medicare entitlement.

You should talk to your family, friends, and caregivers about your future intentions. Some chronically ill people feel they are far more of a burden on their loved ones than they really are. You may decide to postpone **Voluntary Refusal of Food & Fluid** when you begin to discuss it, even though you still feel it will be something you will do in the future. In the meantime, you can continue to enjoy significant meaningful and memorable interaction with your family.

Ask your physician if, when the time comes, he or she will provide sufficient medication to keep you comfortable or whether you will have to ask for pain-relieving medications several times a day. It is usually preferable if your doctor writes orders for the nurse to administer your medications on a routine schedule that keeps ahead of the onset of your pain. Here is why: If you do not ask for more medication until your pain returns, you will suffer as you wait and then you may need more medication for relief. Your doctor may also order a machine that allows you to press a button to receive the next dose of medication, if you are capable of pushing a button, as long as the amount of fluid delivered is small.

Just letting your physician know that you intend to choose **Voluntary Refusal of Food & Fluid** raises the question whether you need more aggressive *Comfort Care* or treatment for depression and anxiety. Ask your doctor about seeing a psychiatrist. An evaluation for depression and your mental capacity to make medical decisions may reassure everyone concerned that your resolve is sound. Laying the groundwork early on is the best way to avoid delays when you are ready to begin **Voluntary Refusal of Food & Fluid**. If aggressive palliative care does reduce your most bothersome symptoms, such as air hunger, physical pain, or nausea—and you can then find meaning in life—you may postpone the time when you **Voluntarily Refuse Food & Fluid**.

Ask your physician to sign a pre-hospital Do Not Attempt to Resuscitate Order (or a POLST, **Physicians' Order for Life-Sustaining Treatment**). Keep that written order near you so that emergency physicians and technicians who do not know your preferences do not employ invasive and burdensome interventions that you do not want. As some of the stories in this book illustrate, despite clearly written instructions in their Advance Directives, some patients were nevertheless whisked away by ambulances to Emergency Departments or ICUs where unwanted procedures such as resuscitation attempts were performed.

If you reside in a long-term care or skilled nursing facility, discuss your intention with its staff. You will need their support and assistance.

Complete all your business and financial tasks, make your funeral and memorial plans, and say your good-byes.

Finally, always remember: Even after you start **Voluntary Refusal of Food & Fluid**, as long as you are conscious, you can change your mind to postpone the process, but do so with the advice of your physician, since your medical condition might be complicated, and blood tests to monitor your potassium level may be necessary. (See also i-FAQ # 8: What if I change my mind? How do I resume intake of Food & Fluid?)

35. Are Relatives Taking a Legal Risk by Helping a Loved One Who Voluntarily Refuses Food & Fluid?

While suicide is legal, assisting suicide is not legal (except as permitted under special circumstances in Oregon). Competent patients have the Constitutional Liberty to refuse medical treatment, including artificial nutrition and hydration, and incompetent patients who have documented their previously expressed wishes *clearly and convincingly* may refuse via a Proxy. For patients who can still swallow, one safeguard for the caregiver is to continue to offer these patient Food & Fluid, in good faith, so they can change their mind, if they wish.

Withholding sustenance can also be in bad faith, and not in the best interest of the patient, who was harmed. The two next cases illustrate how different the intentions and circumstances were, compared to other examples in this book:

SKIP

From Extreme Neglect to Murder

The Cases of Kimberly Loebig and Delores Johnson

In April of 2004, prosecutors in Pittsburgh, Pennsylvania, charged Kimberly Loebig with first-degree murder charges for allegedly starving her disabled brother to death. Her brother, Scott Olsen, was an incapacitated young man who was made a ward of Loebig following a significant brain injury in 1996. When Mr. Olsen's six-foot body was found, he weighed just over 60 pounds. Ms. Loebig now faces life in prison, or the death penalty, if found guilty.

In October of 2004 in Rialto, California, Delores Johnson was sentenced to 29 years to life in prison for the starvation death of her autistic brother, Eric Bland. She also received an additional sentence of 14 years for dependent abuse. Eric Bland, a 38 year-old man, was only 70 pounds when police found him dead in his sister's home. Deputy District Attorney, Tristan Svare told the press: "To see a helpless, developmentally disabled man being starved to death—photos of him on his deathbed, sinking in his bed and his clothes hanging off him—it was like seeing a Holocaust victim." Allegedly, the motivation to neglect Eric Bland was that his sister wanted to feed her own cocaine habit with their brother's social security pension money (SSI) instead of caring for him.

ℝ℞

Attorney Michael Evans, J.D., M.S.W., made these points to make clear that Scott Olsen's act was NOT voluntary: (1) Appointed by the court to provide care for her brother, Ms. Loebig had a court-imposed duty to act on behalf of the State to protect her brother from harm because he could not protect himself. (2) Scott Olsen's refusal of nourishment cannot be considered a "voluntary" choice since he lacked mental capacity. If his condition had deteriorated to a persistent vegetative state, Ms. Loebig could have petitioned the court for permission to cease Food & Fluid. Only if the court had then authorized this course of action would she be allowed to carry it out.

In the Johnson case: (1) Eric probably lacked mental capacity to **Voluntarily Refuse Food & Fluid**. Delores Johnson's role as the caretaker of a dependent adult created a **legal duty** to maintain his sustenance. Failing in that duty makes her **negligent** for caring for a person dependent upon on her. Intentionally endangering him creates **criminal liability**. If injury had reduced Eric's functioning to a vegetative state, then his sister, as his caretaker, would be obliged to sustain him. She would *not* have the authority to **Refuse Food & Fluid** for him unless she petitioned a court to issue an order granting that permission. (2) Delores Johnson's action cannot be interpreted as furthering Eric's benefit. Instead she was clearly feeding her own drug habit at his expense, a violation of the trust placed in her. California law imposes a duty of basic care for health and sustenance on persons in the caregiver role. Willful neglect of that duty is grounds for prosecution.

CONTINUE

Both the Loebig and the Johnson cases illustrate that if you are the **caregiver for a dependent person who has expressed the wish to Refuse Food & Fluid, it would be unwise and risky to comply with those wishes** unless you have in your possession: (a) *independent* clinical documentation that the person had decision-making capacity to make such a life-ending choice and (b) *clear and convincing* documentation that the **person voluntarily expressed these specific wishes**, which were *independently* witnessed by others as required to meet the legal standards of your State. In circumstances where these could not be obtained (that is, the person lost decision-making capacity prior to expressing clearly and convincingly, his or her end-of-life wishes), obtain the court's explicit permission.

If you, as a patient, want to effectively empower your **Proxy to Refuse Food & Fluid** on your behalf in the future when you are no longer competent, you can protect your agent or Proxy from criminal accusations by documenting that you possessed decision-making capacity when you clearly and convincingly expressed the voluntary wish that your **Proxy Refuse Food & Fluid** on your behalf under certain conditions in the future.

36. Is There a Legal and Peaceful Alternative to Physician-Assisted Suicide?

[FORM II: I Wish to Voluntarily Refuse Food & Fluid NOW]

Yes there *is* a legal, peaceful alternative. One often-asked question (in addition to arguing about what term to use) is: Why is there so much political controversy over Physician-Aided, Patient-Hastened Dying when the alternative is so simple: to merely Refuse Food & Fluid? The three main reasons are:

A) Lack of information. Terminally ill patients and their families need to know that this method is available. If they knew, mercy killing (see the Prologue), violent ways of dying, and premature dying would not seem necessary. Broad educational programs are necessary for the general public and professionals. There is also misinformation: Refusal of Food & Fluid is *not* "barbaric starvation."

B) Fear that hunger or thirst is so uncomfortable that great discipline will be required for the process to succeed. The staff of Caring Advocates has developed a **TRAK** (**T**hirst **R**eduction **A**id **K**it), has created an instructional DVD, and hosts the sharing of new information and success stories to overcome the symptom of thirst on www.ThirstControl.com, which offers a toll-free phone number: 888-THIRST-0 (888-844-7780). (Basic information is provided on pages 97-111.)

C) Fear of sabotage. Many people who Refuse Food & Fluid will not encounter any conflict as they experience a legal peaceful transition, especially if they remain at home with family members who accept their decision. Yet others have worries that are similar to the anonymous person who wrote, "But They Just Want To Save Me" (page 226) or to Gus, who was resuscitated (page 316). To gain more confidence that their Last Wishes will be fulfilled after they loose consciousness, some may appoint a trusted person to be their "Caring Advocates Guard." All should complete a strongly-worded document similar to the one offered next.

I Wish to Voluntarily Refuse Food & Fluid NOW

This document expresses my **Constitutional right to decide what happens to my body**. In the area of end-of-life decision-making, the practical application of this right leads to a well-known standard of practice in both medicine and the law:

> Any adult whose judgment is not impaired by mental illness may refuse any medical treatment, even if such refusal hastens dying.

I am aware of this ethical position stated by the American Medical Association: "The social commitment of the physician is to sustain life and relieve suffering. Where the performance of one duty conflicts with the other, **the preferences of the patient should prevail**." In that spirit, I request my physicians to provide me with the best available *Comfort Care* regardless of any other decision I make about what happens to my body (even if they personally disagree with my decisions), and even if they hold the opinion that, because of those decisions, I need additional *Comfort Care*.

I am aware of research by Dr. Linda Ganzini and others that was published in 2003. They asked experienced hospice nurses to rate the quality of dying for their last competent patient who was capable of drinking fluids but chose to **Voluntary Refusal of Food & Fluid** at the end of their lives. On average, these patients experienced a **good death**, with a score of **8**, where "**9**" was the highest score for "a very good death," and "**0**" was a very bad death. They rated their **peace** higher, and their **suffering** lower, than those patients who opted for physician-assisted suicide (which was legal in Oregon). Moreover, 70% of surveyed nurses stated they would choose **Voluntary Refusal of Food & Fluid** for themselves if they were terminally ill.

Based on what I consider a realistic view of my current and future medical and mental conditions, I have therefore made the decision detailed below. The first part my decision is indicated by my writing my initials in one of the boxes below (or by directing someone to do so for me, with witnesses, if I am physically unable to initial):

|_____| (*Your initials*) I have decided **NOT to enroll in hospice** but I am willing to discuss both my decision not to enroll in hospice and my decision to **Voluntarily Refuse Food & Fluid** with a psychiatrist. I will also permit this psychiatrist to evaluate my capacity to make these medical decisions and to rule out the possibility that a mental illness is affecting my judgment.   **OR**

|_____| (*Your initials*) I **have enrolled in hospice** with the hope that their team of palliative care doctors and nurses, who are expert at delivering *Comfort Care*, can reduce my pain and suffering to the point where I will want to continue living. After I have given the hospice staff what I consider is a reasonable amount of time for this last treatment effort however, if I still feel my condition is unbearable and intolerable, I may then want to **Voluntarily Refuse Food & Fluid**.

Regardless of whether or not I have chosen to enroll in hospice (as indicated above), I am willing to cooperate with a psychiatrist to evaluate these beliefs: My decision to **Voluntarily Refuse Food & Fluid** does not arise out of my being depressed, anorexic, angry, or suicidal in the usual sense. To explain: I would love to go on living if I felt better, but in my present condition, I find my continued existence intolerable. I also believe that I possess the mental capacity to make sound medical decisions. **If any person, agency, or facility doubts the validity of these beliefs, I am willing to have a psychiatrist verify them, as long as the process of evaluation is completed within seven days of my signing below**. (If I disagree with the first psychiatric evaluation, I can request a second evaluation. If these two opinions disagree, then I can request a consultation from a third psychiatrist, or ask for a consultation from an ethics committee.)

I have had the opportunity to discuss the options of further aggressive palliative care with my physicians, to make final arrangements with my legal and financial advisors, to make my peace with my spiritual and pastoral counselors, and to resolve emotional issues from my past regrets and disappointments with my psychological counselors. I also have had an opportunity to make amends and say good-byes to as many friends and relatives as is reasonably possible. For them, as well as for those whom I have not had a chance to talk to directly, I have had an opportunity to consider creating an *ethical will* that can serve as my *loving legacy* as it contains my personal expression of values; that is, what I have learned in life. The statements in my *ethical will* are the essence of what I want people to remember about me.

As I begin my **Voluntary Refusal of Food & Fluid**, I hope that those who care about me will find comfort in knowing that I can change my mind to postpone the process to hasten my dying as long as I remain conscious (which is typically a few days). While I might need additional care from my physician, I realize that I can reverse the process to hasten my dying merely by asking for something to eat and to drink. I know there is a limit to how long I can wait to change my mind, beyond which time I may experience irreversible organ damage or become unconscious. But the potential for reversibility is one reason why I chose **Voluntary Refusal of Food & Fluid** to hasten my dying over physician-hastened dying, and why I have notified the people who care about me about my specific Last Wishes.

Important: I wish to be clear about one point: **I authorize no one to reverse my decision or to alter the course of my decision after I can no longer speak for myself**; for example, after I slip into a coma. To those lay or professional people, or institutions and agencies who would try to reverse my decision, read this: I emphatically state that my wish to Refuse Food & Fluid is **DURABLE**, by which I mean I want this decision to remain as the final statement of my end-of-life wishes that transcends my mental competence. After I lapse into unconsciousness, I forbid anyone from attempting to reverse my decision by going to a court of law or to an ethics committee to argue that placing a feeding tube or an intravenous line in me would be in my "best interest." I want to avoid such attempts since I consider such attempts **To Delay** as tantamount **To Deny** my Last Wish.

I now list those people I wish to be present at my bedside if they are available and able. They can remain at my bedside for as long as *they wish* |__| or as long as *I remain conscious* |__|. I look forward to our final opportunity to dialogue in general. I understand that some of them may feel a moral obligation to persuade me to change my resolve to continue **Voluntarily Refusing Food & Fluid**. While I will permit them to talk to me, I ask them to balance their attempts to persuade with **respect** for my wishes so that these discussions do not turn into arguments that cause me further anguish. If that situation should arise, I reserve the right to ask others to honor my request to remove them from my bedside. The people whom I want at my bedside are:

_____, _____,

_____, _____,

_____, _____.

Below, I list some individuals whom I wish to explicitly *exclude* from having any power to reverse my **durable** decision to **Voluntarily Refuse Food & Fluid**. (I may make additions to this list orally at any time.) They are entitled to follow their own beliefs for themselves, but I insist that they respect mine:

_____, _____,

_____, _____.

To overcome potential logistic problems such as unwanted resuscitation, rehydration, or transfer to an acute care hospital for any medical treatment, I have appointed the following person to be my "Caring Advocate Guard," whose role is TO FACILITATE my stated wishes, but has NO authority to make medical decisions on my behalf:

_____

Signed: _____ Dated: __ / __ / __

Note: In most states, documents such as this become valid when signed and stamped by a Notary Public, some of whom make home or institutional visits. If you prefer to have your signature witnessed, check with the specific requirements of your State, which may be strict. (Your doctor, those who will inherit your estate, and the owner of your institution are typically excluded.)

This form could refer to three attached statements (if desired):

First are my written suggestions for *Comfort Care* to specifically reduce suffering as I **Voluntarily Refuse Food & Fluid**. I encourage my caregivers to refer to www.ThirstControl.com and to call 888-THIRST-0 (888-844-7780).

The second document illustrates my own personal experiences or those of others of which I am aware, which provide the basis for why I have made the decision to Voluntarily Refuse Food & Fluid **now**. (Some of these experiences may be selected from the stories in the book, **The BEST WAY to Say Goodbye: A Legal Peaceful Choice at the End of Life**.)

The third document is a form that may be named, or is similar to a **Physician's Order for Life-Sustaining Treatment (POLST),** which my personal physician signed. (The exact name of the document will depend upon the State in which I live.) This form is a communication **from my doctor** to other health care providers that it is my wish to refuse emergency life-sustaining treatments such as Cardio-Pulmonary Resuscitation and transfer to an acute care hospital. (See page 316.)

Chapter 11

QUESTIONS THAT RELATE TO THE ROLE OF PHYSICIANS

The Important Roles of Doctors

They can facilitate...

                but they can also obstruct.

They can decrease guilt...

                but they can also increase guilt.

---

37. What Qualities Should I Look For, or Avoid, in My "Last Treating Physician?" and
How Can I Involve My Doctor in Advance Care Planning?

1. General Qualities: It is not realistic to expect one physician to possess all the ideal qualities that we could list for our "last treating physician." One reason is the lack of continuity in the way medical care is delivered in the United States. Many of us visit clinics where we see different physicians each time, or various physicians for a variety of complaints. Even when there is one doctor whom we call "our" primary care physician, we still cannot be sure that she or he will be "on call" for minor emergencies. So how much confidence can we have in predicting the identity of our last treating physician—whom we hope we will not need for several years or decades?

Furthermore, the best end-of-life treatment requires the skills of specialists whom we may meet for the first time in the last chapters of our lives. These specialists include the fields of oncology, cardiology, neurology, pulmonology, and nephrology. Yet it is our long-term primary care physician who is most likely to know about our life history, our family values, and our religious leanings, and who therefore would know whether or not we would rather leave our estate to our grandchildren rather than spend our assets on medical treatment in an Intensive

Care Unit if such treatment is unlikely to extend the quality of our lives. Primary care physicians, who are usually generalists in the fields of family medicine, internal medicine, geriatric medicine, and gynecology, will often defer treatment to our last physician(s). Finally and very importantly, among the ideal qualities of one of our last physicians is specific training in palliative care medicine to reduce our suffering, and either to be associated with, or to know when and how to refer us to hospice.

2. Essential Qualities: There are still certain traits that are reasonable to expect from any doctor involved in planning or administering our end-of-life care. Ronald Baker Miller, M.D., states that first, physicians must be committed to their patient's welfare. To dialogue well about end-of-life decisions, they should strive to be non-judgmental. Doctors need to be conscious of their own values so they can set them aside and accept their patient's preferences for end-of-life treatment. The duties of physicians are not limited to diagnosis and treatment, as Frances Peabody [1927] taught: the best way to care FOR a patient is to care ABOUT the patient. In sharing the decision-making process, physicians should discuss the possible treatment alternatives along with their risks, benefits, and probable outcomes. They should describe the possible scenarios with empathy and then allow patients, or other decision-makers, sufficient time to absorb the material and to ask additional questions before requiring them to finalize such difficult and often irreversible decisions. When the decision is made to choose *Comfort Care* over **aggressive care**, physicians must make it deliberately clear that efforts "to cure" have been replaced with other important goals. They should NEVER say, "There is nothing more we can do for you." Caring never stops even though the modality and goals of treatment may change.

Sometimes the best person to designate as your Proxy is someone who knows and cares about you, who can be objective, and who knows how the world of medicine works, but is not directly related to you. A doctor who is a friend of the family or moderately distant relative might meet all these criteria.

3. Time: Ideally, physicians should be involved in advance care planning with both the patient and Proxy. Yet a doctor's time is limited and few insurance companies have billing codes that pay for the time of such discussions. Research studies show that many doctors also lack the training or inclination to discuss these difficult issues. Even when doctors do discuss these issues adequately, additional steps are usually required. For legal effect, the decisions must be put in writing, and in some States, the document must be appropriately witnessed or notarized. Some States grant physicians the authority to make their patients' orally expressed wishes legally binding merely by writing their wishes in their medical charts, however. This is so, in California. Yet such expediency may preempt a wider discussion and dissemination of their wishes among interested parties. Some knowledgeable patients are effectively proactive by first creating their Advance Directives and then presenting the document to their doctors, as they remain open to accepting suggestions and revisions. Often, the challenge is to get the doctor to listen, as the next story illustrates:

"Doctor, please listen and comment on my plan."

At a meeting of the San Diego chapter of *End Of Life Choices* in 2005, the chapter president, Kenneth Fousel, said, "When I visited my doctor, I asked him if he would be willing to sit down with me to discuss the end-of-life preferences that I had written in my Advance Directives and make them part of my medical chart. I realized that my insurance company might not reimburse him for his time and that it would take us at least a half-hour, so I offered to pay him for his time at $300 per hour. Previously I had decided that if he refused, I would select another doctor. Fortunately, he agreed. So I handed my doctor a copy of my Advance Directives and as I looked at my copy, we went through the document together, line-by-line. I considered his suggestions, and, at the end of the visit, my doctor filed his copy in my medical chart."

Mr. Fousel advised those in the audience to consider a similar strategy. While some doctors may still not be willing to talk about Advance Directives, this tactic could eliminate the financial hurdle. (One problem still remains: to get that medical chart or at least the copy of this relevant section to the Emergency Department or Intensive Care Unit when a critical decision must be made. That function could be facilitated by a *Living Will Advocate*.)

❦

Does a half-hour sound like a reasonable amount of time to discuss the complexities and contingencies to make future life-or-death decisions? Readers of this book will have already put in several times that amount of time to arrive at this page. Yet in one study, Dr. James Tulsky and others [1998] learned that, in discussions about advance care planning during regular office visits, physicians spoke for only about 4 minutes, and they allowed their patients to speak for less than 2 minutes. Furthermore, these doctors were judged to be vague about outcomes. While one-quarter of the patients expressed a desire not to be maintained as a "**vegetable**," no physician in the study asked any patient what he or she meant by this statement. Only 25% of the doctors mentioned the decision about initiating or withdrawing **artificial nutrition or hydration**. The authors concluded, "Physicians may not have addressed the topic in a way that would be of substantial use in future decision-making, and these discussions did not meet the standards proposed in the literature."

Subsequent published comments about Dr. Tulsky's research finding raised the doubt that additional time might not, by itself, suffice to improve the quality of communication (see the story below).

4. Quality of Communication: The closer researchers looked, the more problems they found in doctors' communication with patients. Even when the focus was only on patients' consent for "routine clinical decisions," Braddock and others [1997] showed that physicians **rarely** assessed their patients' understanding of the decision.

Returning specifically to Advance Directives, Roter and others [2000] compared experts (those who had published in the field) with community physicians—regarding their initial discussions with a group of patients who were either over the age of 65 or had serious illnesses. The experts spent almost twice as long as did community physicians in these discussions: 15 minutes compared to 8 minutes. Experts emphasized the psychosocial and lifestyle areas and engaged more in partnership-building than did community physicians. While communication was still far from perfect, it is significant to note the context of this research study: All the physicians were aware that their discussions were being audiotaped for research analysis. That condition should have encouraged the doctors to communicate their best, or better than they typically would have.

How important are such discussions? One of the coauthors of the last study, Dr. James Tulsky, published a "Perspectives" essay that indicated how much progress this area still needs [2005]. Part of it is summarized below.

Tragedy on the ICU

An Unnecessary and Traumatic Resuscitation

Surgeons discovered that a 55 year-old man's cecum (lower bowel) had perforated. Cancer had spread throughout his abdomen, which they could not close before they transferred him to the Medical Intensive Care Unit. When his daughter saw him in that state, she was distraught. "They were hooking him up to everything and they couldn't give him pain meds because... his heart would stop. They just kept him hanging on in agonizing pain... " She stated her father would not have wanted to be kept alive in this situation and that he had completed an Advance Directive ten days earlier. The primary physician returned to his office where he hoped that, by then, he would have received a FAX from the patient's attorney —the Advance Directive that designated the daughter as his Proxy. Until this point, the patient had not signed a DNR, but his medical status kept on changing.

Meanwhile, the patient had a cardiac arrest to which the Medical ICU team responded by beginning efforts to resuscitate.

His daughter objected vigorously as she stood between her father and the code team. She recalled screaming, "Why won't you listen? I am giving [you] the document that says he does not want this. He is in pain. He's talking through morphine telling you to let him die and you're ignoring his wishes."

Only after resuscitation did a physician write the "Do Not [Attempt to] Resuscitate (DNR)" order. Later, in referring to "one of the most horrendous experiences of my time as a physician," he recalled how his patient gestured to the endotracheal tube (that kept him breathing) and "kept trying to pull the tube out, saying that he was in a great deal of pain... The tube was removed and he died not long after that." (The patient was sedated before removing the tube.)

The experience also led the daughter to lose trust: "I think, in all honesty, that [the physicians] were more interested in protecting their own jobs, not wanting to be responsible for my father's death... It wasn't until I got emotional and started screaming and crying that anyone noticed... We had discussed over and over again my father's wish for a good quality of life. It kind of goes null and void when you have a whole new set of doctors who just come in and start treating the patient."

After the patient died, one physician explained that, although it was clear that the patient valued quality over quantity of life, he was still unsure from reading the patient's written Advance Directive whether a "perforated bowel" met the patient's criteria for withholding aggressive treatment. (Note: This is a typical problem: How to interpret the Living Will.) Yet this doctor did agree that he could have been more forceful in recommending that the attempt to resuscitate be withheld, since he knew that such attempts were rarely successful in patients with advanced cancer.

The author of the article, Dr. Tulsky, explained that while Advance Directives are NOT the equivalent to DNR orders, there was no reason to wait to receive the Advance Directive to write the DNR order. He also stated, "Misunderstandings remain about the role and applicability of Advance Directive documents, and interpretation of preferences may be difficult when overshadowed by questions of uncertainty, trust, affect, and hope."

Dr. Tulsky concluded, "This case is an extreme example of what can go wrong when advance care planning takes the form of nonspecific discussions and documentation as opposed to directed discussions with the physician about the patient's condition and facts of the case."

☙❧

This story also illustrates the limitation of the "**Directive to Physician**" (Living Will) as a NON-self-enforcing document that CANNOT anticipate changes as they occur. Ultimately, the daughter had to make decisions on behalf of her father as more information became available. Dr. Tulsky wrote she apparently "acted as her father would have, in consenting to the surgery, but then wanting withdrawal of support." In other words, she met the criteria for Substituted Judgment. Yet by relying on the **Directive to Physician**, a "tragedy occurred when the withdrawal of support was delayed, and the patient underwent an unnecessary and traumatic resuscitation attempt."

Strategies to Help Avoid Unnecessary and Traumatic Resuscitations

(Note: The points below can be generalized, but for purposes of illustration, refer to the case above.)

A) The father could have designated his daughter as his Proxy in a written **Proxy Directive**, which gave her immediate power as his co-decision maker, even if he was still competent to make his own medical decisions.

B) The daughter could have brought this empowering document to the hospital, to prove her authority to any physician who became involved in her father's care.

C) In that case, physicians who felt that his life could be saved only by taking immediate action could have felt comfortable in following the daughter's decisions. They would not need to wait for a FAX, or feel they needed to interpret the nuances of the father's intentions from what he wrote when he did *not* know his exact present circumstances.

D) Had an empowering **Proxy Directive** been in place, the daughter would have asked her father's physicians about the likely risks and benefits of the treatment options (including no treatment), and then strived to make the decision that she felt her father would have made under those conditions.

E) Had there been two documents—a **Directive to Physician** (Living Will) and a **Proxy Directive**—then one additional statement, as to which had priority would also be necessary. In this case, the better outcome would have been to prioritize the Proxy's decision.

F) Even if the daughter had placed the patient's treatment-refusing documents in front of the doctor's face, the patient could still insist that the doctor "err on the side of life." Neither the law nor doctors' ethics requires patients possess ability to make medical decisions for them to override a Living Will or a Proxy's current decision—if they wish to continue treatment to sustain their lives. This priority reduces the risk of *immediately* authorizing another person to serve as one's Proxy.

After Dr. James Tulsky read the strategy above, he made this comment: "People should definitely choose health care Proxies, but they must have in-depth discussions about their values, priorities, and preferences, so that their designated Proxies (often, their loved ones) can avoid misinterpreting their preferences. If a patient also completes a Living Will, this document should be more focused on values, goals, and general preferences rather than on specific treatments—all of which should be discussed with the Proxy."

Given such real-life communication problems between doctors and patients, it is not surprising that the arts rarely encourage such dialogues. Actually, art often portrays physicians in an unkind manner. In the play and movie, "Whose Life Is It Anyway?" discussed above, the treating physician never stopped worshipping the "god" of preserving life, regardless of the patient's clearly expressed wishes.

The next example from the arts makes its impact via omission. The play "Vesta" by Bryan Harentiaux [2002] is becoming a popular means to introduce lay people to end-of-life issues.

Vesta's Story

Vesta recovered from a stroke and then from the side effects of cancer chemotherapy after she refused further chemotherapy. After she regained her strength, the elderly woman could again enjoy walks with her granddaughter, Kelly. One afternoon, to Kelly's surprise, they arrived at a lawyer's office where Vesta talked a bit and then signed a Living Will. As dinner ended that evening, Vesta read the "no nutrition or hydration" and "do not resuscitate parts" to her family.

Although several doctors had, or were treating, Vesta for her stroke, cancer, and heart failure—Vesta consulted none of them about her end-of-life wishes. So the play implicitly discouraged such discussions with physicians.

The play portrayed well how family members can struggle to let go. Near the end, Vesta's daughter said, "She's my mother... I'm not going to watch her starve [sic] in my own home. No food or water. Just watching. I can't do it." The granddaughter responded, "It's not about us, Mom. Gramma did a strong thing... She sat at the dinner table and told us what she wanted. She said 'No' to all that." Kelly ended the play by informing the audience that Vesta received hospice care in their home and that she died peacefully three days later—as her mother, Vesta's daughter, stood at her bedside and held her hand.

5. How accurate is the art of prognosis?: Dr. James Bernat wrote, "Physicians have an ethical duty to accurately determine and clearly communicate a patient's prognosis because a patient's or surrogate's decision whether to consent for aggressive treatment rests largely on their understanding of the patient's diagnosis and prognosis" [2004]. Dr. James Tulsky [2000] reviewed a book written by Nicholas Christakis [1999] as "the most scholarly analysis ever written on prognosis." Both a physician and a sociologist, Dr. Christakis revealed how doctors tend to overestimate survival and future quality of life, which is called the optimistic bias. He noted that some doctors behave as if they believe in the "self-fulfilling prophecy"—that merely predicting good outcomes will cause them to happen. Dr. Christakis cautioned, "Patients may be twice removed from the truth of their disease and its prognosis: first, because physicians themselves generally believe the prognosis to be more favorable than it is, and second because they generally do not communicate their actual beliefs to the patient" [*Page 123*].

Not all physicians estimate too high when it comes to survival prognosis. The president of the Canadian Critical Care Society, Dr. Graeme Rocker, led a multi-centered study that included 15 ICUs in 4 countries [2004]. Their results showed a strong pessimistic bias that this table summarizes:

Predicted *Versus* Actual Survival on the ICU

Prediction by Physicians	Actual Survival
Predicted "less than 10%"	29%
Predicted "10 to 40%" survival	79%
Predicted "41 to 60%" survival	91%
Predicted "61 to 90%" survival	96%

For every category of prognosis, actual survival on the ICU was higher than the physicians' predictions. While the accuracy of prognosis was greater when physicians visited patients more than once to form their opinions, and while some of the patients who were discharged from the ICU later died in other areas of the hospital, the discrepancy between prediction and actual was still greater than two-fold for those patients who were most seriously ill (e.g., predicted as "less than 10%").

If family members were aware of such discrepancies, it is possible that they might have less confidence in trusting physicians who predict a poor prognosis for their loved ones when asked to make an irreversible treatment decision. Physicians play an important role in determining the fate of seriously ill patients. Dr. Rocker shared this view: "Patients do not want their fate determined by the serendipity of the ICU in which they land, or the ICU team to which their care is entrusted."

6. Other kinds of bias: In addition to the optimistic bias and the pessimistic bias, other kinds of bias can influence doctors' behaviors and decisions. Some are subtle or unconscious, but none have been quantitatively researched to my knowledge. The novel *Lethal Choice* [Terman, 2007] considers these types:

"Dr. Wallet" includes physicians who work in a doctor-owned HMO where the less money the corporation spends on treating patients, the larger their salary or bonus.

"Dr. Burn-out" is so emotionally drained and tired from overwork that he might unconsciously be more eager to agree with decisions to hasten dying so that he would have fewer middle-of-the-night calls and be less frustrated by having to perform procedures that turn out to be futile.

"Dr. Religious" includes physicians who believe that only God can decide when a biologic existence should end (notwithstanding the ability of modern technology to prolong the process of dying or even to keep neurologically brain-dead bodies functioning). Some doctors may believe suffering is necessary for salvation. Such biases can prolong the process of dying, increase suffering by under-treating pain, increase the psychological burden of the family members, and drain the financial resources of the patient's estate and of society.

Another label that applies to some physicians is "Dr. Scared." These doctors fear malpractice suits brought by vocal family members who survive after their patients die so they follow the family members' requests even when they know the patient would have chosen differently. Another type of fear plagues physicians who aggressively treat end-of-life pain: the fear of accusations that they overdosed their patients to hasten dying, which could lead to criminal charges, loss of their licenses, or imprisonment. The failure of Gonzales v. Oregon in the 2006 U.S. Supreme Court decreased this fear for physicians in all States.

The bias of "Dr. Hero" can seem consistent with the concept of a "good" doctor so many people may not be aware that some doctors can be too zealous in their attempts to treat patients to get well. Such efforts may only increase and prolong physical and mental suffering. Other physicians qualify for the term, "Dr. Hope." These doctors may be in denial because they are reluctant to reveal bad or disappointing news to their patients or their families.

"Situational" bias can arise for any outside factor that has a significant impact on the physician's mood. For example, if the physician has just experienced a great personal or business loss, he might express more pessimism about a patient's prognosis than at other times, for example: "Dr. Bad-Hair Day"

Still another type of potential bias is relational. The better and longer a physician knows his patient, the more likely the doctor will predict a high likelihood for survival and quality of life. For this type of bias, the term, "Dr. Friend," may be appropriate.

Although not strictly a bias, some doctors can be described as "Dr. Avoidant" or "Dr. (too) Sensitive," if they decline the opportunity to relate to their patients on the deepest human level, as discussed next:

Dr. Beck and others [2005] began their article entitled, "On Saying Goodbye: Acknowledging the end of the patient-physician relationship with patients who are near death," with this typical quote: "... You'll be in good hands with hospice. I'll see you later." This "goodbye" is not appropriate if the doctor's true expectation is that he or she will never see the patient again. Dr. Beck's paper suggests that engaging as a human being in the reality of the impending loss of the doctor-patient relationship can "create an opening for physicians to hear and receive the deep appreciation that patients and their loved ones often express and gives physicians a chance to reflect on the meaning of their work in a way that may enhance their resilience." The authors conclude that the challenging practice of saying goodbye "requires that the physician be mindful, authentic, and willing to lead" [the patient].

7. Cultural competence: Physicians must be sensitive to patients' particular cultural mores. Dr. Alex Green and others [2003] defined cultural competence as, "providing health care that takes into account the unique sociocultural based perspective of the patient / family / community, focusing on effective communication, trust building, and a sensitivity to differences in attitude, custom, and belief." The authors urged transcending the reductionistic oversimplification of stereotypes while keeping relevant themes in mind. Most health care providers trained in the Western tradition place a high value on autonomy, the rights of the individual, and full disclosure to the patient. Yet some cultures have different priorities. In such cases these authors suggest asking the patient to state his or her preferences about who should receive medical information and who is the decision-maker. If possible, discussion about this issue should occur prior to forming life-threatening diagnoses.

Betancourt, Green, and others [2000] give several examples: "Certain Navajos consider it inappropriate to make mention of any negative future events because voicing them is akin to wishing for their occurrence." People from "countries such as Japan, China, and the United Arab Emirates" may prefer doctors to withhold information from patients if the diagnosis is terminal. Even in the United States, some subcultures have "a more family-centered approach to decision-making" or "believe in the power of hope, and the negative consequences of losing hope."

Paul Rousseau [1999] reviewed the racial disparity in advance care planning. His article has many citations to studies which indicate that African Americans are more likely to request aggressive treatment, and are less likely to complete Advance Directives, when compared to white contemporaries—even if they are reside in nursing homes, where the patients are older and more often afflicted with chronic and terminal maladies. One study, for example, revealed that 53% of whites intended to complete a living will compared to 24% of non-whites.

While understanding the reasons for such differences is still an area that deserves further investigation, Dr. Rousseau cited some interesting findings: In one survey, 14% of African Americans believe that such documents would decrease the quality of medical care compared to 4% of whites; and 18% believed these documents would promote a feeling of hopelessness compared to 9% of whites. Another study showed that 25% of African American patients felt *how long they lived* was more important than *how well they lived*, compared with only 6% of white patients. Another factor may be the race of the doctor with whom the patient communicates. Among young nonwhite patients with acquired immunodeficiency syndrome, 56% discussed resuscitative measures with nonwhite physicians but only 22% discussed them with white physicians. Although distrust is frequently cited, one large study that Dr. Rousseau cited showed no differences in the "stated degree of distrust" of the medical system or fear of inadequate medical treatment.

Certainly, mistrust is warranted among African American patients given the infamous Tuskegee Study of Untreated Syphilis. Some studies have shown that Latinos are more likely than whites to feel they are treated unfairly as cited by Betancourt and others [2000]. These last authors conclude with a statement on "the ethics of caring" that adds to what qualities to look for in physicians: "incorporate attributes of attentiveness, honesty, patience, respect, compassion, trustworthiness, and sensitivity, into all acts of behavior."

Given all the potential conflicts of interests due to physician bias, some States, including California, exclude any treating physician from qualifying as eligible to serve as your designated health care power of attorney (Proxy). They also often require at least one of the witnesses to your Advance Directive to have no interest in your estate, which usually excludes their being a close genetic relative. While some professional associations discourage "dual relationships"—defined as having more than one relationship with a patient—such relationships may work well at times. Often the key to success is the professional's awareness of conflicts of interest. Professional standards that forbid dual relationships are designed to protect vulnerable patients from potential harm, but that does not necessarily mean that dual relationships cannot work well in some case, as illustrated in the next story. I believe Dr. Ronald Baker Miller responded to the medical and emotional needs of his mother as he recognized and overcame his possible bias due to their other relationship.

A Peaceful End to a Beautiful Life

© Ronald Baker Miller, M.D.

My mother, Virginia Gordon Wilson Miller, was born in 1911 in Swarthmore, Pennsylvania. Even before she married my father at the age of 16, she was an actress and a dancer. But she gave up that career in New York City to raise three children, and moved to California. When the youngest began kindergarten, my mother taught in a psychoanalytically-oriented nursery school. She then became the director of a second nursery school, undertook research on the therapy of autistic children, taught underprivileged children in the Head Start program, and volunteered at a State hospital for children. In her 60s, she went to college and received an AA degree. Her favorite retirement activities were family celebrations, traveling, and bird watching. Her greatest interests were the environment and national and foreign affairs. But above all, she was a nurturing, nonjudgmental, encouraging mother, grandmother, and great grandmother.

In her 70s, she fractured her hip, which ended her ability to enjoy "square dancing on horseback." She required months of hospitalization because of additional falls, a fractured pelvis and femur, removal of an artificial hip for infection, and later, a second artificial hip. She was so disabled from these injuries and from unrelenting pain from arthritis that it took her five minutes and great effort just to walk across a room. Yet she rarely complained. Instead, she remained cheerful and optimistic about the futures of the world and of her family and friends, even though she outlived many of them. She was never quite the same after she lost the independence afforded by her driver's license and the ability to drive friends to the theater and to musical performances. She refused to live with any of her children or in an assisted-living facility.

Her most threatening medical problems were chronic lung disease and congestive heart failure. I recommended hospice to improve the quality of her care, but her internist, who was the director of a home-health agency and hospice, thought the timing was premature. However he gladly directed her care in hospice after the cardiologist concurred that hospice was appropriate. Hospice provided outstanding care and support for my mother, my two sisters, and me. My older sister left her home 400 miles away from my mother in order to care for her. She prepared meals and helped with dressing, toileting, and bathing. She also drove my mother to physician visits and helped fill out innumerable insurance forms and pay medical bills.

Since I am a nephrologist and internist, my mother's physician asked me to adjust her medications, especially diuretics to control the congestive heart failure. This was not uncomfortable for me since, over many months of hospitalization over two decades, I had often attended to my mother's basic comfort and minor medical needs (e.g., diet, stool softeners, sleeping medications) allowing her surgeons and physicians to attend to important postoperative and other medical needs. To my dismay, the high doses of potent diuretics needed to remove excessive body fluid also impaired my mother's kidney function. When resultant waste-product retention (her BUN was 105 mg per 100 ml.) threatened symptoms, I felt compelled to discuss the option of dialysis for kidney failure with my mother. Dialysis would not only prevent uremic symptoms of kidney failure, but could also control body fluids and thereby prevent heart failure and shortness of breath.

When I presented this "bad news," my mother was obviously distraught—but not for the reason I assumed. Rather than being concerned about the medical consequences of kidney failure, she was upset because she thought that I was recommending dialysis, rather than merely informing her of this treatment option. Previously, my mother had begun to hint that she hoped she would die of natural causes soon. Now, she stated firmly that she did not want to undergo dialysis because of her increasing disability and dependence, and the added burdens she knew dialysis would impose. By then, she was suffering the indignity of bowel incontinence. Although it was only occasional, she found it quite embarrassing and especially problematic since she could not bathe without great effort and the risk of physical injury.

I expressed relief when my mother refused dialysis, understanding that, from her perspective, the burdens of this treatment would outweigh the benefits, and be intolerable even though dialysis might be needed only temporarily. Fortunately, reducing the dose of diuretics alone was sufficient to allow her kidney function to return to its previous asymptomatic level without an increase in shortness of breath.

Unfortunately, she then developed uncontrollable muscle contractions with jerking movements in her arms. They could be controlled only with medication that also caused sedation. She was either awake and jerking, or asleep. Worse, my mother considered this problem to herald further loss of control of her own body and further dependence on others. Despite her active and inquisitive mind, as she approached her 91st year, she decided it was time to "surrender."

When my mother asked me to help her end her life, I procrastinated since selfishly I wished her to live longer, and I knew that her daughters, my children, and her other grandchildren all wished to visit her. But I was ambivalent since I could appreciate her existential suffering and exhaustion from the involuntary movements that needed daytime sedation despite her nighttime insomnia. After her physician prescribed a sedative medication, it was temporarily impossible to rouse my mother. Her breathing was so reduced that, at one point, my sister thought she had died. Since her physician was out of town, I discontinued the sedative.

By the next morning, my mother was fully awake and again she asked me to hasten her dying. I informed her that if she **ceased intake of all food & fluid**, she would die in a week or two. She had no hesitation in deciding to do this, even though one of her excellent hospice nurses thought it was immoral. At my request, my mother agreed to defer her fast for one day, to get up out of her hospital-type bed and sit in her lounge chair so that she could visit with family and friends who wished to celebrate her life.

Several years before, my mother had written a 350-page autobiography, and in the few months preceding her death, my sister had videotaped interviews in which my mother expressed her values and her hopes for the world and for the preservation of the environment. We had previously hosted a lovely and well-attended 90th birthday party for my mother, and that assuaged some of our guilt in helping her to depart. Although she was not religious and did not believe in an afterlife, several times in her final weeks as she awoke from a nap, she reported "visions" of friendly strangers who beckoned her to join them. My wife suggested that, if there were an afterlife, my mother might be able to debate politics with former presidents and world leaders. My mother found that suggestion pleasant and comforting.

After an exhausting day of visiting with family and friends (including an attempt by a friend to shake her resolve to **cease intake of food & fluid**), my mother returned to bed. We all came to realize that having done everything we could to express our love, it was now time to honor my mother's decision.

The following morning, however, she awoke and asked for breakfast. I wondered if she had changed her mind. Given my unintended influence when I had mentioned the possibility of dialysis, I was mindful that it was important for me to be neutral when asking her about this apparent change of mind. My facial expression must have revealed my concern as well as consternation when I said, "You may eat and drink whatever you wish, but remember if you eat and drink it will delay your dying." Without hesitation, she made it clear that she had simply forgotten. She was resolved to **forgo food & fluid**. She also commented that it must be very difficult for me to discuss her wish to die, but she appreciated my helping her. To the very end, my mother was nurturing, nonjudgmental, and encouraging. As I look back on that moment, it seems that my mother had reversed our roles: Whereas I was trying to be the counseling physician, she became the healer: affirming my feelings and attempting to relieve me of future guilt.

So my mother refrained from eating breakfast and continued her fast. She slept almost constantly for three days, and died quietly in her sleep on the fourth day. So ended a beautiful, devoted, nurturing, exemplary life.

My mother had all her financial affairs in order and had planned cremation with scattering of her ashes at sea. Although she preferred no funeral, she nevertheless consented to a memorial service when we explained that it would help bring closure for family and friends. Despite the passage of time and my solace in having facilitated a peaceful death for my mother who was suffering unbearably, I continue to find her death extremely sad and painful. —Even though she was blessed with a long and happy life that was meaningful not only to her but to countless others.

Afterthoughts: Why have I chosen to write about such personal matters?

My mother taught me, in the most personal way, that the decision to end one's life may be rational—even when one is not imminently terminal. She was depressed by her loss of independence in life, by her increasing lack of control of her own body and dependence on others, and by oppressive fatigue. Her psychological and existential suffering were not the typical symptoms that physicians and psychologists treat, and the symptoms may be less obvious than physical pain, but they are real, deserve our compassion, and can form a reasonable basis for the decision to **forgo food & fluid** if there is no other life-sustaining treatment that can be discontinued to hasten dying.

It is important that the refusal of life-sustaining treatment is not contaminated by lack of information, misinformation, treatable depression, or coercion, and to ascertain that such a decision is authentic, consistent, and persistent. **Forgoing food & fluid** can be relatively comfortable, and dying can be peaceful. The initial several days during which one is fully conscious provide an opportunity not only for a change of mind, but also for meaningful good-byes, amends, apologies, tributes, and an opportunity to leave a legacy of wisdom and love. My son said to me: "Your remorse over helping to facilitate the final transition of someone you loved so dearly, while taking pride that she achieved a desired and peaceful end, is one of the most important lessons that you have to share."

Ronald Baker Miller, M.D.
August 16, 2005, the 94th anniversary of my mother's birth.

38. What are My Options if My Physician Will Not Support My Decision to Voluntarily Refuse Food & Fluid?

If your physician is not willing to grant your wish for **Voluntary Refusal of Food & Fluid**, ask why. If your physician has no experience with the process or is not aware that exercising this option is legal and peaceful, ask him or her to call one of the organizations or clinicians who have knowledge about and experience with **Voluntary Refusal of Food & Fluid**.

The ethical guidelines of the American Medical Association do not require physicians to perform procedures that they feel are in conflict with their personal, moral, or religious values. But at the same time, these guidelines and some State laws DO REQUIRE the declining physician to refer the requesting patient to another physician or facility that may honor his or her legal request so you should ask for a referral. Sometimes patients must know and insist on their rights since some doctors will not volunteer this information. Some may even feel culpable for referring you to another doctor who will perform a procedure they believe is immoral. (The same applies to institutions and facilities.) To be more optimistic, some physicians may change their minds if you ask for a second opinion from a physician on staff, or for a consultation from the institution's ethics committee.

Consider this humorous story before reading the next one:

Who Can You Trust?

A gang leader finds out that his bookkeeper has cheated him out of ten million bucks.

This bookkeeper is deaf, so the gangster brings along his attorney, who happens to know sign language.

The gangster asks the attorney to ask the bookkeeper: "Where is the 10 million bucks you embezzled from me?"

Using sign language, the attorney asks the bookkeeper where he hid the 10 million dollars.

The bookkeeper is tied to a chair but still able to use his arms and signs back: "I don't know what you are talking about."

The attorney tells the gangster: "He says he doesn't know what you're talking about."

The gangster pulls out a 9 mm pistol, puts it to the bookkeeper's temple, cocks it, and says: "Ask him again!"

The attorney signs to the bookkeeper who is now shaking badly: "He'll kill you for sure if you don't tell him!"

The bookkeeper signs back with broad gestures: "OK! You win! The money is in a brown briefcase, buried behind the shed in the southeast corner of my cousin Enzo's backyard in Queens!"

For a while, the attorney doesn't say anything so the gangster has to ask: "Well, what'd he say?"

The attorney shrugs his shoulders and replies: "He says you don't have the guts to pull the trigger!"

The next story may be hard to believe, but it is true. I met "Jack" at a writers' conference where he shared this personal experience. It explained why he was so interested in the subject of this book.

Jack From Brooklyn Has "a Way" With Doctors

After my father had his third heart attack in two years, we both knew that his next could well be his last. We talked about it, but only a few words. Dad wasn't one for gab. He took pride in being a man of action, a quality that I tried to emulate.

I wasn't home the day Dad collapsed. In a state of emotional crisis, his friend called 9-1-1 before trying to reach me, and no one could find Dad's pre-hospital "Do Not Attempt to Resuscitate Order." As I sped to the hospital where he was being taken, I hoped that his medical evaluation would quickly determine whether or not there was a chance for Dad to recover to his previous level of functioning.

The doctor wouldn't let me see him for an hour. Then he told me Dad was in severe heart failure. As I entered the room I could see that he was receiving oxygen from a mask that covered his nose and mouth. The head of his bed was tilted down, and mechanical pumps were squeezing his legs. —All this to send enough blood with oxygen to his brain. In addition, the nurses said he was on a dozen medications. I had never seen anyone connected to so many tubes.

The nurses said the doctor would return in a few hours. I said, I'd wait, that I had something important to talk to him about. When he returned, I asked him what Dad's potential for recovery was. The doctor was evasive. I assured him I could handle bad news. I explained that Dad and I had discussed this before. The doctor was still vague. I wondered whether the doctor had a bad bedside manner or whether it was hard for him to share bad news. Either way, I assumed the unspoken message was that the news was bad.

That night, I slept on the couch in Dad's room. The next morning, I took a short break to get a cup of coffee. As I went through the cafeteria line, I overheard two medical students chatting in white coats. One said, "So this afternoon, we'll learn how to do peritoneal dialysis on that old man in 528."

Dad's room! I almost dropped my coffee. I left the cup on the tray and ran to the elevator. As I rode up, my teeth were clenched.

I looked down the hall and saw Dad's doctor come out of another patient's room. I dashed toward him, and stopped, planting myself in front of him. I tried to be calm as I asked, "How's my father doing?"

"I haven't seen him yet. I was just now going to his room," the doctor replied.

"Well, I'll wait, because I need to talk to you about him." I walked slowly to the plastic chairs at the end of the hall. After the doctor went in the room, I positioned myself directly in front of the door so that when the doctor exited we would be face-to-face. About ten minutes later, when he opened the door, I stood up so he had to stop short. I asked, "Well?"

"I'm sorry but there's not much to say. He's about the same."

"He looks worse to me," I said. "I still want an answer to the question I asked you yesterday—Does he, or doesn't he, have a chance of making a good recovery? You were vague then. Please tell me now."

"I wish I could say, but it's hard to tell," he replied.

"Look," I said, "this is Dad's fourth heart attack and it's obvious he needs many more tubes and machines than last time. Dad and I discussed this possibility. If he won't get better, Dad would say it's time to let him go. As his closest relative, I speak for him."

"I'd like to try a few more procedures and tests first," the doctor said.

"Like what?" I bit my tongue as I wondered if the doctor had to ask my permission to start peritoneal dialysis.

"Well his kidneys are not working all that well. He needs another machine to make up for it."

"What's the point?" I asked. "Will it make any long-term difference? You still have not answered my question: What exactly is his potential for recovering useful function?"

"You never know."

"Do you mean you don't KNOW? Or you won't SAY?" The doctor tried to walk around me, but I blocked him. "Tell me straight, right now." I was right in his face. His forehead had beads of sweat.

"Excuse me, please," he said. "I must see other patients. I'm doing all I can for your father."

I didn't budge. I raised my voice, "Is this a teaching hospital?"

"Yes, University Hospital trains many residents and interns."

"Be honest, Doc. What's the real reason you're keeping my father alive? Is it to train these young doctors?"

At that point, the doctor's face got red, but he managed to say, "We just want to be sure that we've given him every possible chance."

I took a step to the right and put my hand on his shoulder, then moved it across his back. One second later, I had the doctor in a Half-Nelson. "Look Doc! In my humble opinion, I think Dad would want you to let him go."

I restrained myself from squeezing too hard as I waited for an answer. None came, so I said, "Dad and I discussed what he would want when this time came. I ask you again, Doc, will you let Dad go?"

Silence.

"Okay Doc, maybe you need to think about it a little while. But as you do, remember two things: First, I know where you park your car. Second, I can be more convincing in a parking lot." I let him go.

The doctor stumbled forward. He turned back to glance at me, looked stunned, and ran across the hall to the staff toilet.

Dad was never dialyzed. That night, as I sat by his bed and gently held his hand, Dad died peacefully.

∽❧

While it is rare for a member of a patient's family to physically threaten a doctor, it is not uncommon for them to threaten lawsuits. Often they try to put it mildly by saying, "I'll make sure that you are held liable for the extra cost and his indignity." Although the high court in the Jean Elbaum case agreed with the husband to discontinue the feeding tube, it still held the husband responsible for the cost of care—$100,000 in 1980 dollars. Still, it is hard to convince a jury that a doctor did anything wrong by trying to keep a patient alive, as in the Furlong case. "Jack from Brooklyn" may have been generally aware of this.

Doctors who are threatened usually try to transfer the patient to another doctor. That can take considerable time, however. The State of Texas allows ten days. In this case, however, the doctor had reason to worry that Jack would not have much patience when it was possible to let Nature take its course. After four heart attacks, his father had little healthy heart muscle left, so all his doctors had to do was to stop some medications or mechanical support, and his blood pressure would drop and he would pass on peacefully. Consistent with that treatment plan, the doctor could also have written an order not to attempt resuscitation.

39. Can Doctors Significantly Affect the Guilt of Patients and Family Members?

"Sometimes, it is not so much what a doctor says... as when the doctor says it."

A woman who had attended one of our lectures called me on a Sunday evening. She wanted to discuss a challenging decision.

Her husband had suffered from Alzheimer's disease for 16 years. During the last 5, he seemed miserable, living in an "Alzheimer's only" institution. She was calling since he had a stroke the previous day and had not been able to eat or drink for 18 hours. The staff had suggested she consent to a Speech Pathologist consult to determine if her husband could still swallow. She talked with her son who saw no problem in asking for a consult.

Before this woman could ask me for my opinion on whether or not to have a Speech Pathologist evaluate her husband's ability to swallow, I blurted out, "If my husband or father were in that condition, I would NOT consent to have a Speech Pathologist's evaluation."

I not only broke with the usual "psychiatric protocol" to fulfill my profession's stereotype by answering a question with another question, I did not even wait for her to ask me the question!

She immediately agreed and recalled from my lecture that the time for any mild discomfort from not eating and drinking that some people experience had already passed. In her husband's case, he might not be aware enough to experience anything from his long-term deterioration from Alzheimer's. She also briefly reviewed the major surgeries and medical interventions her husband had undergone over the past few years, and then stated that if the time had come to let Nature take its course, she could accept that as long as she knew her husband was comfortable.

The bottom line was that she did not want to know whether or not her husband could swallow. She thanked me for expressing my opinion since it would help her explain how she felt to her son. It made no sense to consent to such an evaluation when the results would not change the inevitable course of events.

I asked her how she felt about my voicing my opinion BEFORE she asked for it, or even before she told me hers. She said the timing led her to believe that I had stated my true personal and professional opinions. Otherwise, she would have considered my stated opinion more skeptically, knowing that people pay psychiatrists to be supportive and nonjudgmental.

When I thought about it later, I realized that there had been a whole range of possible options, each of which had a different potential to cause guilt. In the continuum below, given the wife's beliefs, her guilt would increase with higher numbered options:

1. Express my opinion without waiting for her to ask (as above).

2. Agree with her opinion, after she had expressed it, risking her skepticism.

3. Not expressing my own opinion, or stating that either option—to consult or not to consult—would be acceptable.

4. Agree with her son by stating it would do no harm to consent to an evaluation by the Speech Pathologist.

5. State that an evaluation by a Speech Pathologist was necessary because if her husband could swallow, then he should be spoon-fed; otherwise, she could let Nature takes its course.

6. State that if the Speech Pathologist found that her husband could NOT swallow, then she should consent to insert a PEG tube through his stomach since such minor surgery is not a burden.

7. Tell her that tube feeding via a PEG tube is always "basic care" that "every human being deserves."

While I could have communicated options # 2, or 3, or 4, the first option reduced her guilt the most. I responded as I did to not aggravate her feelings of guilt. Other professionals whose values differ from mine could have endorsed # 5, 6, or 7, with increasing guilt—if she decided *not* to follow their advice. She would have felt badly in other ways, had she followed their advice.

The next story is about an infant, which makes doctors' roles more complicated since parents generally make decisions for their infants, but the State shares the duty to protect all children. [See also, Disclaimer # 8 in Chapter 1.]

Doctors' Fear of Investigation Leads to Increasing Parents' Guilt

My daughter seemed normal when she was born. However when Yvette was two months old, she had a series of strange seizures. She would jackknife at the waist, extend her neck, and her arms would wrap around herself in a tight self-hug. The neurologist called them "Infantile Spasms." After a thorough evaluation, the cause was determined to be a rare gene. Her prognosis was grim. She would never develop beyond the six-month milestones. The best my wife and I could hope for was that she would be able to hold her head up, grasp a toy, and roll over. —The most severe developmental arrest I had ever heard of.

I didn't have enough courage to ask how long Yvette might live and how she might die until our third visit. The neurologist was vague. My wife and I had several long, difficult discussions. We concluded that when Yvette could no longer take in nutrition, we would let Nature take its course. My wife's mother had a long, drawn-out process of dying from end-stage Alzheimer's, and that experience taught us a lot. It didn't do her any good to put in a PEG tube to feed her artificially. We agreed not to put Yvette through that.

The next time we saw the neurologist, we watched him examine Yvette and write notes in her chart, and then, as we had planned, we asked him, when Yvette could **no longer take in Food & Fluid**, could we expect his support to just keep her comfortable? His exact words were, "Don't worry. I'll do exactly what you want." It was strange to realize that I felt relief when we all agreed to let my daughter die. But I knew the reason was compelling: I did not want her suffering to be prolonged. With the toughest decision behind us, we could deal with the day-to-day details of her care and make her as comfortable as possible. We would not have to worry about how we would grapple with the ultimate decision, if there were a crisis. We could begin the mental process to let her go.

I still felt a bit unsettled. As I drove home from the neurologist's office, I had the vague feeling that something was incomplete. Many months later, I was able to pinpoint where this feeling came from: The neurologist had not re-opened Yvette's chart to document our momentous discussion.

At the age of sixteen months, Yvette developed serious bowel issues. A complete block would cause her colon to enlarge, burst, and lead to a blood infection that would be lethal. To avoid such dire consequences, we used increasingly vigorous bowel regimens. Twice a day, we placed Yvette on a mesh chair with small legs in a tub so she could stay out of the water as my wife and I kneeled on each side. We gently inserted a Fleet enema through an infant-size rectal tube and pushed it up about 12 inches to get above the stool. Then, I would rock Yvette side-to-side and massage her abdomen to gently push the stool down, as my wife removed stool with her gloved fingers.

Yvette hated this ordeal; she opened her mouth as if to scream, kicked her legs, made terrible faces, and cried nonstop. The procedure was physically and emotionally exhausting. So was the all-day process of feeding. On her worse days, Yvette would not open her mouth. She just moaned for hours. Nothing helped.

Exhausted from not sleeping for weeks, my wife and I went to the neurologist to learn if there was any way to reduce Yvette's suffering. We did not go to this visit consciously thinking perhaps "that time" had come. We waited patiently as he performed a physical examination, and ran an EEG and other tests. We sat in his office as he looked up after reviewing her medical chart. "Your daughter hasn't gained any weight in the last six months," he said. "Maybe it's time to start a feeding tube."

Stunned, I asked myself, how could he make this recommendation after our previous conversation? Had he forgotten his promise? Was this his way of informing us that he would renege and withdraw his support?

When I reminded him about our previous discussion to which he had agreed, he stated he personally had no problem with letting Nature take its course, but others might accuse us of child neglect or abuse.

Child neglect? Abuse? After all our extraordinary effort to avoid bowel complications, how could anyone accuse us of neglect or abuse? I was speechless, but my wife managed to ask the neurologist what he would recommend. He referred Yvette to a pediatric GI physician.

Prior to the appointment, I felt confident that this specialist would understand the total problem, that Yvette's entire GI tract was not functioning. So what good would it do, to insert a feeding tube? I was so wrong. The doctor's words were, "You can't let her starve to death. That would be a horrible death. A feeding tube is your only choice."

I felt beaten down and emotionally overwhelmed. I was so drained of energy from Yvette's daily ordeal and almost no sleep. I could not even imagine battling with two doctors. I knew they were wrong, but who would take care of Yvette if I had to meet with attorney several times, and spend time preparing for, waiting, and then, appearing in court? After discussing the options with my wife, we opted for the path of least resistance: to consent to the feeding tube.

For the next seven months, we watched Yvette struggle to absorb her feedings. At best she took in 25 ml, compared to the 80 ml that the doctor prescribed. She never smiled. Her little body filled up with secretions. She perspired profusely. Her skin developed terrible sores, especially around the entry site of the PEG tube. We used silver nitrate to disinfect, but that chemical stings even healthy skin. I knew that, from personal experience.

Tube feeding did little good in terms of Yvette's weight. Her skin color paled. She looked sickly. Desperate, I asked a hospice program to help us manage her care at home. Fortunately, the staff recognized how much emotional support my wife and I needed.

A few months after Yvette died, my wife and I were still very depressed. We went to see a family counselor who helped us distinguish our feelings of loss from our feelings of guilt. She confirmed our impression that the doctors had forced us to prolong Yvette's suffering, and that doing so had, in turn, increased our guilt.

To this day, because of what both doctors said, my wife struggles with intense guilt. Her thoughts follow this path: A mother should never consider letting her child go. She feels guilt even though, on an intellectual level, she knows that it would have decreased Yvette's suffering and definitely been in her best interest.

My guilt has another source: I repeatedly ask myself if I could have fought harder with these two doctors; if I could have advocated more vehemently for what was clearly in Yvette's best interest.

A year later, we reviewed the facts of Yvette's case with an end-of-life bioethicist. He gave us insight into why the doctors behaved as they did. The neurologist might have been afraid that the State's Child Protective Service would accuse him of neglect or abuse, so the safest option for him was to refer Yvette to a GI specialist. The bioethicist knew the GI specialist; he was a devout Catholic who believed that doctors should always try to preserve life.

According to the bioethicist, both doctors should have informed us that we had the right to ask for additional medical opinions, and they should also have referred Yvette to a physician whose moral, personal, and professional beliefs were not in conflict with our stated choice: to let Nature take its course. Even the strictest interpretation of the teachings of Pope John Paul II were in line with discontinuing or not initiating tube feeding since Yvette could not absorb enough fluid to maintain life (the Pope used the words, "proper finality"), and tube feeding definitely increased her suffering.

The State's obligation to provide an extra layer of "protection" to sick children, which leads to dozens of investigations of doctors every year, did not apply in Yvette's case since her prognosis was terminal. What difference did it make if she gained weight before she died? Why put her through so much more suffering for such a longer time?

I am still angry with these two doctors. They prolonged my daughter's suffering; they did not tell us we had other options; they did not refer us to other physicians. Clearly, one's motivation was to protect himself from an investigation and the other's was based on his religious beliefs. Neither disclosed their real reasons, and that caused months of suffering for my daughter, for my wife, and for me.

I did not pursue a lawsuit because the laws of my State give immunity to doctors if they act in good faith to preserve life. Attorneys told me it is always extremely difficult to prove that doctors did not act in good faith. Certainly, they did not gain financially from prolonging Yvette's suffering.

Eventually, I got the courage to request a copy of the neurologist's medical chart. Just as I feared, it did *not* include a note to memorialize our conversation to let Nature take its course. Thus in a court of law, it would have been our word against his.

Instead of stewing in anger, I now volunteer some of my time trying to teach other parents and patients about how to get professional help. I wish we had known that hospice offers respite care so we could have had the time and energy to check out other sources of support and advice. The right advice at the right time could have reduced how long and how much we all suffered. The other message I want to convey is to make sure your physician has recorded your last wishes.

Be Sure Your Physician Records Your Last Wishes

If honoring your end-of-life wishes will depend upon what the doctor writes in his chart, then if possible, have a impartial witness observe your verbal request to him or her. After the doctor finishes writing, ask him or her to read back to you exactly what he or she wrote in the medical chart, so you can make sure it reflects what you wanted, and if not, apologize for *your* not being more clear and politely ask your doctor to revise what he wrote and read it to you again, with your revisions or additions. Finally, ask for a photocopy *before* your leave the office.

If your doctor seems uncomfortable with the process or complains that you seem rather "pushy," explain that you want those words to clearly represent your Last Wishes, just in case he or she is not available when a critical life-or-death decision must be made and other clinical providers must depend on what was just written down. The decision they make may determine whether you live or die. Could anything be more important?

In retrospect, Yvette's parents did have some alternatives: One was to contact hospice earlier and to take advantage of their support, especially "respite care." A few days of desperately needed rest might have restored their energy sufficiently to consult with other medical and legal experts. Their advice might have led then to welcome an investigation by the State's Child Protective Service for possible "abuse." Why welcome? Because none would have been found. Or they could have requested a consultation by members of an ethics committee, who would likely have found that the burden of suffering far outweighed the potential benefit of inserting a PEG tube, and therefore would not be in Yvette's BEST INTEREST. Even the last resort—to have a judge hear the merits of the case—could have had a major benefit: A judge's ruling could have relieved the doctors' worries about losing their licenses, and lessened the parents' guilt as they struggled with the decision to discontinue treatment.

As much as Yvette's story exemplifies how doctors can *increase* guilt, the next story shows how an empathic doctor can significantly *decrease* guilt.

This story is modified slightly from one written by Lance Davis, M.D., that appeared in his informative book, *At The Close Of Day* [2004]. This story now represents a composite of several patients. Dr. Davis was sensitive to the needs of the spouse. He risked thinking outside the narrow role of "modern medicine," to focus *only* on the patient and treat whatever *can* be treated. He listened and responded to both the needy spouse and the identified patient who was lying in the hospital bed. Medical schools rarely teach the skillful way that Dr. Davis responded. Hopefully, that will change soon.

Doctors Can Minimize Family Members' Guilt

© 2005 Lance Lee Davis, M.D.

The day I met a couple whom I will call Fred and Jane was early in my career, when I was a resident, training in Family Medicine. I was on duty in the Emergency Department. At sixty-nine, Fred had spent three years in bed after a massive stroke. His wife called the Emergency Medical Service that day. She was desperate after Fred had unconsciously pulled the feeding tube out of his stomach since it was his only source of fluid and nutrition. Emergency Medical Services brought Fred to the hospital wearing only a diaper and a coat. He was gaunt, dehydrated, and contracted. He could respond only to painful stimuli. Before I saw Fred, another physician had admitted him and started an IV with antibiotics as the laboratory reports indicated he had a urinary tract infection.

Jane looked so haggard and depressed that I told her to take her time and tell me the whole story. The couple had been married for thirty-three years, and for most of these years, enjoyed much vitality. Then came Fred's stroke. She grew teary as she recalled how the stroke suddenly caused Fred to go from an active traveler to a completely dependent person. He lost all ability to speak and could not even follow simple instructions. Despite her great efforts to provide the best care, a year later Fred started to develop recurrent pneumonias and urinary tract infections, and the sores in the skin over his buttocks and heels refused to heal. He could not feed himself or indicate if he was hungry or thirsty, although he cooperated as Jane continued to spoon-feed him.

After a year of spoon-feeding however, Fred simply stopped chewing and swallowing. Jane felt Fred was ready and prepared to pass on. But when she asked his physician for advice he said, "If we don't put a feeding tube in place, Fred will die." Jane stared hard at me as she recalled, "Those were his exact words. I will never forget them." Jane stated that she doubted Fred would want to be kept alive by artificial means if he was totally dependent and had no ability to interact with others. Yet how could SHE choose to say "No" to a feeding tube? How could she sentence her husband to die? The guilt would be unbearable. So she authorized inserting a feeding tube through Fred's abdominal wall into his stomach and learned how to administer liquid nutrition through it.

Over the next year, complications related to the feeding tube and recurrent infections led to more frequent visits to the hospital. Each time, a different doctor solved the presenting problem, but none helped her plan for Fred's inevitable death. Too guilty to ask for advice on how to let Fred die naturally, Jane became depressed and socially isolated. Her own medical condition worsened.

As I listened to her story, I imagined that today, Jane again lacked the courage to request that treatment not be started as she silently watched the admitting physician start the IV and antibiotics. I guessed this scenario had been repeated several times, which was confirmed as I reviewed Fred's thick medical chart. As I performed a physical exam, I came to the conclusion that Fred was a victim of the system. What he really needed was *Comfort Care* during his impending natural death. But what he had received instead was *inappropriate life-sustaining interventions*.

I recognized that further medical interventions would be futile because they would only prolong Fred's suffering and might even increase it, without any hope of benefit. But at my early stage in the practice of medicine, my experience and confidence were still limited. So I wrote orders to continue Fred's IV and antibiotics and made this promise to Jane: "I will do all I can for your husband."

Although I sensed that Jane also felt that Fred was ready to pass on, my six years of education in medical school, internship, and residency training had never taught me that it could be appropriate to let a patient die of a treatable medical condition.

Later that day, Fred's infection began to improve with antibiotics and hydration, but his mental and physical state remained the same. The next step would have been to replace his feeding tube and send him home. Yet my instincts were screaming that doing so would be wrong. With no experience to guide me on how to address this issue with Jane, several questions buzzed in my mind: If I suggested discontinuing the IV and antibiotics, would she accuse me of being unfeeling? Was that suggestion equivalent to euthanizing her husband? What if I was guessing wrong about what Fred really wanted? After all, I had just met the two of them, so who was I to decide? Was I contemplating "playing God"? If so, what right did I have to do so?

After much turmoil, I looked inside myself. I came to this conclusion: I was not only Fred's doctor; I was also a human being with my own personal sense of what seemed morally right. So I decided that I would express both my doctor side and my human side to Jane.

Jane was at Fred's bedside as I asked, "May I speak to you outside?" We walked down the hall to the "quiet room." First I let the "doctor" part of me speak, as I said, "The surgeons can replace the feeding tube tomorrow, and the we can send Fred home on antibiotics." I watched her careful, minimal nod. I inferred that she might be reluctantly resigned.

So I went on to express my human side. "I hope I don't offend you by what I will say next... but... I am not sure that reinserting the feeding tube would be the correct thing to do, for Fred."

Jane's eyes burned, eager to hear what I would say next.

"Fred has basically been in this non-responsive state a long time. And he seems to be getting worse, not better." Her next nod was far more definite. So I continued. "At this point, in his present state, do you think Fred would want to continue to exist?"

Jane's exhausted face showed anguish, guilt, and ambivalence. "What else can we do?" She asked.

I took her question as indicating she was open to consider other options. I responded by a general statement that at some point, patients need *Comfort Care* instead of *aggressive treatment*. She agreed. That gave me the courage to proceed. I took a deep breath and said something I had never said or heard before, yet I did so with such a tone of confidence that it even surprised me: **"Fred is my patient and I am his doctor. My decision, at this point in his long and unrelenting illness... MY decision is to allow Fred to die peacefully."** I studied her face for any reaction, ready to withdraw or revise my offer... if she showed the slightest objection.

For a moment, Jane seemed stunned. Then she broke down. Her tears seemed to reflect relief more than sadness. She thanked me repeatedly for bringing up a subject that she had long wondered about. She asked me why no other doctor ever discussed this option. She admitted she felt frustrated and profoundly guilty as she watched Fred suffer as she passively went along with so many medical decisions that only prolonged his suffering. As she studied my face for a reaction, she must have sensed this was new territory for me also, because she stood up and hugged me in a grandmotherly way and said, "You did the right thing, Dr. Davis. Thank you for offering this option to me. Thank you for making this choice possible for Fred. Thank you, especially, for making the decision for me. Thank you... for me. And thank you, for Fred."

For the next few minutes, it felt like I was operating on automatic pilot. Although it was the first time I ever did anything like this, it felt so right that I had no further hesitation. I stopped Fred's IV and antibiotics. I canceled the order to consult the gastroenterologist who would have replaced his feeding tube. I wrote several prescriptions to keep Fred comfortable at home, such as morphine and sedatives. Finally, I suggested that Jane call hospice so one of their nurses could make a home visit soon after Fred returned.

Over the next couple of hours, however, Fred's condition declined. His infection returned and his blood pressure dropped. Jane approached me with an assertiveness I had not seen in her before. She requested that I let Fred remain in the hospital until the end came. She explained that she wished he were already at home, of course, but she feared the ambulance transfer would be quite uncomfortable.

That evening, I was at the bedside with Jane as her husband took his last breath. He was comfortable as his lips were moist since he was receiving excellent nursing care. His body simply came to a halt. He took one last, slow breath and then slowly lost his color. My attending physician teacher also happened to be present. He gave me a nod and then left the room. Jane watched me as I bent down over Fred. I listened for a heartbeat, felt for a pulse, and checked for a pupil response to light. As I expected, none were there. I looked up at Jane and took her hand. "I'm sorry, but Fred is gone." She gave a squeeze, another hug, and then asked to be alone with Fred. I left the room and waited outside.

When Jane emerged from Fred's hospital room, her face looked calm and less sad than before. She seemed to feel peace. I wondered if it arose from this quiet victory. As a team, we had accomplished a challenging task and carried it out in harmony. For Fred's sake, we had succeeded.

Jane and Fred taught me something very important that day. It is something that I will never forget.

Since Fred's passing seven years ago, I have seen many bed-bound and neurologically devastated individuals die naturally after withdrawing artificial feeding and hydration. Their deaths have always been peaceful and not prolonged. On the other hand, I have seen many other patients kept alive long past their natural lifespans via feeding tubes or IVs. If they were alert to any extent, they suffered as their skin broke down, infections set in, and muscles withered and contracted—despite their caregivers' best efforts. Theirs was a cruel and nightmarish reality, and the more awareness they had, the worse it was for them. I cannot believe that forcing such a fate on someone is the morally correct course.

[Dr. Lance Davis continues:] I feel compelled to offer my perspective, as a physician:

It is a common misconception that it is cruel or painful to allow a person to die from starvation and dehydration. Based on my clinical observations, this is simply not true. Hunger pangs pass after the first several hours, and the sensation of thirst is markedly diminished by good mouth care. I understand that society uses food to nurture and to please another on a daily basis. —Even more, for special occasions. I appreciate that most Americans assume that the experience of initial hunger pangs and thirst worsen with time if they are not fed or given fluid. Yet when a human being reaches the point where he or she cannot or will **not accept fluid & food by mouth**, he or she is approaching a peaceful death. If artificial feeding and hydration are not initiated, the person will fall quietly asleep over a period of hours to days. All life processes will slow down gradually. Eventually, a peaceful death occurs.

Some people of religious faith insist that removing life-supporting medical interventions from a patient is "playing God." I strongly believe otherwise. **Keeping someone alive against the Forces of Nature when, without modern medical technology, his or her life would have ended, IS playing God**. Surrendering control by withdrawing a patient's life support releases this control to higher forces beyond oneself. In contrast, attempting to control bodily functions creates a man-made artificial situation. We must realize that advances in medicine come in two forms: We have the technology to prolong existence for years beyond what was possible a couple of generations ago. But technology can also provide exquisite *Comfort Care* to make people's final transitions more peaceful.

Prolonging life beyond the Forces of Nature not only drains loved ones' emotions, as it did for Jane. A lifetime of savings can be exhausted to pay for medical expenses as scarce medical resources are squandered on someone who not only has passed the time of their natural life, but also may be living in bed-bound misery with no hope of returning to anywhere near normal functioning. To be clear: I am certainly not suggesting that we put our most vulnerable people "out to pasture" so they will die and we can collect their inheritance. Nor am I offering a way to avert the coming financial crisis of Medicare. I am suggesting only that we be honest by accepting that everyone's life must someday come to a natural end. I am also suggesting that we use modern medical technology appropriately by exercising responsible financial stewardship by directing our resources to keep dying individuals comfortable and peaceful rather than to fight Nature and prolong suffering.

This story of Dr. Lance Davis illustrates how the doctor's role can be expanded from focusing on only prolonging life of the designated patient to reducing the guilt and suffering of a family members by providing them with the critical information they are so desperate to learn. In Latin, "doctor" means "teacher," and **teaching heals**. Doctors who withhold the knowledge they possess instead of reducing suffering are not just being paternalistic; their acts of omission can be considered morally wrong. What is right? Doctors can minimize expressing their personal bias as they present information in a non-judgmental way and leave the final decision to patients or patients' loved ones. Some patients or family members will directly ask doctors to inform them of their options. But other patients or family members may be too guilty, too scared, or too naïve to ask. We believe doctors should take the initiative to teach, to heal, and thus to inform.

Dr. Davis' sensitivity led him to present the option of discontinuing hydration and antibiotics in a manner that would relieve Jane from feeling that only she could bear that awesome responsibility—a decision that might have left her with life-long guilt. Dr. Davis' words stated it as HIS decision: "Fred is **my** patient and **I** am his doctor. **My** decision, at this point in his long and unrelenting illness, would be to allow Fred to die peacefully." Out of context, others might criticize these words as paternalistic or controlling, but they were part of an intimate exchange during which Dr. Davis closely watched Jane to assess her reaction. He always remained willing to accept what she decided. Thus he provides a fine example of a morally correct response that reduced Jane's suffering as well as Fred's.

For doctors not as sensitive as Dr. Lance Davis, another family member could request considering this approach. Jane's adult daughter, for example, could inform "Fred's" doctor how much anguish Jane has already endured and how guilty she would feel if she felt it was her decision to withdraw treatment.

If the intent to provide information on **Voluntary Refusal of Food & Fluid** effectively reduces the suffering of both patients and their loved ones, then many people would consider the act of providing this information as morally good, even if the patient did not spontaneously request it. The experiences of patients like Fred and Jane thus provide compelling arguments in response to the criticisms of Loewy [2001] and of Sulmasy [2002] who state they feel it is morally wrong— unless patients first ask—for physicians to inform patients about **Voluntary Refusal of Food & Fluid**. The clinical experience and comments of Dr. Davis can also serve as a response to the March 2004 Allocution of the Pope, in which he insisted that patients in the Permanent Vegetative State must be indefinitely provided artificially administered Food & Fluid.

40. Can Doctors Help Prevent Unwanted Resuscitations at Home? [FORM III: I Wish to Decline Emergency Resuscitation Attempts and Transfer to a Hospital]

When patients are in hospitals, they or members of their family can usually discuss the potential for recovery with the doctor. Such conversations may result in the doctor writing a **DNR** order. The more accurate term is "Do-Not-*Attempt*-to-Resuscitate order" or **DNAR** since most attempts fail. A more positive term is "**PND**" (**P**ermit **N**atural **D**ying), which also includes Withholding Food & Fluid. **DNAR** orders are usually both written and flagged in the patient's medical chart, which may be placed prominently near the hospital bed (HIPAA permitting). Most people prefer to die at home, however. Unless enrolled in hospice or home health care, there may be no medical chart. Some States have approved "pre-hospital" order forms to alert personnel from Emergency Medical Services (Emergency Medical Technicians) that the doctor has written an order that reflects the patient's wishes for NO resuscitation attempt. Even in States where standard approved forms have been distributed as a POLST (Physician's Orders for Life-Sustaining Treatment), many doctors and patients are not aware that they exist.

People often call **9-1-1** because they do not know what else to do if there is a sudden medical crisis. Yet their loved one may only need *Comfort Care*. Others call to make sure their relative has really died or because they need emotional support from a professional. Too often such calls results in unwanted resuscitation attempts or transfer to a hospital, which can sadly can cause physical trauma to the patient whose unwanted suffering is greater as well as unnecessarily prolonged. Reviving patients can also cause emotional trauma to survivors, who may suffer from horrific memories. Then they have reason to worry if, in their last chapter of their own lives, they will be subjected to unwanted resuscitation attempts. Finally, unwanted **DNAR**s are a waste of medical and economic resources.

For 70% of dementia patients, their final months to years will be in nursing homes where **DNH** (**D**o **N**ot **H**ospitalize) orders are uncommon. Mitchell and others [2007] found that **DNH** orders average 7%, but vary from 0.7% to 25% depending on the State. Black residents and those residing in regions with more ICUs are less likely to have DNH orders. Demented patients find medical interventions distressing. "Hospital transfer is seldom consistent with a palliative approach." One exception is *Comfort Care from* repairing broken hips. Others have reported the cost of one week in an ICU can be as high as $100,000. The presence of an Advance Directive increase the percentage of **DNR**s, but few standard forms prompt asking the question specifically.

The horror of dialing 9-1-1: Gus received resuscitation and IVs that he clearly did not want.

By the time Uncle Gus made his decision to **Refuse Food & Fluid**, he had engaged in lengthy deliberation with all his close relatives. Given his long medical ordeal, the details of which I will spare, his choice seemed reasonable. When he set the date to begin his fast, no one who lived nearby disagreed. His favorite cousin Sandra lived 3000 miles away. Bad weather delayed their air flights so that she and her husband, Vince, arrived the day after my uncle began his final fast. Fortunately, Gus was still lucid when they arrived and they were all able to exchange meaningful good-byes.

Given Vince's belief system, I was not surprised as he tried to persuade Uncle Gus to resume eating and drinking. Gus remained determined, however.

Three days later, Gus lapsed into a very deep sleep. That's when Vince really mobilized into action. He began by questioning how we could be *so sure* that Gus was really comfortable. To my ears, his style was designed to incite argument rather than seek possible resolution. The next day, as voices were rising and our attention was focused on Vince, he abruptly left the room in a huff. Later I realized that he had chosen that very moment to distract our attention from Gus, who had stopped breathing. The reason he left the room just then was to call Emergency Medical Services. He did so secretly, without asking for our consent since he knew the rest of us would have objected.

Less than five minutes later, two huge firemen appeared at the door. One carried a wood board. The other carried a white molded plastic case. Before we realized what was happening, these men had pushed us all aside. They refused to listen to our pleas as they pounded on Gus' chest and broke some of his ribs. Then they used a giant syringe to inject some medication directly into his heart. Finally, they applied electrodes to his chest that made his body jerk up sharply. A few moments later, two more men arrived. They introduced themselves as the Advanced Medical Support Team. One mumbled how dehydrated Gus appeared. Then they started an IV in each arm. After adjusting the flow to run fast, they finally turned around to us. That was the first time we were given the opportunity to reveal what we knew about what medical treatment Gus preferred not to receive. But it was too late.

In our State, once someone dials 9-1-1, even if seeking advice on *Comfort Care* or for family support and to confirm a recent death, resuscitation attempts are often on "automatic." Patients like Gus cannot have their Last Wishes honored unless legal forms signed by a physician convince the Emergency Medical Services (EMTs) to abandon their urgent focused mission to save lives. Action-oriented, these dedicated men and women know that every second counts so they have minimal time to read documents with contingent treatment options, no time to read Proxy-empowering statements that contain reasons and examples, and certainly no time to resolve conflicts if there are differences of opinion among family members. Their Number One Rule is: To save the patient's life—try *now,* talk *later.* But Number Two Rule could be, Is there a POLST or the equivalent? In addition, these experienced professionals have a lot more than resuscitation to offer: they provide needed compassion at moments of existential crises.

I asked them what strategy might have worked to honor the Last Wishes that Gus had so clearly expressed. In some States, there are approved forms to refuse resuscitation attempts that EMS personnel are trained to honor—provided that, like DNAR forms in hospitals, a doctor has signed them. So I asked, "If Gus had such a form signed by his doctor, would they honor it in our State?" I had to respect the way one answered: "Only if I could reach the doctor immediately on the phone. Otherwise... the answer would be 'No.' Delaying would be the same as not attempting to save that life."

The response made me ask, "Why must you be so cautious?" They explained that it is more than just doing the job they were trained for, although that is a large part of it. They also fear that, if even one family member disagreed with their decision not to attempt resuscitation, there might be a lawsuit. So my question was, "Have you ever been sued?" The answer was predictable: "No, but maybe that's because we also almost always attempt to resuscitate." (Yet professionals who act in good faith usually do not get sued.)

Without much hope that I'd get a useful answer, I finally asked, "Was there any hope of honoring the Last Wishes of Gus if he had clearly stated them in writing?" Their response: "Find out the agencies nearby that are likely to respond to 9-1-1, call the supervisor of each one, and ask them for their cooperation. You're trying to break new ground here."

As the Emergency Medical Technicians were leaving, they asked, "What will you do now?" I turned around and looked back at my poor uncle slumped in his bed. I just felt sad. The only thing I could think of was how attempts to resuscitate sometimes turn out badly for everyone. This time, especially for Gus: an unwanted attempt to resuscitate violated and disrupted his chance for a peaceful transition.

ఛ౿౿

The key to dissuading EMTs from attempting their goal of resuscitation is a valid order from the attending doctor. Sometimes this is not possible, however. The form suggested below combines words from several approved State forms. It provides alternatives when no physician's signature is available. A study by Feder and others [2006] showed that when Emergency Medical Services agencies agreed to participate in adopting new guidelines and to train their EMTs on the new guidelines, the probability of withholding resuscitation increased more than six-fold for verbal requests made by patients, caregivers, or family. Overall, for both written and verbal requests, the rate of withholding resuscitations was about twice in the study group, even without using doctors' orders.

*It is best to have your doctor sign your State-approved form (if your State has one). If your State has no approved form, ask your physician to sign the form below. Until your physician is available to sign the form, you may choose one or more of the other options under "Documentation" at the end of the form but you can only **hope** it will work. EMTs may not respond to your Last Wish not to attempt resuscitation or to be transferred to a hospital since they are trained to TRY FIRST, and ask questions later. They may insist on knowing who has legal standing and if the patient had sound judgment when the form was signed.*

I Wish to Decline Emergency Resuscitation Attempts and Transfer to a Hospital

Section 1. My intent and the purpose of this form:

I may use this form for several reasons: A) If my State does not recognize any form called "POLST" or "MOLST" (Physician's/Medical Orders for Life-Sustaining Treatment), then I hope that Emergency Medical Technicians will honor this form instead; B) If my physician or nurse practitioner or physician's assistant has not yet signed the State-approved form to certify my wishes, then I hope Emergency Medical Technicians will still honor this (temporary) form; and/or, C) If my State-approved form does not clearly cover this point, I want to indicate for what specific conditions I do NOT want to be transferred to a hospital.

Section 2. Why I wish EMS personnel and paramedics to honor my wishes:

My life condition and/or my potential for treatment is one of the following:

A) I have a terminal condition;

B) I am now permanently unconscious, in a persistent vegetative state, in a minimally conscious state, or have advanced irreversible dementia;

C) Attempts to resuscitate would almost certainly not succeed; or

D) Attempts to resuscitate would impose an extraordinary burden on me or my loved ones, after taking into consideration my current medical condition and the expected limited benefit from resuscitation or of hospitalization.

Section 3. What Kinds of Emergency Treatment I Do Not Want:

I wish to decline ALL resuscitation attempts offered by emergency medical services (EMS) personnel, including but not limited to:

1. Cardiopulmonary resuscitation and cardiac defibrillation:

2. Transfer to a hospital or other facility that provides emergency services and aggressive medical treatment aimed at curing disease;
or

3. Administration of food & fluids, whether by tubes that go directly into my circulatory system or gastrointestinal system, or by manual assistance through my mouth.

Section 4. Disclaimer:

I hope that EMS personnel who are concerned about following my above **written** request will consider the results of a research study conducted in Washington State by Sylvia Feder and others [2006]. In this study, similar requests were honored even though over half were **not written** but only stated verbally by the patient, caregivers, or family members. While EMS personnel in the "research" agencies had supplemental training to acquaint them with newly implemented guidelines, I offer this alternative: My signature below represents my competent request to ask my survivors to hold harmless any and all EMS personnel who respectfully honor the wishes I have stated above.

My signature:_____ Date: _____

Section 5. Documentation:

My physician's signature: _____ Date: _____

Printed name of Physician: _____ Phone #s: _____

Until my physician signs above, please honor the following:

A) A valid Advance Directive (Proxy Directive) which authorizes a sequence of individuals to speak for me, is |__|, is not |__| attached.

C) Signatures of unrelated witnesses, who know my end-of-life treatment values and preferences and who have read my statement above, are |__|, are not |__| below:

D) The signature of a supervising representative from my local Emergency Medical Services agency is |__|, is not |__| below:

E) A Notary's signature and stamp is |__|, is not |__| below:

After reviewing this form, author Sylvia Feder commented, "Most firefighters/ EMTs will be reluctant to honor such a form unless their local guidelines have addressed it. In a resuscitation scenario, they won't take the time to read it and they won't feel comfortable honoring it." The Seattle Times [Ostrum, 2006] quoted one EMT: "We wouldn't even talk to the family member. We'd rush in, rush right past them, throw down our equipment and get to work. We're really good at pushing people out of the way and just taking over."

What is the solution? Ms. Feder suggested a four-point plan:

1. Encourage states to adopt directives that can be honored by EMS personnel.

2. Encourage families to obtain those forms.

3. Educate physicians about the forms.

4. Allow EMS providers to honor verbal requests if written forms are not present."

Ms. Feder noted: "Clearly, one challenge to bring about change is that you need to approach the task from many different levels: lawmakers, family, physicians, and EMS providers and their agencies who train personnel on how to follow the guidelines." The good news is that some but not all of the *other* agencies (those that served as "controls" in Feder's research) are now adopting the new guidelines in a program called "Compelling Reasons." This innovation shows that change at *any* level may improve honoring of this Last Wish.

Ms. Feder's experience of working in the field for 25 years is supported by others' research: A national survey of EMTs [Marco and others, 2003] showed that while nine out of ten would honor a state-approved advance directive, only one out of ten would honor a verbal report of an advance directive, and only one out of twenty-five would honor an "unofficial" document. Clearly, educating physicians is important: 6 years after implementation of the POLST in Washington State, 6 out of 10 physicians still did not know that it was required in the prehospital setting [Silveira and others, 2003]. In Feder's study, for those patients for whom resuscitation was withheld, only 1 in 25 had the State-approved form.

Based on the lack of physician knowledge and patient acceptance, as well as the fact that people travel to other States, I therefore add one more recommendation to those of Ms. Feder: **State laws and agency guidelines should permit EMTs and paramedics to honor forms that are *similar* to those that are "approved."**

Lance Davis, M.D., points out [2004], "Remember that the Living Will and Health Care Power of Attorney are generated by the patient and their surrogate, expressing their wishes for end-of-life care... The Do Not Resuscitate order is signed by the patient's physician to prevent hospital staff or EMS workers from actually performing unwanted interventions... Even though a person may have a Living Will, Health Care Power of Attorney, and a DNR order in their hospital chart, one still needs the Out-of-Hospital DNR form, or unwanted CPR or intubations may occur during transport to or from the hospital... It is imperative to keep the Out-of-Hospital DNR order or identification with the patient at all times. EMS personnel in every state will perform CPR until they see the valid DNR." Dr. Davis' "staff has researched each state's policies on this matter." For each state, http://www.atthecloseofday.com/outofhospitalDNR.htm lists: Specific title of document; How to obtain document; Means of identification; Informational Links; Link to State EMS Office; and Special notes/considerations.

The tragic story of Gus indicates how important it is for everyone to agree on the same treatment plan. Include all relevant staff if your loved one is in an institution. Consider this experience: A friend of mine stayed up all night with his father as he died in a nursing home. The next morning, as my friend was reflecting in a solemn moment of deep love and memories on the side of his father's bed, the door suddenly flew open. Two men in fireman's boots charged in. My friend recovered from his shock and pointed to the DNAR order posted above his father's bed. Although the firemen left immediately, the damage had already been done: They had interrupted a precious moment that could never be retrieved. Later, my friend found out who and why 9-1-1 had been called: the night-time receptionist was merely following the "general policy" of his institution.

Obviously, it is time for a change in policy. But the experience of Gus and my friend both illustrate the same point: If anyone does call 9-1-1, the most powerful signature that can prevent an unwanted resuscitation is always the one penned by a physician.

Chapter 12

QUESTIONS THAT RELATE TO OBTAINING ADVICE,
TO SECURING A PROXY, AND TO FEELING SECURE THAT OTHERS
WILL HONOR YOUR LAST WISHES

Our Society Has Done Nothing to Deal With One of Our Two Greatest Fears

If our brains are so devastated by trauma or dementia that we are not aware of our environment and cannot respond to our loved ones, we fear being forced to exist in a prolonged state of increasing indignity and total dependency.

This fear can result in premature dying if those in the early stages of dementia choose to die when they CAN, instead of when they WANT TO.

Attempts to legalize Physician-Aided, Patient-Hastened Dying cannot, nor are they intended to help demented or brain-injured patients. Yet there are thousands of times more brain-impaired patients than terminally ill patients who retain the mental competency and physical ability to hasten their dying.

If we cannot depend on individuals whom we know and trust to be willing, available, and able to carry out our future wishes, perhaps we can instead depend on an organization of professionals to serve as our future Proxies, and entrust them to honor our end-of-life values and preferences.

---

41. To Live as Long as Possible, How Can I be Assured That My Existence Will Not be Prolonged if My Condition Deteriorates to Indignity and Dependency? and
What are My Options if I Do Not Know Someone I Can Trust to Serve Effectively as My Proxy or Advocate?

Robert Hammerman's sad story has been briefly mentioned twice before in this book. His **premature** death was based on the realistic fear of his impending dementia. The method he chose was **legal but not peaceful**.

Judge Robert Hammerman had no children and he never married. His only sibling was a sister who was one year older than he. He had many devoted friends and "thousands of surrogate sons and daughters" he came to know from 60 years of guiding a community service group that he founded, The Lancers Club. Still, he felt that no one could serve as his effective Proxy, to prevent him from enduring what he believed could be as long as a decade of indignity...

"Many care about me—but none will take care of me."

On November 11, 2004, Maryland's longest serving Supreme Court Judge, Robert Hammerman, died at the age of 76. He died from a self-inflicted gunshot wound to his chest, across the street from the skilled nursing home he never wanted to enter. Far from impulsive, he had made the decision to commit suicide 16 months before. The night before he died, he sent a 10-page letter to over 2000 people. The letter that he had been composing and revising for months was long, rambling, and confusing. For purposes of clarity, I have added emphasis to selected excerpts, below:

Dear friends and family, I owe you an explanation...
The reason is simple—my health. The fear [is] that in the not too distant future I **might be committed** to a nursing home or an assisted living facility—a **fate I am not prepared to accept**... Alzheimer's has attacked me. There has been no formal evaluation. I fear it and have not sought one.... . [Yet] all the symptoms are in place. For one who all of his life has enjoyed an exceptional **memory**, it **has seen degeneration** at a quicker and quicker pace for two or three years or so.... . This has been **embarrassing and difficult** to deal with in **all aspects of my life**. The most common things—every day—I find great difficulty with.... . What particularly grieves me is the loss of memory.... . My mind was a total blank as to a letter [I planned to write]—and still is to this day.... . I thought of a perfect meeting for the Lancers Club. Try as I might, I have yet to remember it.... . I could cite so many more [examples].
"The **simplest tasks** are now becoming more and **more difficult** to do. **Confusion is my daily companion**... I am in a **constant state of worrying about my forgetfulness**... For a long time [a neighbor] was forgetful—and then like a light bulb—it was full blown Alzheimer's... The thought of **Alzheimer's is dreadful to me. I'd need institutionalization**."

Convinced he would follow the same fate as his blind mother, Judge Hammerman wrote, "Her Alzheimer's developed to the ultimate stage. She could see nothing and knew nothing."

"There are happily certain people who care about me—but none able to care for me... In truth, it is breathing, not really living... To be institutionalized for a period anywhere approaching 10 years would be extraordinarily expensive—**a total and tragic waste of 'living' and of resources**... 'the slippery slope to darkness'... the slope is *there*, with me on it..."

Judge Hammerman also noted, "The sight of [my judge friend] helpless, **being strapped into the bed** was more than I could take. Our [mutual] close friend told me, '**If** [Judge _____] **knew what lay ahead of him, he would never have let it happen**' ... . The awareness that I could become disabled that would require me to be shipped out to assisted living or worse... I could not accept.

"I love life deeply... There is so very, very much that I want to see unfold, **but it is time to leave.**"

~❧~

I consider it unlikely that Judge Hammerman committed suicide due to a Depressive Disorder. He still loved life and found satisfaction in supporting the Lancers Club. The hopelessness of the future he perceived caused him more anguish than his present degree of impaired mental functioning, but that was significant, also. As a medical doctor, I think there was a slight chance that a thorough evaluation would have uncovered a treatable cause for his memory problems, most likely his symptoms were due to irreversible dementia. His fear of testing and resignation were understandable. After all, nothing could be done for his neighbor, his mother, his judge friend, or millions of others.

Some might consider Hammerman's explanation as an effective argument for "rational suicide." His letter documented his knowledge, appreciation, and logical reasoning, as well as his wish to avoid the ravages of Alzheimer's disease that had remained consistent for 16 months.

On the other hand, Hammerman's letter and suicide were tragic calls for a need that our society does not yet meet. With no close relatives expected to outlive him, there was no place Hammerman could turn if he wanted to live as long as possible, but still wanted to be certain that he would avoid prolonged institutionalization in a state of indignity. If society continues to neglect the need created by the increasing burden of people with progressive and irreversible dementias, the consequences will be emotional "bankruptcy" to caregivers, and financial bankruptcy to society. (Discussed in greater detail, later.)

The most tragic aspect of suicide is when it leads to a premature death. Oregon's Death with Dignity Act was acceptable to lawmakers and voters because it requires two doctors to certify that the patient is terminal, which is defined as having a life expectancy of less than six months. In contrast, when a teenager commits suicide, the grief is intensified by the loss of an entire adulthood. Yet to patients with terminal diagnoses, every month, even every day, is valuable.

Recall the question, "Who would want to live to the age of 90?" The usual answer is, "Everybody who is 89!" But in reality, not always.

Dr. Sherwin Nuland related a widow's reflections about her incontinent husband before he died [1994, *Page 101*]: Previously dignified and modest, he had always been proud of his appearance. Now, he had "to be undressed to clean off the filth that profaned the pittance of humanness still left to him... It's such a degrading sickness! **If there was any way he could have known what was happening to him, he wouldn't have wanted to live**." In contrast to quoting rabbis who typically end memorial services with, "May his memory be for a blessing" [*Page 242*], Dr. Nuland wrote this about the indignity of end-stage Alzheimer's disease: "A life that has been well lived and a shared sense of happiness and accomplishment are **ever after seen through the smudged glass of its last few years**" [*Page 105*]. {Emphasis added.}

So, why did Judge Robert Hammerman act on his words, "**it is time to leave**"? Only because "There are happily certain people who care *about* me—but none able to care *for* me." In other words, only because society had no mechanism to assure him that he would not be forced to live in a prolonged state of indignity.

The judge's story is similar to the premature death of 54 year-old Janet Adkins, who died a decade earlier. Although Alzheimer's afflicted America's "great communicator," Ronald Reagan, nothing has yet reduced this end-of-life fear: If our brains are so devastated by trauma or dementia that we are not aware of our environment and cannot respond to our loved ones, will we be forced to exist in a state of indignity and total dependency?

As baby boomers age, millions of people may wish there were mechanisms in place to assure them that society will "**care for them**" in a *special way*. When they reach a point they decide is far enough down that trajectory of irreversible and progressive indignity and dependency, many will want their **Proxies** to have the power to **Refuse Food & Fluid** on their behalf. If those diagnosed with early Alzheimer's have confidence in their Proxies' future effectiveness, then they can choose to live as long as possible rather than to die prematurely. Ironic, but true: Knowing you can exercise control over *when* you die can lead you to decide to live *longer*. Meanwhile, your anxiety and worry about being trapped will be lower.

Patients fearful of dementia may comprise the majority of those who wish such assurance, but there are others, as well. Similarly, having several family members is necessary, but may not be sufficient to allay a person's fears of a dismal future. Both of these concerns are illustrated in the next true story.

"The Self-Made Man"

Bob Stern had a large and devoted family. They were all in good health and most lived near him: his devoted wife, two adult daughters, and an adult son. After he died, his daughter Susan spent three years creating an award-winning documentary, *The Self-Made Man* [2005]. A central part of the film is the home video that Bob Stern made of himself. On it, he explains why he decided to shoot himself the next morning: He was unwilling to risk surgery and cancer treatment because the procedures might leave him dependent and he did not want others to let him linger and die slowly... suffering... without dignity—as was the fate of his son's father-in-law.

This emotionally engaging film leaves many questions unanswered. Did Bob Stern shoot himself because he was "not strong enough to be weak"? That is, was he afraid of becoming ill and dependent? Perhaps. Yet a more likely possibility arises from this hint: He chose to create a video instead of having a family discussion. That decision intentionally excluded input from his two daughters. If he chose the video option so he could avoid an emotional struggle about their letting him go, how he could feel he could ask any family member to guarantee not to let him linger in a state of suffering and indignity? Absent the confidence that he would be spared the kind of dying he most feared, this "self-made man" felt compelled to bet on a "sure thing" while he still had the physical and mental ability to remain in control. So, instead of risking medical treatment and surgery, he affected his own "self-made death."

What kind of mechanism could provide assurance for patients who are at high risk for Alzheimer's disease, who were recently diagnosed with dementia, or who are medical or surgical patients whose interventions involve high risks? Is there an alternative for patients who cannot identify **Proxies** they can trust to **Refuse Food & Fluid** on their behalf at some defined future point?

One possible alternative is this: People can form small groups where each person selects some of the others to be their Proxies. The awesome responsibility to make life-determining decisions will seem less daunting if group members can seek advice and support from a professional end-of-life organization. This organization could also provide guidance as people create or revise their Advance Directives, as it would ideally consist of several professionals whose backgrounds are in the fields of end-of-life law, medicine, and ethics, and who have had experience working as a team with terminal patients and their families.

For people like Robert Hammerman who know of no individuals who can serve as their Proxies, and for people like Bob Stern who fear their family members love them too much to ever let them go—the professional staff members of the local organization could agree to serve as Proxies. In some ways, their role would be similar to that of bank trustees who offer an alternative to designating a close relative as the Durable Power of Attorney for making financial decisions. An individual's Advance Directive could authorize the professional group to permit an alternate staff person as a successor Proxy if necessary, to make sure that someone in the organization is willing, able, and available to serve as the patient's Proxy. Before a professional could accept the role of Proxy for an individual, this person would need to impart sufficient knowledge about his or her end-of-life values and preferences so the designated Proxy would understand how to make decisions based on the "Substituted Judgment" standard. The guiding principle would be to respect her views and to honor his or her Last Wishes. Depending on the person's specific wishes, the **Proxy** might or might not be authorized to **Refuse Food and Fluid**, and to refuse aggressive treatment for such terminal diseases as pneumonia, heart disease, cancer, or kidney failure, if the patient is also suffering from late-stage dementia.

Designating a stranger may at first sound somewhat impersonal. Granted, end-of-life wishes are very private. They reflect the patients' beliefs about religion and the afterlife, obligations and wishes for heirs, and concepts about personhood versus biologic existence. Yet it is possible to respectfully acquire knowledge about person through semi-structured interviews and focused questionnaires. Other family members and friends may also be interviewed. A narrative summary of all interviews and questionnaires could be placed on file so that another professional in the organization can become quickly informed, if necessary. The process is analogous to sharing your secrets with a psychotherapist who starts out being a stranger and soon knows some of your deepest secrets, but who may need to pass on the essence of this knowledge to your next therapist, someday.

There are two advantages to selecting an organization of professionals: assurance that a professional will in the future, be able, willing, and available; and, the patient need not worry about causing their loved ones so much emotional toll that they become unwilling to carry out their end-of-life wishes because they "love them too much."

Perhaps... if Janet Adkins had confidence in such a professional organization, she would have chosen to live several more useful and pleasurable years, and have played many more sets of tennis with her son. Perhaps Judge Robert Hammerman would have chosen to live and remain active in the Lancers Club. And perhaps

Bob Stern might have risked the downside of surgery and cancer treatment, survived, and enjoyed another few years of quality life.

We would like to end **The *BEST WAY* to Say Goodbye: A Legal Peaceful Choice at the End of Life** with the above proposal to extend life by establishing an effective social mechanism so that people who suffer from terminal or devastating chronic illnesses can have their fears replaced by confidence, so that no one ever feels it necessary to end his or her life prematurely. Patients should not have to worry about being forced to endure years of suffering and indignity. Nor should they fear becoming an extreme burden on their families and society. Instead, they should feel certain that others will respect and honor their Last Wishes to end their existence in a legal peaceful way. When relieved of these worries and fears, they can turn their energy to battling their underlying diseases and be free to enjoy their last months or years as much as possible. Under these circumstances, many will willingly prolong their lives. It is both ironic and poorly understood that assuring patients that they can exercise their freedom to control when they die can set the stage for them to enjoy life *longer* as well as *more*.

We began the last paragraph with the words, "We would like to end..." Unfortunately, politics is intruding into the realm of end-of-life decision-making in America today. Those in power feel it is their duty to impose their morality on ***your*** BEST WAY to say goodbye. They have created a strong statement of their arguments. One way it took form is The President's Council on Bioethics' report on "Taking Care," discussed next. Its goal is to influence your caregivers (as well as policymakers including legislators) on how to make medical decisions for you, if you no longer can make your own. They insist on treatment choices that will **"extend the life that still remains,"** even if such decisions disrespect your previously written instructions. As the most formidable challenge to honoring your Last Wishes since Living Wills were first proposed, the next **i-FAQ** considers in detail, counterarguments and strategies to effectively overcome its challenges.

42. How Can I Overcome the Challenges to Honoring My Advance Directives from the President's Council on Bioethics report, "Taking Care: Ethical Caregiving In Our Aging Society"?

Overview: *Taking Care: Ethical Caregiving In Our Aging Society*, a report **The President's Council on Bioethics** ("The Council") was released on September 29, 2005. Well-written, it presents convincing data establishing the enormous economic, emotional, and cultural challenges that will inevitably result from huge increases in the number of elderly and especially demented people, whose need for total care for years before they die may well overwhelm our resources. The report's moralistic concepts and recommendations threaten every individual's right to create Advance Directives, and they weaken assurance that others will ultimately respond to them.

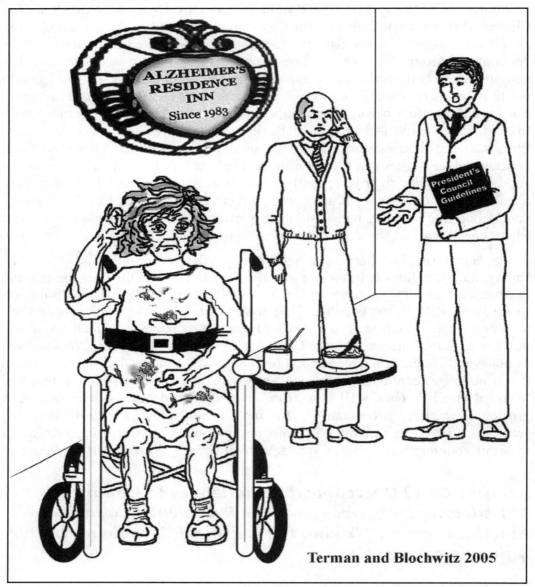

ALZHEIMER'S RESIDENCE INN Since 1983

President's Council Guidelines

Terman and Blochwitz 2005

"I'm sorry, the President's Council on Bioethics considers her Living Will as NOT moral."

The Council's report agrees with some conclusions presented in **The *BEST WAY* To Say Goodbye**; for example, **Proxy Directives** are generally superior to **Living Wills**. Some of The Council's presentation is based on clinical science, but its conclusions and recommendations are skewed by a moralistic motivation. Their arguments have the ultimate intent to undermine the primary goal of advance care documents, which is to assure people that others will honor their end-of-life decisions. The Council's report challenges the basic right of each person to decide in advance, how they want to die. If followed, the report's strongly worded recommendations would deprive patients of basic rights that have been repeatedly and consistently affirmed by court rulings and that are the current standard of clinical practice. The Council's arguments may initially seem reasonable, but further analysis leads to the conclusion that some are logically invalid and contrived to convince readers to adopt The Council's view of morality as their guide to end-of-life advance care planning and decision-making.

The chapter titled, *The Limited Wisdom of Advance Directives,* succinctly states The Council's negative perspective: "**No legal instrument** can substitute for wise and loving choices, made on the spot, when the precise treatment dilemma is clear and care decisions are needed. Proxy directives can appoint decision-makers, but **only ethical reflection and prudent judgment** can guide them at the bedside." Councilmember Professor Rebecca Dresser states in the Appendix: "The standard legal and ethical approaches to treatment decision-making for incapacitated patients supply **insufficient guidance** to loved ones and clinicians responsible **for dementia** patient care [where] advance instructions are of limited use." {Emphasis added in both quotes.}

The Council's report states that **our primary moral task** is to ask what we owe patients in their current state, even if so doing requires that we *not* honor the patient's previously expressed wishes. The report casts doubt on the validity of granting "informed consent" years before potential treatment decisions must be made. Yet people *are* fully informed when they create their Advance Directives; they realize they are engaging in an exercise that focuses on future medical treatment decisions. In fact, people create Proxy Directives and Living Wills *precisely* because they hope that the wishes they can express when they are competent will be respected as *durable* if and when they can no longer make their own medical decisions.

The President's Council of Bioethics states that the "text constitutes the official body of this report; it stands as the work of the entire Council" and the report gives no hint of any dissent. Yet Councilmember Dr. Janet Rowley's statement in the Appendix concludes with these words: "For me, this report on the care of the demented aging is a scary document... [since the report states] Advance Directives can and should be ignored depending on the situation at the time."

The Council's report clearly defines four competing domains of what constitutes humanity or personhood. But then it selects one as primary without acknowledging the possibility that some individuals might prefer to ascribe to others as their guide to end-of-life decision-making. Furthermore, The Council's report barely cites the principle of medical ethics called "social fairness" or "social justice." Instead, the report explains, "there will always be large disparities in the economic conditions of the elderly; this fact is unavoidable in any free society" [*Page 26*]. But The Council's preferred domain of *human equality* actually exists in a world of *gross inequality of available resources*: "Three billion people exist on less than $2 per day," and "30,000 children die every day due to hunger and diseases related to utterly preventable causes (such as lack of clean drinking water)," according to data quoted by Reverend Jim Wallis [*God's Politics*, 2005]. Rev. Wallis wrote [*Page 47*], "Just to decry these facts has not solved the scandal of poverty" and noted, "the prosperity of the 1990s sent a financial windfall straight to the very top, while leaving those at the bottom even farther behind and creating a new middle-class anxiety" [*Page 236*].

To argue against current legal and medical practice, and to single out dementia as a condition that defies advance care planning, many of the 333 pages of The President's Council on Bioethics' report are devoted to justifying its basic recommendation **to transform the role** of Proxies, caregivers, and policy makers... *from* showing patients respect by honoring their previously expressed end-of-life decisions... **to** performing as if Proxies and caregivers were the patients' duly appointed **moral agents** who must feel obligated to disregard, rather than to honor their previously expressed Last Wishes [cartoon, page 330].

The Council would have "Prudence" and "Best Care" [defined in the report's Glossary and discussed further below] effectively replace "Substituted Judgment," the standard of decision-making where the designated Proxy has learned enough about the patient's values and wishes to feel confident he or she can make the decision the patient would have made. The Council's message *permits* future physicians to *consider* patient's Advance Directives, but explicitly *forbids* granting these documents priority, even if they are clearly and convincingly written.

The Council's report first confuses and then ignores the "Best Interest" standard of decision-making. No data are presented about what "reasonable people" would want, in terms of surveys that asked people if they would want medical treatment to maintain their existence if they were permanently unconscious or suffering from advanced dementia, had no hope of recovery, faced further indignity, and became a burden to their family and society by requiring total care. A few representative surveys cited here show that The Council's recommendations vary markedly from what the vast majority of people want.

The Council's arguments that Advance Directives do not and cannot work for patients who suffer from dementia are seriously flawed. The report starts with "Two Moments" from a semi-hypothetical clinical case, but then it inappropriately extrapolates to reach conclusions that are neither logically nor clinically valid.

Accepting The Council's recommendations would have widespread and dire consequences: Patients' intensity and duration of suffering would increase, as would caregivers and families' financial strain and emotional burden. The probability that Medicare and Medicaid will be destroyed will increase or be greatly hastened. Liberty and privacy would be restricted despite guarantees in our Constitution. The poor and uninsured in this country will be further neglected as will efforts to reduce preventable dying of children in developing countries, if medical and financial resources are allocated, as The Council insists, to patients who cannot even appreciate that sacrifices are being made for them.

Reverend Jim Wallis [2005] popularized the idea that the U.S. budget is a "moral document" that "expresses our priorities as a culture." Similarly, every individual's advance directive includes his or her personal decisions about end-of-life options that can also be considered a moral document. This perspective extends the notion of "heroic" dying described by Dr. Jack McCue [1995]. In contrast, the trend of the recent Federal budgets have consequences that are antithetical to the espoused values of The Council's report and its claimed motivational basis: to care for our vulnerable and needy.

Adept politicians know that merely citing true and compelling facts that are connected by sound logic is often inadequate to convince people to endorse policies that are clearly in their best interests. The strategy to overcome the challenges of The Council's recommendations is based on Dr. George Lakoff's approach to influence moral politics [2002, 2004]. A cognitive scientist and linguist, Dr. Lakoff teaches that to be effective, arguments must appeal to people's sense of identity and basic values. Memoirs will illustrate these values.

1. Summary of the future crisis

The Council's report provides an abundance of facts to document this awesome statement: "We seem to be on the cusp of an historically unprecedented situation, both in the degree of care that elderly individuals will need and in the proportion of society's resources that will have to be devoted to such care." Here are a few relevant "highlights":

The success of modern medicine has created an enormous problem. The consequence of keeping people alive to old age, according to a study by the Rand Corporation, is that 40% of us will now die "only after *prolonged dwindling, usually lasting many years*; this is the typical course of death from dementia (including Alzheimer's disease or disabling stroke) or generalized frailty of multiple body systems. This trajectory toward death is gradual but unrelenting, with steady decline, enfeeblement, and growing dependency, often lasting a decade or longer." Unless pandemics and huge natural disasters kill people more quickly, this figure of 4 out of 10 will increase.

❧ *SKIP*

Alzheimer's disease usually "runs a course from onset to death of about 6 to 10 years, although it may last up to twice as long." The "period of dementia could stretch out ten years, the last five of which require nonstop nursing care." Putting it succinctly, David Brooks wrote in the New York Times [2005]: "the Kass report is a declaration of dependence." (Dr. Leon Kass stepped down as The Council's chairman soon after The Council's report was published.)

The future crisis will affect most of us, even those who are lucky enough to not be among the **4 out of 10** who will die slowly with total dependence. A married couple whose four parents are alive has a **7 out of 8** chance that at least one parent will die from the ravages of dementia. The chance that at least two parents will die this way is about 1 in 2. Few will escape the ravages of dementia. Worse, changes in demographics will put burdens of unprecedented proportions on the dwindling number of available lay caregivers. The ratio of potential caregivers in the prime years for family caregiving (between 50 and 64) compared to the number of people who will need care (those over 85), is expected to decrease by more than two-thirds in one generation. In 1990, there were **21** potential caregivers for each person over 85; in 2030, there will be only **6**. The demanding job of caregiving leads to a high burnout rate. Hence the number of professional caregivers will decrease as need for their services increases dramatically.

The stark truth is that "roughly **half the people over 85** will suffer major cognitive impairment or dementia as part of their final phase of life. At present, according to the Alzheimer's Association, an estimated 4.5 million Americans have Alzheimer's disease; by 2050, the number of Americans with Alzheimer's disease is estimated to range between 11 million and 16 million." Furthermore, "even with new treatment modalities that might slow the onset of [Alzheimer's] disease, none of the projections expects less than a **three-fold rise** in prevalence in 2050."

"The Congressional Budget Office forecasts that the cost of long-term care, roughly $123 billion in 2000, will reach $207 billion in 2020, and $346 billion in 2040. These extraordinary costs risk bankrupting State budgets, which currently devote 20 percent of expenditures to Medicaid." The strain on the Federal budget is also enormous. Compare the estimates for long-term care above with the total requested in fiscal year 2004 for Health and Human Welfare of $66 billion, with the Department of Education's $53 billion, and with the 2004 budget deficit forecast of $521 million—according to data quoted in *God's Politics* [2005].

The Council's report also considers the non-economic burdens of caregiving. Caregivers have high rates of clinical depression and physical illness. Often, they are forced to give up other life interests and family obligations so they can provide 24/7 care for loved ones who, despite their best efforts, still progressively and hopelessly decline. Their loved ones cannot appreciate the sacrifices being made for them. With little or no relief for years as they provide care, caregivers simultaneously grieve for loved ones who are both "there and not there": They are "there" in body, but "not there" in mind. Meanwhile, caregivers may experience guilt for neglecting other family members, feel unfulfilled by not having time or energy to pursue their own interests, and feel helpless for not being able to contribute economically as their family's assets are drained.

✑ CONTINUE

2. What the President's Council on Bioethics report does not consider

The Council's report does state, "Feeding tubes and respirators are not always obligatory... . And if these measures are used for a time, there are circumstances when it is morally permissible—and even, perhaps, morally required—to desist. Dying as well as possible—or, more modestly, in as little misery as possible—is also one of our concerns and cares." Yet the report does NOT consider the **overuse of feeding tubes** in the United States, or that many States impose higher standards of proof of a Proxy's authority to refuse nutrition and hydration. Some of these laws "exert the practical effect of clouding and confusing the legally permissible boundaries of end-of-life care" according to Kapp [2002], who delineated the sources of legislative harm in an editorial that referred to the research article by Sieger and others [2002].

✑ SKIP

To add to the studies cited about feeding tubes in Chapter 5, these four articles are relevant to patients with dementia: In the Netherlands, for those nursing home patients with dementia for whom decisions concerning artificial nutrition and hydration (ANH) were made, only 6% had feeding tubes [Pasman and others, 2004]. In contrast, at a New York hospital, in the two months before the authors offered an educational program designed to change physicians' behavior, 40 out of 58 dementia patients received feeding tubes (69%). This percentage decreased to 30% after the education program, although statisticians would not consider the numbers significant. What did **not change** was the percentage of dementia patients given feeding tubes even though their Advance Directives **refused** tube feeding. This figure remained the same: 15% [Monteleoni and Clark, 2004]. The trainers/authors presented facts to the physicians that should have been convincing; for example: "Studies have found no evidence that feeding tubes in this population prevent aspiration, prolong life, improve overall function, or reduce pressure sores. Additionally, the quality of life of a patient with advanced dementia can be adversely affected when a feeding tube is inserted. The patient may require wrist restraints to prevent pulling on the tube or may develop cellulitis at the gastrostomy site, develop decubitus ulcers, be deprived of the social interaction and pleasure surrounding meals, and require placement in a nursing home." Monteleoni and Clark concluded, "Unfortunately, many doctors are unfamiliar with this literature or face barriers—attitudinal, institutional, or imposed by the health care industry—to applying its findings to their practice."

Doctors Casarett, Kapo, and Caplan noted that short-term tube feeding can benefit certain types of patients. Tube feeding probably extends life for patients in the permanent vegetative state but does not benefit or extend life for patients with severe dementia. (I have not seen the reasons for this difference discussed but two come to my mind: First, PVS patients can be young when their brains experienced trauma or lack of oxygen while demented patients are usually old. Second, PVS patients need tube feeding immediately while dementia patients have a longer window to change the route of supplying nutrition. Once a tube is implanted, however, new risks suddenly increase for dementia patients. They have increased infections due to more bedsores from restraints to prevent them from removing the feeding tubes.) Clinical data led Dr. Casarett to conclude [2005]: "Artificial Nutrition and Hydration is a medical therapy with substantial risks and burdens, which must be administered using technical medical procedures. In addition, it has no role in palliative care, since it does not promote patient comfort or ease suffering."

Doctors Truog and Cochrane [2005] not only agreed that tube feeding is often inappropriate, they extended the argument to include **oral** administration of nutrition and hydration by writing, "All medical choices that are available to competent patients must also be available to incompetent patients.... Surrogates are asked... to make decisions based on how they think the patient would have weighed the burdens of an intervention against its benefits... Different jurisdictions may apply certain evidentiary thresholds for these decisions, but in principle **the withdrawal of oral nutrition and hydration from patients who are capable of eating and drinking has a firm ethical and legal basis**." They thus endorsed the "right to refuse any unwanted intervention, medical or otherwise [which is] grounded in the fundamental rights to self-determination and bodily integrity that are deeply rooted in the American legal tradition, which prohibits any unwanted touching as battery."

Another topic that The Council did not consider deeply is the potential benefit from medical treatment. The report does state, "Medications that slow the breakdown of acetylcholine... [have] been demonstrated to slow the progress of the disease [Alzheimer's] in some patients in the early first phase often by as much as a year or more." But the report does not mention the potential benefit of **early diagnosis** and **treatment**, that these same medications may **delay the onset** of dementia, and that slowing down the progression of symptoms can postpone the need for institutional care, which is more expensive than home care.

While the report mentions that **caregivers need extra support and treatment**, it does not state that doing so would not only provide direct benefit to caregivers, but would also be **cost-effective** since it would postpone the time of starting professional caregiving, which is more expensive than care provided by loved ones that is often given "free."

The Council's report does admit that it has not considered how to manage society's future financial burden of increasing numbers of dementia cases, but it does not estimate the **additional cost or who would pay for following its recommendations to prolong the existence of patients with advanced dementia**. Councilmember Dr. Janet Rowley poignantly asks (in the report's Appendix), "Where will that money come from? Might it not come from programs that help needy infants receive better health care and early childhood education so that some of the disadvantages associated with being born in poverty might be ameliorated by an enriched early childhood? If you asked them bluntly, would grandparents really want to steal from their grandchildren?"

In contrast, Britain's National Institute for Health and Clinical Excellence (NICE) asks their health economists to evaluate the cost effectiveness of various therapies by comparing cost with benefit. Implicit in their calculations is the recognition that the value of life is lower with illnesses. NICE uses a parameter called **Quality-Adjusted Life Year** or **QALY**. Here is how the weighting scale works: a QALY of 0 = dead, while a QALY of 1 = perfect health. This analysis recognizes that resources are limited, so they should be used where they can do the most good. Britain's health care system usually approves of therapeutic interventions only when the benefit is greater than 1 QALY for spending $50,000 [Whalen, 2005]. In contrast, The President's Council on Bioethics' report does not consider the possibility of using similar guidelines. Instead, it argues against the evaluation of quality of life based on its view of morality and personhood (see below). The report states, "rationing resources for debilitated or demented persons risks dehumanizing them… and "might perversely alter the role of the State, by making certain therapies illegal across the board for certain classes of patients, **rich and poor alike**… The principle that persons with dementia have human dignity equal to non-demented persons provides an essential moral foundation for a caring and caregiving society" and dementia should not be "a reason for discrimination or a legitimate grounds for the denial of equal treatment" [*Pages 126-127*]. The Council's report mentions only briefly "what obligations persons with dementia (in its early stages) may still have to the society of which they are part, including generosity toward and concern for generations yet to come" [*Page 128*]. {Emphasis added since the poor are denied care anyway.}

Granted, in countries such as Great Britain or Canada, where the budget for health care funds is fixed, funds not used to pay for one disease may automatically become available for another disease. In the United States, money saved from not prolonging the dying of severely demented patients does not automatically become available for other worthy causes, but it would only become possible if those funds were not spent. Some of the savings might even be used in developing countries. One great need is to decrease the number of preventable deaths from malaria among African children under the age of five. The point is, now is the time to start increasing public's awareness, to take steps to help others around the globe. Otherwise, we will become exclusively concerned with our own actual or impending bankruptcy. We must therefore design our Advance Directives keeping in mind that the aggregation of our specific requests can have great impact both on our American "budget as a moral document" and around the world.

With respect to more fortunate individuals and countries, The Council's report states [*Page 198*]: "Those with unlimited resources might owe their loved ones more in terms of medical care; those nations with greater wealth might owe their citizens more public assistance and support." However The Council's report does not consider the option of **using our individual or national resources elsewhere**. Starting in 1993 with the World Bank Development Report, economists have used a parameter to assess the burden of disease called **DALY** or **Disability-Adjusted Life Years**, which combines years of potential life lost owing to premature death with years of productive life lost due to disability. The burden of both years and disability can then be compared with the cost of clinical interventions or the amount of money spent on research. The first detailed comprehensive estimate of using DALYs conditions in the United States was quite recent [McKenna and others, 2005]. In Europe, Dr. Essink-Bat and others [2002] are still working on establishing DALYs for dementia and other disease states. Yet the President's Council on Bioethics' report entirely rejects the concept of judging quality of life. The report ignores the fact that the term "**quality of life**" is used in almost 75,000 citations in the database of the National Library of Medicine. The Council insists instead on "the **equality** of human life."

The Council's report does not consider global comparisons of "good"; for example: To maintain one severely demented patient in a skilled nursing home, who cannot recognize her loved ones and has no awareness of the sacrifices being made for her, costs about $100,000 per year. In contrast, to reduce substantially the risk of malaria that kills millions of African children under the age of 5 would cost only $4 per year per family (slightly higher for chemically treated insect nets that do not require periodic re-treatment with insecticide). According to Stephen Magesa [quoted by Michael Specter in The New Yorker, 2005], such nets are 30 to 50% effective in saving lives. So, as a global society we have a theoretical choice that could be put into practice: spend $100,000 to maintain "one unaware unconscious body, for one year," or to buy approximately 10,000 (upgraded) nets to effectively insure the lives of about 4000 young children (assuming the nets are 40% effective). The European Disability Weights Projects is unlikely to assign a value as high as 0.1 for the last year of life with dementia, while the average 5 year-old who has not succumbed to malaria will have acquired enough immunity to live 40 years or more at reasonable, if not perfect health (for purposes of an example, assuming a disability weight of 0.8) to be able to compare two DALYs: For 1 person for 1 year whose disability weight is 0.1 (really less) *with* DALYs for as many as 4000 people for 40 years whose average disability is 0.8. Very roughly, then, for the same $100,000, we have this astounding difference:

Two Choices on How to Allocate Resources

(4000 times 0.8 times 40) divided by (0.1 times 1 times 1) = **1.3 million**

This is a **1.3 million times more effective** use of money to save DALYs.

Of course, some African children will survive even without insect nets, but I still asked Robert H. Frank, H. J. Louis Professor of Management and Professor of Economics at Cornell University and columnist for the *New York Times,* "Economic Scene," to review this numerical comparison. Dr. Frank had engaged economist Dr. Landsburg in an argument about the economics of life-sustaining treatment, which is discussed on page 26. Dr. Frank clarified concepts [2005] introduced by Thomas Schelling, who won the 2005 Nobel Prize in economics. Dr. Schelling distinguished between a "statistical life" and an "identified life" by observing the apparent paradox that communities often spend millions of dollars to save the life of a known victim yet are, at the same time, often unwilling to spend much less on prevention of accidents before they happen. I wonder if a similar mentality may be in effect when strapped down in a hospital bed is a body that looks like your father or mother, in contrast to the theoretical savings of hundreds of lives on another continent.

Dr. Frank explained, "Schelling's point is not that a single identified life trumps any arbitrary number of statistical lives. It's just that we are especially motivated to intervene in cases in which a known life is at stake. Schelling's discussion also did not address the issue of demented or comatose persons. These are not the kinds of 'identified lives' with which people readily identify or experience empathy. Personally, if I were in such a state, I would not want anyone to spend a nickel to keep me alive. So by all means, save the money spent on late-stage dementia patients and spend it instead on mosquito nets or something else in health care or education, which has the potential to do some real good."

Rev. Cecil L. "Chip" Murray, Tanzy Chair of Christian Ethics, School of Religion, University of Southern California and Pastor Emeritus of the First African Methodist Episcopal Church, had these words of spiritual wisdom at the California Science Center in Los Angeles [2006]. {Title from a previous sermon.}

When You're Down to Nothing (but Dry Bones), God is UP to Something!

If we believe in God and think of ourselves as spiritual beings, then we will have to consider what is *meaningful* existence compared to *mere* existence. Presently, the right wing fundamentalist church is holding hard on existence, no matter what, not meaningful existence, but mere existence...

Yet 45 million Americans have no health insurance and 37 million live in poverty... 470 million people in the world suffer from malnutrition... that's mere existence... and 70 million die every year. Aren't we going to care about the "living dead" as well as about the "dead living"? Can't we say, you do your best, you fix what you can, and let God fix the rest? You take care of those whom we call the living, and let God use a magnetic power to somehow pull us through the curtain of death to a curtain of life (if we choose to believe that way). But no matter what we believe about death, we all must ponder the question about life: *meaningful existence* versus *mere existence*.

Beyond *mere* faith or common sense, Professor Jeff McMahan's sophisticated metaphysical/philosophical analysis of death may convince some readers (including me) why a *person's* death is distinct from the death of a human biological *organism'*. He states, "According to the Embodied Mind Account of Identity, there are no cases in which progressive dementia results in a different individual, much less different person," and the "series of 'discreet and mutually irrelevant episodes' do not offer a strong reason for sustaining the Demented Patient's life" [*Pages 494, 503; 2002*].

Consider the recommendations of the President's Commission for the Study of Ethical Problems in Medicine and Biomedical and Behavioral Research [1983]: "Access to costly care for patients who have permanently lost consciousness may justifiably be restricted on the basis of resource use in two ways: by a physician or institution that otherwise would have to deny significantly beneficial care to another specific patient, or by legitimate mechanisms of policy formulation and application if and only if the provision of certain kinds of care to these patients were clearly causing serious inequities in the use of community resources." Twenty-two years after the Commission's statement, The Council's report still ignores the inequities in providing health care.

While The Council's report of 2005 vividly describes the burdens of caregivers, and it notes the strain on our society's resources, it does not admit that its recommendations would increase the suffering of patients and families, or that it would make it more likely that the medical crisis of caring for Alzheimer's disease and other dementias will destroy not only our ability to provide adequate health care for those who are mentally aware of its benefits, but many other "goods" in our society. (These important areas are discussed later.)

Although The Council's report was published one week prior to oral hearings, it does not consider the U.S. Supreme Court case of Gonzales v. Oregon (04-623), which threatened the viability of the Death With Dignity Act, which State law voters in Oregon twice approved. Many people—whether or not they believe it should be legal for physicians to prescribe medications to help terminally ill patients with unbearable suffering hasten their dying—believe strongly that the more fundamental issue is one of personal freedom, which should be protected from the imposition of the values of others. (The Council's only oblique reference to the Oregon law is the report's comment that "six months" is a long time, discussed further below.)

The Council's report devotes only one sentence to the **causes of death in dementia patients**: "In the end, an overwhelming infection, a stroke, or some other insult that a severely weakened body cannot handle becomes the proximate cause of death." This is consistent with the investigation of the immediate causes of death by Kammoun and others [2000], who concluded that "Dementia was an underlying but never a primary cause of death." However, in a series of over 300 demented patients, Attems and others [2005] found that the main causes of death were **pneumonia** (46%) and **cardiovascular disease** (31%).

The more general and important truth about dying is this: All of us, whether we are demented or not, must die. About that, we have no choice. Yet some of us would prefer to have the right to choose HOW we will die while we are still competent to make those decisions, especially since some ways of dying involve less suffering than others. In Oregon, for example, cancer is more painful a way to die than an overdose of sleeping pills. And for an overwhelming majority of "reasonable people," death is preferable to continued existence in end-stage dementia (which data are presented, below).

A decade ago, Dr. Jack McCue wrote, "Loss of motivation to eat and drink—whether volitional or a result of neurological or psychiatric changes with aging—may thus be an important component of natural dying," and "Making *dying* a diagnosis recognizes it as a chronic and incurable condition—an inevitable process that is independent of underlying diseases [that] requires acceptance and accommodation, not fruitless attempts at diagnosis and cure." Dr. McCue noted, "Death makes way for the birth of children... Dying bravely is heroic, and a heroic death may be the most intense memory that we can pass to posterity" [1995].

The President's Council on Bioethics' report includes one clinical case where the decision pending was whether or not to treat pneumonia aggressively in a patient with dementia. Continued survival would likely lead to more suffering in the future from a painful death from cancer. The discussion about the decision reveals how high The Council sets the bar for treatment refusal. In contrast, they would readily accept the decision for treatment if the patient previously held a religious belief in the redemptive power of suffering.   (More details, later.)

CONTINUE

Councilmember Dr. Janet Rowley writes the report "takes a very draconian view of dying. The more painful it is made to be by applying rigid ethical rules, the more ennobling it is for both the patient and the caregiver." Not surprisingly, the Council's report does not consider the legal peaceful way to die by **Refusing Food & Fluid by Proxy**—which for some patients may be their only way out. Instead, it presents general values, guidelines, and specific examples that others could quote to support the view that **Refusing Food & Fluid by Proxy** is morally wrong. The Council's report thus fails to accept both the possible means and the philosophy as stated in the concluding words of Dr. McCue in his article, "The Naturalness of Dying" [1995]: "On its simplest human level, for many very elderly persons, death is an undeniably desirable relief from suffering."

3. What is the basis for the President's Council on Bioethics' recommendations?

Councilmember Dr. Janet Rowley noted that The Council's report used the word "compassion" only 5 times in two key chapters. Aside from Dr. Rowley's statement, the word "compassion" appeared 8 times in the entire report of 333 pages. In contrast, the report used the word "moral" 262 times. (The word "never" was used 96 times.)

What is The President's Council on Bioethics moral position? "In matters regarding life, death, and basic rights, the most basic commitment of our society is and has been to **human equality**.... The commitment to equal human worth stands as the basis of a welcoming community—one that assures all living human beings, even those in a disabled or diminished state, that their lives still have meaning, worth, and value for **all of us**...."

ॐSKIP

The report acknowledges the existence of four domains of human worth, but it considers them to be in conflict: "The '**ethic of equality**' (valuing all human beings in light of their common humanity) exists in deep tension with the '**ethic of utility**' (measuring lives by what they are worth to oneself or others), with the '**ethic of quality**' (valuing life when it embodies certain humanly fitting characteristics or enables certain humanly satisfying experiences), and with the '**ethic of autonomy**' (valuing each person's freedom to decide what sort of life has worth for us as individuals). If the worth of a human life depends entirely on a person's utility, then some lives are clearly more valuable than others... If the worth of a human life depends upon the presence of certain uniquely human qualities (such as, for example, memory, understanding, and self-command), then we may judge that some lives never had such worth and others (such as those with advanced dementia) no longer do. If the worth of a human life depends on one's 'autonomous' assessment of self-worth, then clearly some... lives (such as those incapable of autonomous choice) may seem to lack human worth altogether."

The Council's report then preaches: "Against these dangerous and erroneous temptations, the 'ethic of equality' defends the floor of human dignity, ensuring that *even the most diminished among us is not denied the respect and care that all human beings are owed*. The Council embraces this teaching as the first principle of ethical caregiving. Yet, in some respects, equality will always stand in tension with what may seem to mark the *height* of human dignity: the qualities that distinguish our humanity, that make us useful to others, and that we freely choose and affirm for ourselves. That tension will always mark our thinking about the process of aging and the ravages of dementia." [*Pages 106-107.*]

❧*CONTINUE*

The Council's report harshly denounces attempts to prioritize the other domains of personhood as "dangerous and erroneous temptations" [*Page 106*]. Later, it uses the word "discrimination" in a startling context, "Discrimination by a past self against a future self" [*Page 170*]. The Council's report thus demeans both the process of creating and of honoring Advance Directives.

The Council defines Ronald Dworkin's competing principle of "precedent autonomy," as, "All individuals should have the freedom to decide for themselves, while they are still competent, whether (later) life with dementia would have any meaning or dignity *for them*, and what kinds of treatment should be pursued or rejected on their behalf." While the Council judges Dworkin's principle as having "partial wisdom," it does not apply them as it deliberates its clinical examples or presents its general guidelines.

Clarifying note: The principle of "human equality" is both worthy and dignified; it recognizes the fundamental truth that every human being deserves considered care and respect. However, if the demented person, when previously competent, made a diligent decision to prioritize the other three ethics of human life, then the crucial question about end-of-life decision-making comes down to this: Who decides? Can each individual decide for herself what principle(s) shall prevail? Or must we accept the recommendations of The President's Council?

To argue its point of view, The President's Council on Bioethics' report quotes clinical outcome data from which they draw reasonable and logical conclusions. For example, use of Living Wills has failed to have great impact on how physicians make end-of-life decisions. Yet the main basis of The Council's philosophy is a two-part premise for which no scientific evidence could be presented. —Nor could there be, since this premise is based on faith rather than observation:

A. There is a **continuity** of "being human" that resides in the body; and,

B. There is a **discontinuity** of "being human" that resides in the rational, thinking, decision-making mind.

The implicit adoption of this premise is necessary to support The Council's diatribe against both creating and implementing Advance Directives, to support their mandate to set aside the previously expressed wishes of individuals as written in their Living Wills; to have other priorities override the content of discussions of Last Wishes with designated Proxies; and to transform the roles of professionals, of lay caregivers, of policy makers and legislators, and of designated Proxies... **from advocates of precedent autonomy... to moral arbitrators of previously expressed end-of-life decisions**. In other words, The Council's recommendation is to "Err on the side of life." The only reason to **disallow decisions to forgo treatment** is if the burden of the treatment itself is too great, or the treatment will not work. Otherwise, The Council would prolong the process of dying.

4. What are the logical consequences of believing in the continuity of the body and the discontinuity of the mind?

One is obvious: under most circumstances, caregivers are obligated to maintain "life" as long as the body and medical technology will permit. Councilmember Professor Gómez-Lobo states in the Appendix, "A demented person is a severely handicapped individual who does not thereby cease to be a person. To think otherwise is to embrace **a radical form of dualism** that leads to the positing of two deaths: one for the mind and one for the body. But this does **not match our unified experience** of ourselves and of others." {Emphasis added.}—Or does it? The Greeks contrasted *zoe* (physical or biological life) with *bios* (a life as lived, made up of actions, decisions, motives, and events creating a biography). Doesn't modern medicine often prolong *zoe* after *bios* has ended? What about the neurological criteria of brain death that was first defined by a Harvard Committee [1968] and has since received further consensus in the journal, Neurology [1995]? (Citations are in the Glossary under Brain Death.)

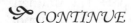*SKIP*

The precedent to honor Advance Directives is not a new idea. Its origins can be traced to the late 1960s. A President's Commission for the Study of Ethical Problems in Medicine and Biomedical and Behavioral Research [1983] concluded "that the authority of competent, informed patients to decide about their health care encompasses the decision to forego treatment and allow death to occur." This Commission also stated, "When patients are incompetent to make their own decisions, others must act on their behalf." The Commission considered "existing legal procedures can be adapted for the purpose of allowing people while competent to designate someone to act in their stead and to express their wishes about treatment." (For this reason, the framed sign in the cartoon on page 330 includes the words, "Since 1983.")

CONTINUE

Another consequence of adopting The Council's premise is to justify the assertion that the mind that could once think rationally and make decisions, has no legal standing in terms of speaking for the future body. The belief that the mind is discontinuous justifies The Council's report's use of highly charged language: the report repeatedly states that attempts by an earlier thinking self to request refusal of life-sustaining treatment for the future demented self **discriminates** against a **disabled** person. The Council's two-part premise justifies setting aside previously expressed wishes and replacing them with The Council's moral and ethical guidelines, which The Council has decided must be based on the current circumstances of what is it right for the body.

Below is a selection of excerpts from The Council's report. [Some were modified very slightly for grammatical consistency.] Some values are generally sound, but they can be misapplied to restrict individual Liberty since The Council insists on OVERRIDING the previously expressed wishes of the patient to apply their *first principle of human equality.*

❧ *SKIP*

A. Regarding the moral responsibility of competent individuals as they create their Advance Directives, and as others consider honoring their directives:

- The fundamental limitations and shortcomings of advance instruction directives can never replace prudent **judgment by devoted caregivers** about what a patient **now needs**.

- As caregivers, decisions about treatment always fall within the realm of our moral responsibility; it is the realm in which **we decide** what **we owe** the patient. It is the realm in which **we exert** greatest control and therefore have greatest responsibility..."

- Living Wills can never relieve us of the responsibility **we have to care** for one another **as best we can**, even in difficult circumstances such as those dementia creates.

- Responsible caregivers should **not** acquiesce in **denying the worth of the person** entrusted to their care.

- Competent individuals should **resist** making **a priori negative judgments** about the **disabled person they might become**.

- Only by making an all-encompassing determination that his life with (more than minimal) dementia would never be worth sustaining might the competent individual rule out in advance all future treatments should he become demented. But such a blanket assertion about the worth of a future self **denies the**

intrinsic dignity of embodied life even when one's cognition is impaired; it discriminates against an imaginary future self long before the true well-being of that future self is really imaginable [*Page 194*].

• **We** are **obligated to treat** [patients with dementia] with respect and to seek their well-being, **here and now**.

• But even such improvements [in Living Wills] do not address the **fundamental limitations and shortcomings of advance instruction directives**... Ethics committees, drafters of professional guidelines, policy-makers, and legislators at both the state and federal levels should address these **failings** and search for more practical and **responsible alternatives**.

B. Regarding The Council's moral guidelines that could restrict exercising the option of Refusal of Food & Fluid by Proxy:

• Our primary goal is to do everything we reasonably can to benefit their lives— from **meeting basic needs and sustaining life**, to easing pain and curing ailments, to offering comfort in difficult times and, in the end, keeping company in the face of looming death.

• We should always **seek to benefit the life** incapacitated persons **still have**, and never treat even the most diminished individuals as unworthy of our company and care.

• Caregivers in particular and society as a whole must **never lose sight of the humanity** of those persons with dementia entrusted to their care.

• The shared moral framework recognizes the deprivations of dementia, the limitations on family and social resources, and the significance of a person's prior wishes, but never defines life with dementia as "life unworthy of life" and **never sees causing death as a morally choiceworthy means** to the end of easing suffering. After all, it is self-contradictory to propose to "care" for any patient by making him dead.

• We should remember that **aiming at a person's death is always a kind of betrayal**.

• Ethically responsible caregivers operate within certain firm moral boundaries— central among them the obligation **never to seek a patient's death in making decisions about a person's care**... The aim is always to care and **never to kill**, always to benefit the life the patient still has.

- Caring wholeheartedly for a frail patient or a disabled loved one is **incompatible** with thinking that **engineering their death is an acceptable** therapeutic option.

- We emphasize both the singular importance of seeking to serve the life the patient still has and the **moral necessity of never seeking a person's death as a means of relieving his suffering.**"

- We abandon them if, even with the best of intentions, we do not do what we can to **benefit the life they still have**.

- Lasting moral duties **never [include] withholding effective and non-burdensome treatments** from patients who are not already irretrievably dying.

- For responsible caregivers, death itself will never become the means to relieving suffering, and life itself will never be treated as the burden to be relieved. **We cannot, after all, serve the well-being of a person's life by seeking his death**.

℘ CONTINUE

Semantics is pragmatically important. The word "care" can mean to honor the patient's previous request OR it can mean to decrease the patient's suffering. The words "effective treatment" and "benefit" do not necessarily compel incurring great economic and emotional burdens to prolong the existence of a body that will be remembered in increasing states of indignity, and that will never regain the abilities to think, to know oneself, and to recognize loved ones.

In terms of how the above principles are applied, consider one of the clinical cases that the President's Council on Bioethics presented and discussed.

Would the President's Council on Bioethics Recommend Treating Pneumonia in an Alzheimer's Patient Who Was Also Suffering from Terminal, Painful Cancer?

A woman with middle-stage Alzheimer's disease—disordered speech and some disorientation, sometimes emotionally overwrought, sometimes withdrawn, and only occasionally able to recognize her close family members— is also suffering from a rare form of cancer, already widely spread.

There is no hope of cure, invasive treatments aimed at slowing down the disease are no longer an option, and the patient is already experiencing pain from the bony metastases. The cancer will almost certainly lead to a painful decline and excruciating death over the next three to six months, where pain can be controlled only by constant and heavy sedation, and even then not completely short of inducing coma. Concurrently, the patient contracts a treatable bacterial pneumonia, and a decision needs to be made about whether to treat it. [No changes were made in the case description, from *Page 187.*]

❧ *SKIP*

Excerpts from The Council's discussion:

"The treatment itself [antibiotics and hydration] is non-burdensome: it does not involve moving or violating the patient, or causing her new kinds of discomfort or distress. As caregivers, however, we must think about the future as well as the present, about future burdens as well as present needs. In treating her pneumonia—even if we assume it is the right thing to do—we make it more likely that she will endure more future pain than she would were the pneumonia to take her life. We cannot avoid that stark reality." [and] "The demented person may reach a point—if she is not already there—where the pain is so awful and her cognitive capacities are so limited that life with cancer is sheer and incomprehensible misery, with nothing positive in her subjective experience to compensate or sustain her." [and] "**As caregivers, we do not want to refuse treatment as a way of getting the patient to die.**" [and] "**Our most fundamental commitment is not to minimize suffering but to maximize care**—never to abandon care for another human being." [Note:] "Six months is not a short time; it allows for her life to be touched by loved ones (though her capacity for interaction is already severely limited by her dementia), or it gives time to enjoy whatever simple pleasures (if any) still mean something to her." [so:] "This is surely a hard and puzzling case with no easy answers. It appears to be a case in which the distinction between "active killing" and "letting die" might take on real significance: which is to say, **we appear to possess the moral discretion**, as caregivers, to let pneumonia take its course, but (as always) never the moral freedom to kill the patient directly." [however:] "If the patient was or is a religious person with a redemptive understanding of suffering, this fact might move **loving caregivers to treat**." [so:] "In the end, we believe that **the moral *argument* could go either way** in this case, depending in part on many personal and medical particulars... it seems wise to leave family members and doctors some leeway to decide, lovingly and prudently, when to surrender to Nature." {Note the use of charged language: "loving caregivers."}

Comment: Again, note how high The Council sets the bar of current and future potential suffering for its report to consider it "wise to leave family members and doctors some leeway to decide" [so that] "the moral *argument* could go either way." Other experts have different opinions; for example, van der Steen and others wrote [2005]: "The frequent withholding of antibiotics with an intention to hasten death may reflect a willingness to abandon a cure-oriented approach in dying patients for whom prolongation of life is not an aim." [and] "In patients with end-stage dementia... **life-prolonging treatments may be seen as prolonging suffering**." {Emphasis added.}

Other clinical examples in the report reveal The Council's principle is that treatment refusal is morally permissible only if the treatment itself is likely to cause a "great burden." While The Council considers, "Forgoing treatment might allow the patient to live out *her last days* with the happiness that her relatively stable and peaceful home life still permits—with minimum disruption or struggle, and without being treated as a mere object of care requiring permanent coercion," {emphasis added}, the report adds, "With possibly six months left to live, one must be hesitant about seizing an occasion for death by leaving the pneumonia untreated. But as six months becomes six weeks or six days, the case for surrender strengthens, especially as the debility of the cancer gets worse."

Comment: In distinguishing between "six months" and "six weeks or six days," The Council **explicitly imposes *its* moral view** regarding the expected length of time to death on end-of-life decision-making. Obviously, The Council feels that longer times preclude the decision to withhold treatment. Others may disagree: for patients with unbearable suffering, the longer they must suffer, the greater the unwanted burden of continued existence, so it would be an act of compassion to allow Nature to take its course earlier. But the supreme ethical principle here is not which argument is more convincing about six months versus six days, but **who should decide**—The Council, or the previously competent patient? (The next paragraph describes the common standard of practice, as I understand it.)

✑ CONTINUE

If this terminally ill woman—who suffered from dementia, cancer, and pneumonia—had created a Living Will or had designated a Proxy, according to many medical ethicists, the Living Will or the Proxy's decision should be honored. If neither existed, most American physicians would consult with family members and close friends in a hierarchal sequence that starts with the person closest, in order, to decide whether or not to treat her pneumonia. If the woman had no one to speak for her, or if those close to her revealed they did not know whether she would have accepted or refused treatment, or if several people said they knew her well but disagreed, then many medical ethicists would recommend applying the "Best Interest" standard, which is discussed in the next section.

5. How ignoring data relevant to the "Best Interest" standard of decision-making allows The Council's report to "Err on the side of life"

The Council's report considers the challenge of decision-making by stating, in a footnote on *Page 64*, that the "crucial distinction is between trying to discern what the person would want if the competent self of the past could speak and trying to do what is best for the incapacitated patient here-and-now." While both are worthy of consideration, the report does not, as the courts have done, consider a conflict exists only when there is no or little information about the wishes of the patient. Instead the report blurs the relevant standard of decision-making. In its Glossary, The Council provides these two definitions [*Page 231*]:

"**Best Care**" is defined as the "standard for caregiving that always seeks to serve the patient's current welfare. It emphasizes benefiting the life the person now has, while considering also his own earlier ideals, preferences, and values as an integral part of his current well-being."

"**Best Interest**" has a three-part definition that I separate, label, and highlight to discuss: (A) "A legal standard of **caregiving** for incompetent patients," (B) "defined by the courts in terms of what a "**reasonable person**" would **decide** in a similar situation," and (C) "generally attempts to weigh the burdens and benefits of treatment **to the patient** *in his present* condition." {Bold emphasis added; Italics emphasis, original.}

Comments: With respect to end-of-life decision-making, the words of the first definition, "Best Care," have *not* been codified in either clinical or legal practice—to the best of my knowledge or that of several colleagues whom I surveyed. Yet the words, *Comfort Care*, and Palliative Care, and even the word "care" itself, are universally agreed upon as obligatory standard of practice. In contrast, the term "treatment" implies a curative goal.

"Best Interests" is a well-recognized standard of **decision-making**, *not* of **caregiving** (A). While courts defined it as a standard, it is also used clinically (B). Weighing the burdens and benefits of treatment **to the patient** *in his present* condition is certainly a major consideration, but not the overriding consideration (C) when the patient had previously indicated his Last Wishes by a written document, in a *clear and convincing* way.

The Council's report states [*Page 128*], "to speak of 'interests' alone also seems somewhat impoverished: human beings are not simply collections of interests, but whole persons whose lives are intertwined with others, lives that have meaning even when their interests seem limited... In this, **the proper aim is not simply 'best interests' but 'best care'** for the well-being of this patient, under these circumstances, at this time." {Emphasis added.}

Comment: The Council's tactic is that few would argue against the well-being of a patient. Yet one could argue that there is an unwarranted linking of values here, followed by an unjustified assertion of which values are more dear. Specifically, The Council's goal is to link "best care" with "prudent judgment" and then assert this pair is more noble than considering the pair explicitly expresses Last Wishes and "best interest." The statement of The Council's report on *Page 196* is clear: "**prudent judgment points toward overriding the living will, even when caregivers disagree**" [about forgoing treatment]. Prudent judgment (The Council's view of morality) prevails over all; hence, there is no reason to consider "Best Interest," which large body of data The Council ignores. Its value-based argument looks like this (where **>** means "is more valued than"):

{PRUDENT JUDGMENT = BEST CARE} **>** {LAST WISHES *or* BEST INTERESTS}

The court-accepted definition of "Best Interest" standard of decision-making requires decision-makers to know what "**reasonable people**" would choose if they were in a similar medical condition as the patient. Here is a sample of surveys about what "reasonable" patients and healthy people would choose:

❧*SKIP*

Singer and others [1995] asked over 500 then competent patients who were facing hemodialysis what treatments they would want with coexisting diseases. Only 14% would continue treatment if they also suffered from **severe dementia**.

Dr. Mortimer Gross [1998] examined 343 Advance Directives available from inpatient and outpatient charts of individuals treated in 1994 at a community hospital near Chicago. He concluded, "The overwhelming desire expressed by the patients in their Advance Directives was not to have their lives prolonged if their medical condition were such that treatment would merely delay death. Only a minuscule number of patients, less than 0.7%, wanted everything done to prolong life regardless of the chance for improvement or the cost." Only 3% of the Advance Directives restricted refusal to the state of an irreversible coma. The other 97% specified NO life-sustaining measures "if my agent believes that the burdens of the treatment outweigh the expected benefits [after considering] relief of suffering, the expense involved and the quality as well as the possible extension of life..."

The study by Hammes and others [1998] in La Crosse, Wisconsin, revealed that over eleven months of data collection, "treatment was forgone near the time of death by 98%." In other words, "Only in 2% of cases were there no decisions to withhold treatment. Only 4% indicated they always wanted some form of treatment. (The "Respecting Your Choices" program of La Crosse is known for this success: 85% of the community had Advance Directives, and 95% of these Advance Directive were available to the physicians when needed.)

A study by Gjerdingen and others [1999] surveyed cognitively normal older people. "Approximately three fourths of participants said they would not want cardiopulmonary resuscitation, use of a respirator, or parenteral or enteral tube nutrition with the milder forms of dementia, and 95% or more of participants would not want these procedures with severe dementia."

❧*CONTINUE*

To summarize this sample of clinical surveys, from 86% to 99.3% of "reasonable people" would forgo treatment that may sustain life if their cognition was severely impaired.

❧*SKIP*

Popular polls taken over the TV just before Terri Schiavo's feeding tube was removed for the last time in March, 2005, showed that 87% of those responding would not want their lives prolonged if they were in a similar state. A Gallup poll in May, 2005 [Moore], revealed that 85% of those Americans surveyed said they would want to have their life support removed if they were "in a persistent vegetative state with no hope for significant recovery." Analysis of the results by subgroups revealed that **even those religious people or conservatives who were "most opposed to euthanasia or doctor-assisted suicide, nevertheless would want their life support removed**." {Emphasis added since this striking result implies that the position taken by the President's Council on Bioethics report may reflect a small minority of even those who state they are religious or are politically conservative.} Further details: Among evangelical Christians, 61% support euthanasia; among Catholics, 70%; among conservatives, 63%; among Republicans, 65%. With respect to persisting indefinitely in a vegetative state, the percentage who would want their life support removed was: conservatives, 83%; Republicans, 82%; weekly churchgoers, 75%; and evangelical Christians, 70%.

Several Gallup Polls since 1997 revealed which end-of-life condition most troubled Americans: for 73%, it was "being in a vegetative state." A March 2005, ABC News poll indicated, "only 14% of Americans would want to be kept alive"; a 2003 Fox New poll indicated that "74% would want their guardian to remove the feeding tube." [Saad, 2005] A 2003 Gallup poll [Newport] revealed that 80% support a law to allow a spouse to make a final decision to end a patient's life by some painless means if the patient is in a persistent vegetative state caused by irreversible brain damage. A 2005 Harris poll [Pyhel, Wong, Gullo, 2005] indicated that 78% wanted "the patient's next of kin" to have "the final say about keeping the patient alive or allowing to die," if "in a persistent vegetative state and there is no living will."

Note: Some medical specialists know that patients in the Minimally Conscious State and in advanced stages of dementia experience more suffering than patients in the vegetative state. But other clinicians and the general public may lack this knowledge. This is an important area for future research.

✎ CONTINUE

The conclusions relevant to "Best Interest" is that the vast majority of "reasonable people," including both well people and patients, would not want to be kept alive if they had severe brain disease or damage, and a majority would permit spouses or next of kin to make these end-of-life decisions for them. These results could be considered if there is no specific information about a patient's values and treatment preferences. Yet as important as these data are, they are not included or referred to in The Council's report.

6. How The Council argues to disregard Living Wills

The Council offers this clinical example: A man has a *"written a Living Will [that] stated very clearly that he wants no invasive treatments of any kind once his dementia has progressed to the point where he is no longer self-sufficient and can no longer recognize his family members."*

Yet when he receives the diagnosis of operable cancer in his sigmoid colon, his Proxy/daughter decides not to honor his Living Will.

✎ SKIP

The Council's report argues: "The **primary moral obligation** of caregivers is to serve the well-being of the patient now here, and **to ask not only what the patient would have wanted** but what we owe the person who lies before us... [and] not following its orders regardless of all other circumstances... [When he] wrote his living will, perhaps he could not imagine the desire of his daughter to care for him, or the fact that he would be so cheerful with dementia, or that **he would be willing to endure surgery** of this kind... All of these factors, so difficult to anticipate beforehand, should make us hesitate simply to apply his instructions in a mechanical and thoughtless manner, **as if we were not ourselves reflective moral agents responsible to do the best we can** for the man now before us. In this case, there seem to be **clear and compelling reasons** for caregivers to **override the terms of the advance instruction directive** [Living Will] and to proceed with treatment, understood by both the daughter and the doctors as **the best way possible to benefit the life the patient still has**." {Emphasis added.} The hypothetical example continues: Suppose the patient did NOT want to spend down his financial assets on medical treatment but to leave them to leave to his children and grandchildren. Here again, The Council agrees with the daughter's overriding the reasons that motivated the patient to write his Living Will.

In discarding "the guiding principle of the current legal arrangements governing caregiving for persons with dementia [which] is the obligation to respect the wishes of the competent person the patient once was," the President's Council on Bioethics claimed that the "idea seems to imply that only competent individuals command respect as persons, and, more subtly, that all individuals with dementia are objectively less worthy of care than they were when they were cognitively healthy; or it suggests, at the very least, that there is no obligation to consider their **best interests** [sic] as they are, here and now."

Comments:

A. The daughter should discuss her father's current situation with his doctor; however, she has a [moral] obligation to honor the Last Wishes that her father previously expressed. Her father did not ask her to function as a moral agent to reflect on what she thought would be best IF he reached the conditions he described. Overriding his end-of-life decisions would be presumptuous.

B. "Best Care," if it prolongs the process of dying, is NOT equivalent to, and can sometimes be the opposite of "Best Interests." A person may wish to prioritize the needs of family and society instead of prolonging his dying, his suffering, and depth and time he descends into progressive states of indignity.

C. The subjective standard of the Living Will takes precedence over the "Best Interests" objective standard since in this case, the father's wishes are known.

D. The Council's report is **wrong** when it states that the patient "would be willing to endure surgery of this kind." This is **wrong**. The patient does NOT possess decision-making capacity. If he were competent, there would be nothing to discuss. His doctor would merely ask him, "Do you, or do you not want surgery?" The Council's report merely presents a scenario in which the patient does not obviously resist *Comfort Care*. It is incorrect and presumptuous to infer from such observations that he would therefore agree to major surgery.

Further Comments:

The patient's Living Will requests applying the "no treatment option" when he "can *no longer* recognize family members." The scenario states he "does not **usually** recognize" his daughter. Hence the "IF" condition of his Living Will does not yet apply.

"Complete obstruction of his bowels" is a great concern of future *Comfort Care*. Since his tumor is currently operable, he should have the operation.

Although I agree with The Council's report that the man should have the operation, it is for a huge difference in reasoning: Based on statements in the patient's Living Will, the "no treatment option" *does not yet apply*. In contrast,

The Council's report presumes that it is **morally appropriate to override statements in Advance Directives even if they DO apply**. The Council subsequently generalizes this conclusion.

✎ *CONTINUE*

Proxy Directives are preferable to Living Wills since the ethical and legal duties of Proxies oblige them to consider current and future clinical and personal interests of the patient as they consult with treating physicians and others, in the context of knowing the patient's previously expressed wishes.

In most American States and some other countries, "a negative living will has been given legal status such that a physician is compelled to follow the will when the patient does not wish curative treatment unless there are sufficient grounds not to do so" [Van der Steen and others, 2000]. Despite problems in gaining wider acceptance and the loopholes of conscience clauses that permit physicians and institutions to transfer patients if acceding to their wishes is against their values, Living Wills have been legally and ethically sanctioned for a generation. Thus The Council was forced to present arguments to encourage its readers to disrespect Advance Directives. The Council's next argument is based on a single clinical anecdote from which they inappropriately generalize. Here, the points from which they extrapolate are called "Two Moments."

Two Outrageous Moments: Did the President's Council on Bioethics Report Use Faulty Logic to Justify NOT Honoring Advance Directives?

About advance care planning, The Council report's goal is to convince us that "No individual can foresee every future circumstance in his or her life; **an individual's best interests and true needs can change over time**; and medical situations are so complex that we can only judge wisely what to do case-by-case and in the moment."

In regard to responding to others' previously expressed wishes, The Council's report states: "Caregivers are obliged to take seriously the instructions [of Living Wills] as such. Seriously, but not slavishly. For past wishes, *as we have explored*, are not always morally decisive in such cases. They [past wishes] are a crucial point of consideration, but not the only, or even the most important one." {Emphasis added.} Just what have they explored? Answer: The semi-hypothetical case on which they base their arguments, discussed next.

Moment One:

"Do Not Honor a Demented Patient's Living Will."

One medical student paid regular visits to *one* patient who suffered from dementia. After several visits with "Margo," the medical student—now elevated to the status of "sage observer"—concluded: "Despite her illness, or maybe somehow because of it, Margo is undeniably one of the happiest people I have ever known." He provided this anecdotal evidence: "She was cheerful and pleased to see him but never knew his name. She enjoyed reading but 'her place in the book jumped randomly from day to day.' She enjoyed music, seemingly unaware that she was listening to the same song over and over. She enjoyed painting, but always painted the same simple pastel shapes day after day."

The President's Council on Bioethics then poses these additional hypothetical facts:

"Suppose Margo executed a Living Will when she was first diagnosed with Alzheimer's, asking that no treatment be given to her if she contracted another serious life-threatening illness. Now Margo contracts pneumonia, which could probably be ameliorated with antibiotic treatment. Should her Living Will be honored and the antibiotics withheld? Or does her present contentment make her continued life worthwhile and override her past misgivings about living with dementia?"

The President's Council on Bioethics judged it would be morally wrong to deny the patient the antibiotics and hydration **at this moment**, since such treatment would be mildly invasive and short-term and therefore a negligible burden, while its benefit would likely permit Margo to resume her contented living in the "here and now."

❧

What reason could any one have to disagree, as long as her life now seems happy? Actually, two groups of people would disagree with aggressive treatment, but their reasons are quite different from The Council's claim that it is not "morally right" for Margo, here and now. The first group is not sufficiently informed about end-of-life options. They DO know that the risk of getting Alzheimer's disease increases with age; that to reach an advanced age, they must be relatively healthy to avoid succumbing to serious illnesses; and that the next opportunity to refuse aggressive treatment for a potentially life-threatening illness might be many months or even years away—by which time, dementia may have progressed to the point that the last several years were spent in abject despondency and total dependency. What does this group of people NOT know? —

That they do need not to wait for the next potentially life-threatening illness if they can trust a caring advocate to **Refuse Food & Fluid** on their behalf at a point in their decline that they previously have clearly defined. (As mentioned above, this group includes the members of The Final Exit Network, among others.)

The second group of people does know that the option to **Refuse Food & Fluid by Proxy** exists, but they cannot identify individuals they trust to carry out this future wish. To quote The Council's report [*Page 88*]: "Trusting others requires the presence of others who are trustworthy—surrogates who are willing to care, able to make wise decisions, and willing to let go when the time comes to do so." The report goes on, however, to criticize **Proxy Directives** on the grounds that "they do not, in themselves, provide ethical guidance about what to do in the face of those dilemmas that devoted Proxies ultimately face." Agreed: This is the precise purpose of the **Empowering Statements for My Proxy** that this book recommends.

As presented, Margo's hypothetical Living Will illustrates a truth: some people do create poorly written Living Wills. In this case, Margo specified only the diagnosis, not how severe her decrease in functioning was required to trigger the "no treatment" option. But the problem is not, as The Council seems to argue, that Living Wills can not be relied upon as a guide to what a person would want. To make that generalization is to invoke the **false logic of extrapolation** from **one** (or some) to **all**. An old saw, amusingly told in a "Robert Ludlum" novel [2005], makes this point well:

✋*SKIP*

The Color of Scottish Cows

You know the old story about an economist, a physicist, and a mathematician driving through Scotland? They see a brown cow out of the window and the economist says, "Fascinating that the cows in Scotland are brown."

The physicist says, "I'm afraid you're over-generalizing from the evidence. All we know is that **some cows** in Scotland are brown."

Finally, the mathematician shakes his head at both of them. "Wrong again; completely unwarranted by the evidence. All we can infer logically is that there exists at least **one cow** in this country, at least **one side** of which is brown."

While no one can predict whether or not Margo will be happy and for how long, after receiving the diagnosis of dementia, Living Wills can take that contingency into consideration either by stating, "I want to continue to receive aggressive medical treatment as long as others consider my behavior as indicating I am happy," or, by describing the negative characteristics of behavior for which further aggressive medical treatment is not desired (as described below). Thus, The Council's report conclusion, that Living Wills "are not always morally decisive" [because] "No individual can foresee every future circumstance in his or her life," which The Council uses to justify setting aside all Living Wills, even those that are well written, is a false conclusion drawn from an inappropriate extrapolation. Similarly, The Council's caution would not apply to a Proxy's decision if the Proxy was well informed and attempted to make decisions according to the "Substituted Judgment" standard.

In a further attempt to justify this extrapolation, The Council's report generalizes their argument with a statement that appears to have been crafted so it would combine generalities with absolutes and thus becomes formally inarguable, regardless of the accuracy of the underlying facts. (These facts are considered, later.) Here is the statement, with emphasis added:

"Patients who complete Living Wills *sometimes* do so without *full* awareness of what life would be like in *all* the various circumstances that might arise."

The report continues with a paternalistic insult to those who do wish to accept the challenge to diligently create their Advance Directives: "**They do not and cannot know** in advance whether the experience of old age with dementia will still seem valuable to a future self, even though it is not the life they would freely choose. Can individuals really know in advance **that such a life would be worse than death**? And, more fundamentally, do **we possess a present right to discriminate** against the very life of a future self, or—even more problematic—**to order others** to do so on our behalf?" {Emphasis added.}

Comments: Of course, no one *really* knows about **death**. So individuals cannot really know that certain degrees of indignity, suffering, or dependency would be worse. Yet "more fundamentally," the consistent legal answer to The Council's question, according to the Patient Self-Determination Act, legislation in every State, and court rulings at every level of government, is a clear "**Yes**." Everyone has the right to create an Advance Directive where her Living Will or the authority she grants to her Proxy can refuse end-of-life treatment.

✒ *CONTINUE*

Note: The Council's report switches from "They" to "we" as it asks, "do **we** possess a present right to **discriminate**." Thus, the report refers to the process of **my** creating Advance Directives; where **I** exercise **my** liberty right to state **my** future wishes for **myself** and then judges some requests as **my immoral order** to others to discriminate against **me**! Again, The Council's report uses charged language: "to order others," when all we are doing is making the request that our Proxies, caregivers, and physicians honor our well-thought out requests. According to The Council, therefore, it could be **immoral** to follow the wishes as expressed in a person's Living Will or learned from discussions with a Proxy, as well as **immoral** to create our Living Will.

I find this position alarming. It is beyond the paternalism of doctors a generation or more ago. Then, paternalism took this form: "Doctors know what is best for patients; therefore they should make their life-or-death decisions." But The Council's moral paternalism goes even further: All decision-makers, including doctors, caregivers, loved ones and designated Proxies, must err on the side of life by following The Council's definition of "Prudence": the "just right" course of action, practical wisdom [*Page 233*] by replacing the "Best Interest" standard of decision-making with their interpretation of what is "Best Care," and that "standard" prioritizes whatever life remains for the patient, no matter how diminished. (**Note**: While this seems to be the moral view of the report, it may not represent the wider range of views held by individual Council members.)

Consider further, the serious implications of the report's semantics by asking: why would The Council's report use the word "***discriminate***"? The reason could be related to the National Right to Life Committee's proposed model State law, which the Committee promoted [May, 2005] after its disappointment with Federal judges who refused to respond to the request of Terri Schiavo's parents, in their attempt to maintain her PVS existence. The "**Model Starvation and Dehydration of Persons with Disabilities Prevention Act**" offers a boilerplate legislation document for States to adopt, which would require all patients to continue artificial nutrition and hydration unless the patient had previously **WRITTEN** *clear and convincing* instructions to the contrary. This model law defines every term it uses—except one: "Persons with Disabilities." Why would the proposed law fail to define the very people it is designed "to help"? Two possibilities are: 1) So that the model law can apply to as many (undefined) people as possible. 2) To invoke sympathy by relating to a class of people who are subject to discrimination.

✑ SKIP

Yet using the term "disabled" to refer to patients with severe brain disease is a gross understatement. It is similar to using the term "being under the weather" to refer to patients with advanced metatstatic terminal cancer. As Lennard Davis wrote, "The aim of making it possible for disabled people to live full lives with their impairments and of ensuring a free and accessible society has little to do with someone who will be dead in six months" [2006]. I would argue similarly: the concept of disability has little to do with someone who is unconscious or severely demented. The Social Security Administration defines disabled people as those who cannot do the work they did before and cannot adjust to other work, for at least one year. The United Nations defines disability as "any restriction or lack of ability to perform an activity in the manner or within the range considered normal for a human being." (Contrast the words "an activity" to "totally unable to respond to the environment," which applies to PVS patients.) Consider the definition established by the American Disabilities Act [1990]: "a physical or mental impairment that **substantially limits one or more of the major life activities**." The U.S. Supreme Court, in Toyota Motor Mfg. Ky. v. Williams, No. 00-1089 [2002] used this definition: a permanent or long-term impairment that prevents or restricts the individual from doing activities that are of "**central importance to most people's daily lives**." Long-term care insurance policies provide benefits if patients need **substantial assistance** with two "Activities of Daily Living," often called **ADL**s: bathing, continence, dressing, eating, toileting, transferring; OR who have lost **some intellectual ability**, which is defined as impaired memory, orientation, judgment as it relates to safety awareness, or deductive or abstract reasoning. The appropriate term for patients in an advanced stage of dementia is NOT "disabled" but "**totally incapacitated**."

Using the words "discrimination" and "disability" together may be designed to create a **mindset for acceptance** for people to overlook the absence of convincing logic and lack of substantiated relevant facts, including the preferences of the overwhelming majority of "reasonable people." Semantics is important and will be discussed in more detail later, in terms of "framing the debate."

Let's consider the facts. The Council's report contends that WE, like the hypothetical "Margo," cannot anticipate any times of pleasure after we receive the diagnosis of dementia because we have not (yet) personally experienced dementia. —Absolutely not true. We have many ways of informing ourselves: we can visit and follow the course of several patients with dementia (for example, our older relatives or the relatives of our friends). We can learn much about the pain and pleasures of their lives—from books, from movies, and from Oprah's interviewing their children on TV. We can read personal accounts of patients who, in brief moments of lucidity, expressed what it was like to suffer from mild to moderate dementia. We can appreciate the reports of psychologists and psychiatrists and other professionals on this devastating illness, as summarized in newspapers, on TV, and in magazines.

Readers of The Council's negative and paternalistic proclamation that we "do not and cannot know" have the right to feel insulted. In our enlightened society, many people actively seek knowledge. The subject of Alzheimer's disease has over 1700 entries on www.Amazon.com, and over 47,000 entries on PubMed (the Internet's free access to the National Library of Medicine). We need not be a bioethicist or a neurologist to learn that at **one moment** in time along their downward trajectory, patients who suffer from brain damage that prevents them from meaningful and responsive speech can still sing the words of songs... and smile with pleasure as they sing. There is much that we **can** therefore know in advance, and such knowledge can form the basis for our exercising a most important Liberty interest guaranteed by the Constitution—to decide what will happen to our bodies, and to make those decisions in the protected privacy of our relationship with our doctor and our Proxy.

Note: By writing this report, The Council obviously assumes its content will enlighten us, that we can learn what we do not already know. Yet this action contradicts their own presumptions that we cannot learn what we need to know.

℘ CONTINUE

More pragmatically, instead of inappropriately extrapolating from **one moment in time**—when Margo was happy—to conclude that previously written Living Wills should not be taken as the primary source for what patients want in the future, The Council could have served its readers better by recommending simply that Living Wills should specify that the stage of dementia must be "severe" to trigger the "no aggressive treatment" options. The study of Singer and others [1995] documented this not surprising but important result: as dementia (or brain function) became more severe, fewer people would want to continue dialysis. Here are the numbers: for mild dementia, **78**%; for moderate, **51**%; for severe, **14**%; and for comatose patients, **10**%. Since categories could possibly be the subject of conflict, this book recommends specific behavioral descriptions instead of categories, to guide your Proxy (or to specify in your Living Will):

Although The Council's logic and facts fail to provide a convincing argument about **one (happy) moment** in the life a hypothetical dementia patient, the report nevertheless expands its recommendation to prolong treatment to other patients by posing this rhetorical question: "Does a person's claim on us for treatment, even if she has a living will requesting that treatment be forgone, depend entirely or primarily on the person's experiential well-being?" Few would argue with the stated value, that happiness is an absolute requirement to remain alive. Hence this argument provides leverage for The Council's report to urge caregivers to consider the **meaning of their role** and **ask** more generally, "Who is this person with dementia now before us, and **what do we owe her** even or especially when her life seems so diminished?" {Emphasis added.}

What does The Council's report fail to consider? Caregivers owe the patient respect by honoring her previously expressed wishes (in her Living Will or in discussions with her Proxy). The Council's report fails to acknowledge this; instead it proclaims that it is the responsibility of caregivers to act as **moral agents** who "cannot simply do what they were told but must also try to do what is **best**," who cannot give those previously expressed "wishes trumping power [if they] force caregivers to forgo doing what is **best** for the person who is now entrusted to their care" [*Page 84*].

To summarize: Yes, it would be inappropriate to deny this one patient, "Margo," treatment at this **one happy moment**. But The Council uses faulty logic to extrapolate a general conclusion so they can recommend putting aside *any* previously expressed set of wishes in *any* Living Will at *any* time, or what was learned in *any* discussions with *any* Proxy. Again, the crucial question is: "Who determines what is *BEST* for you—your previously written documents and the informative discussions with your entrusted Proxy, or the morality espoused by The President's Council on Bioethics in terms of what their report states is morally best?"

Moment Two:

"Do Not Create Advance Directives That Would Discriminate Against Your Future Disabled Self."

To cast doubt on the process of creating Advance Directives, The Council presents this second argument:

"One way to think of Margo as still the same person [meaning the person she was prior to becoming demented] is to focus on the rational will—on the person as one who [by definition] deliberates and chooses. If Margo is the same person she was, and if twenty years ago she chose to enact certain directives about her future care, then one might argue that those directives should now be honored, even if they no longer seem to further the care she most needs. Yet this way of picturing her as the same person over time seems, actually, **to ignore the significance of time**. Instead, it **focuses on a single moment** in Margo's existence—**the moment her living will was enacted**—and gives it governance over all future moments. As her capacity to choose diminishes, she can no longer change her instructions; she is **stuck forever in that timeless point** that is her earlier choice." {The words in brackets were added for clarity. The bold font was added for emphasis.}

❦

Again, The Council's report makes the logical mistake of extrapolating from one instance to all, and adds the dimension of all TIME to all PEOPLE. But it is NOT true that all people make their end-of-life decisions in **a single moment**.

❧ *SKIP*

Before elaborating on this point, note that the clinical example given in The Council's report should have actually begun with a more explicit statement of the hypothetical conditions. Actually, there are two different premises, and both are considered below:

A. "Suppose Margo executed a Living Will when she was **first diagnosed with Alzheimer's**..." [This is consistent with The Council's *prior* hypothetical conditions.]

B. "...if **twenty years ago** she chose to enact certain directives about her future care..." [This reflects The Council's *new* hypothetical conditions.]

First consider hypothesis (A): The Council report is correct in assuming "when she was first diagnosed with Alzheimer's..." that she could still possess decision-making capacity. Her then mild deficit in short-term memory might not prevent her from holding in her mind, the relevant concepts long enough to process them with understanding, appreciation and reasoning so she could arrive at and express a consistent choice. As always, the possession of decision-making capacity depends on the difficulty of the task. It is intellectually demanding to make several treatment decisions about several disease states, which task is required to complete a detailed Living Will. Asking someone in the early stages of Alzheimer's disease to complete this task would be clinically inappropriate. Yet at the same time, it would be quite appropriate to ask Margo to name which close relative or friend she trusts to be her first choice Proxy, and who else she wants to name as alternates. Then, if a few years later, Margo contracted pneumonia but was still happy, her Proxy could, on her behalf, accept treatment for her pneumonia. This hypothetical scenario leads to the conclusion that advance care planning, even when initiated late (after a disease process began to affect her mind), can still be effective in achieving its goals.

With respect to hypothesis (B), The Council's report is making two unkind assumptions. The first is that 20 years ago (six years before the Patient Self-Determination Act!), Margo did not think much about advance care planning before she signed her Advance Directive. The second is that she subsequently never reviewed, let alone revised this document.

Granted, some people do complete "15-minute quickies" downloaded from the Internet or received in the mail. Other patients are handed forms by a clerk as they are admitted to institutions, to comply with protocol to receive Medicare funding. —Certainly not the best time or circumstance to make diligent end-of-life treatment decisions. Some estate attorneys ask their clients to sign forms with little discussion, when the main focus of their work is directed to paying less tax as they distribute their financial assets. The important point is this: Although *some* people will sign Advance Directives with inadequate prior thought, *many* others will diligently consider the execution of such instruments at length **before** they sign, and will also diligently reconsider these documents periodically **after** they sign the first of several drafts, replacing each with an updated revision. The negative and paternalistic tone of The President's Council on Bioethics must again be countered by noting that there are many books, many articles, and many advisors in several disciplines (including law, medicine, religion, and social work) who advise people whose intent is to create an effective document that will be **durable**. So again, extrapolation from one hypothetical patient's single moment in time—to all or even many other patients—is using false logic.

✧ CONTINUE

Moreover, any argument that encourages others to ignore people's previously expressed wishes flies in the face of their precise motivation to create Advance Directives. The reason they created these documents is specifically because they wanted them to be **durable**; that is, the effect of the document will continue even after the person who created it is no longer competent.

The last story in **The *BEST WAY* to Say Goodbye** (prior to the Epilogue) is an idealized illustration of how "Joyce," from the age of 16 to 86, continued to refine her wishes and the means of directing her end-of-life decisions. This story exemplifies how many of the tools and guidelines in this book can be incorporated into one's planning. In this example, Joyce revised her Advance Directives every five to ten years—in contrast to being "stuck forever in [one] timeless point."

So the truth is, instead of a "**single moment** in Margo's [or another patient's] existence—**the moment her living will was enacted**," many people will diligently consider the usual course of the disease of dementia, will consult with legal and medical advisors, and after sufficient reflection, will decide at what point in the downward trajectory of their disease—as described in observable behaviors or recognized stage—they would want to refuse potentially life-sustaining treatment (or invoke **Refusal of Food & Fluid by Proxy**). Many people will then continue to reflect about the decisions they made in their (initial) Advance Directive document, and will revise that document as their circumstances change (e.g., receive a diagnosis) and as they accumulate further knowledge. At some point in time, they may decide they have written the best document they can, and have appointed the best choice of available Proxies. Then they can allow the document to stand as the durable statement of their wishes. So, far from being **a single moment**, the signing of an Advance Directive can be just one point along a rather lengthy and diligent process that could have been preceded by months of prior learning and discussions, and may be succeeded by years of further consideration and revisions.

7. Why The Council's report is so dangerous.

The Council's report represents a significant challenge, one that could destroy people's trust that their Last Wishes, no matter how well considered and clearly expressed in their Advance Directives, will NOT be honored. Current lack of trust could discourage people from creating any Advance Directives and reverse the recent trend of increasing interest that resulted from heightened awareness from the publicized tragedy of Terri Schiavo. Previous surges in public interest, from the sagas of Karen Ann Quinlan, Nancy Beth Cruzan, Robert Wendland, and others, did not succeed in sustaining an increased proportion of people who created Advance Directives. Yet the need for such documents, in light of America's current political and religious polarity, is more important than ever.

Councilmember Janet D. Rowley, M.D., D.Sc., is the Blum-Riese Distinguished Service Professor of Medicine at the University of Chicago. She received the most distinguished American honor, the Albert Lasker Clinical Medicine Research Prize. When I talked to her, she revealed that she and a few other Council Members had fought hard for the right to choose end-of-life options by advance care planning. Despite such efforts however, their lack of success can be gauged by Dr. Rowley's statement that appears in the Appendix of The Council's report:

"The report emphasizes repeatedly that the caregiver's primary responsibility is to the patient 'here and now,' and that Advance Directives can and should be ignored depending on the situation at the time. The clear message from this report is, if you feel strongly about not living in a decerebrate state [where the part of your brain that permits memory, thinking, and reasoning no longer functions], *you better kill yourself* while you have control over your fate!" {Emphasis added.}

Suicide is dangerous and possibly made more likely by The Council's report because it undermines people's faith in a recognized legal mechanism designed to protect the dignity of end-of-life choices.

Readers may recall the tragic scenarios of Janet Adkins, Judge Robert Hammerman, and Bob Stern that this book previously related. The story of Myrna Lebov's premature dying appears in the Epilogue. These few cases exemplify how many thousands of patients may feel. Most will not end their lives prematurely when they still have the mental capacity to carry out the act of suicide, but the quality of the time that remains in their lives will be tarnished by anxiety. They will worry about how long they will be forced to endure a prolonged dying associated with unbearable suffering, or indignity and dependence. They may feel conflicted about draining of the financial resources and stressing the emotions of their families and caregivers. All these burdens will add to the challenge of being terminally ill. For those who do decide to end their lives by premature dying, their loved ones will be deprived of continued enjoyment, sharing, and companionship.

Lack of advance care planning can lead to court battles among family members and to excessive draining of society's medical, financial and caregiving resources.

The Council's report insists that Proxies, caregivers, and healthcare providers follow *their* moral guidelines rather than honor the *patients' expressed wishes*. It expresses its moral premise and guidelines using many admonitions and uses the word "never" 96 times. Statements in the report could be quoted by those whose goal is to prevent others from exercising the option of **Refusal of Food & Fluid by Proxy**, such as *Page X*: "Caring wholeheartedly for a frail patient or a disabled loved one is incompatible with thinking that engineering their death is an acceptable 'therapeutic option.'" I aks, What about how the *patient defined care*?

Patients must become better informed to feel confident that they have created strategic documents that will overcome such challenges, and that they can trust the individuals they selected to serve as their Proxies will make sure that others will honor their Last Wishes. Feelings of confidence can permit patients to enjoy whatever time remains in their lives to the fullest, without worry, fear, guilt, or anxiety. Additional broader effort will still be required to permit society to make more reasonable allocations of scarce medical and financial resources, however.

The Council's harsh recommendations could create dangerous emotional burdens for Proxies, many of whom are already depressed. By *commanding* Proxies to reflect "prudently" and *requiring* them to determine the morality of the patient's wishes, The Council's report could result in Proxies feeling guilt whether or not they remain faithful to their previous promises to follow the patient's end-of-life wishes. One goal of advance care planning is to relieve all concerned of the burden of making decisions based on their own values. Ideally, life-or-death decisions can be based on knowing the patient's values and wishes. Called the "Substituted Judgment" method, the goal is to strive to make the decision that the patient would have made while trying (as much as possible) NOT to impose their own values, preferences, and moral standards. The President's Council insistence on overriding a patient's values and wishes when they are both clearly known and applicable is more than alarming; it violates current legal and clinical practice.

The Council's recommendations also have significant potential to increase the guilt of other survivors. Its report explicitly and repeatedly admonishes caregivers who decide to abandon their vulnerable and needy relatives by hastening their dying, especially if their motivation is relief from extreme burdens of caregiving. From a psychological perspective, however, this admonition is simplistic. The challenging decision to refuse treatment has many dimensions whose underlying motivations are always complex. Caregivers in the "sandwich generation" may generously wish to distribute time, energy, and money to other members of the family who also need attention. The wish for relief from the extreme personal burdens of caring may exist at a subconscious or conscious level even though it accounts for only a small fraction of the whole motivation. The Council's report thus lacks compassion for caregivers who, like other loved ones, almost always ask themselves after someone dies: "Was there anything more I *should* have done, or *could* have done?" The sting of The Council's repetitive suggestions of a selfish motive may long plague the psyche of survivors by adding guilt to their grief.

At a profound level, The Council's recommendation not to honor an individual's written Last Wishes, or clearly expressed values and wishes via a duly authorized Proxy, when the patient's explicit goal was for such wishes to be honored if the ability to make decisions were lost, amounts to the loss of Liberty interest guaranteed as by the 14th Amendment of the U.S. Constitution.

Danger: The Demise of Social Security, Medicare & Medicaid

The most widespread consequence that could result from adopting The Council's recommendations is an increase in poverty due to the enormous burden of the cost of long-term care and medical treatment. The Council's report acknowledged that 20% of State budgets already go to Medicaid; that Alzheimer's cases will increase three-fold; and that caregivers of all types will become more scarce (so the cost of caregiving will increase). The future financial disaster could lead to the bankruptcy of Medicare and Medicaid, which in turn, could result in widespread abandonment of the most needy. If these social programs are destined to be destroyed (as some predict), then adopting The Council's recommendations would hasten their demise. This outcome is particularly disappointing when efforts to delay or prevent their demise would have been consistent with the ethical principle of social justice, which speaks to the fairness of distributing resources—a moral value that The Council's report hardly considered.

SKIP

Consider two statements from The Council's report: "The pursuit of justice begins by trying to see clearly what we owe one another, including what we owe vulnerable members at the end of their lives" [*Page 100*] and "Those nations with greater wealth might owe their citizens more public assistance and support" [*Page 198*].

The first statement sounds honorable, but the second seems antithetical to Lincoln's address at Gettysburg, as if government was not "**of** the people" but only "**for**"—as if government were doing poor people a favor by providing them with benefits. According to the sources that Jim Wallis used for his book, *God's Politics*, our nation—although the richest in history—still leaves one of six American children and one of three American children of color living below the poverty line [2005, *Page 47-48*].

Few people realize that Medicare does NOT pay for long-term care and that for middle-class Americans, Medicaid is NOT insurance. To qualify for Medicaid funding of long-term care as a last resort, middle-class people must "spend down" by losing their life-savings. Yet Medicaid "benefits" are ultimately transformed into a loan; they use your home as collateral. The Medicaid Recovery Act permits the government to take your home to offset the amount they spent on your care, after your surviving spouse dies or your home is sold.

The law about distributing assets prior to spending down for medical care—for example, to your children—was tough, recently got tougher, and may get worse.

At the end of 2005, the Budget Reconciliation Bill (HR 4241/ S 1932) was passed in the Senate when Vice President Cheney vote broke the tie. The bill's terms could be an indication of what direction "our" government will head in.

The Alzheimer's Association summarized its disappointment about this bill's three provisions: "One increases the number of years that a person's finances are subjected to government audit. A second would penalize elderly Medicaid applicants after they've already depleted their resources and are in need of costly care. And, the third denies Medicaid assistance to anyone who happens to own a house that has increased in value beyond an arbitrary amount set by the government." [Alzheimer's media releases, 2005.]

The Wall Street Journal [Lueck, 2005] noted that the new law makes contributions to charity or helping a grandchild pay for college more suspect if the person later attempts, in the following five years, to qualify for Medicaid nursing-home care. The Journal quoted Charles Sabatino, chair of the National Academy of Elder Law Attorneys' public-policy committee, which opposed the changes: "For every case of abuse it is preventing, it's going to hurt ten other sick and frail seniors."

Philip P. Lindsley, a Certified Elder Law Attorney in San Diego, stated in [2005], "The new proposed look back period is so long that it will catch many unaware. The proposed Reconciliation Bill also allows for aggregation of gifts to calculate the penalty. Here is an example: Grandmother gives each of her four grandchildren a gift of $11,000 for college, the sum recommended by her financial advisor as being consistent with the annual gift tax exemption. Her grandchildren are of different ages, so each gift is made in a different year. Four years and ten months after the first gift, Grandma has a stroke. After she runs through her one hundred days of coverage under Medicare, she would face a penalty period about 9 months, beginning when Medicare insurance runs out. This penalty runs regardless of whether or not she had any private resources, which in her case are too little to pay for these 9 months. So the result is that she could be evicted with no alternative care in place. Hardship exemptions, while theoretically possible, are almost never granted."

Attorney Lindsley continued, "In terms of planning, would Grandma ever have contemplated this result when she gave to her grandchildren? Not likely. That's one tragedy. Another is this: If grandparents or elder parents *are* informed about these consequences, they would be less likely to ever help their children get a college education. In middle class size estates, I often advise against such assistance. Similarly, if the estate tax is significantly reduced or eliminated, the greatest incentive to contribute to charities will be lost, in service to the wealthiest

Americans keeping their wealth in their estates for use by their own families."

The Alzheimer's Association noted, "These changes may put nursing homes in the position of kicking out residents who are declared ineligible after they have been admitted. It also may prevent people from getting into nursing care facilities in the first place or from receiving necessary care at home and in the community." The great magnitude of this tragedy is that for these people, Medicaid-funded nursing homes are their last resort.

How bad could it get? The New York Times quoted Lawrence E. Davidow of Suffolk County, N.Y., president of the National Academy of Elder Law Attorneys, as saying, "I'm horrified and surprised that Congress would turn its back on middle-class senior citizens who look to Medicaid as a safety net to pay for long-term care," and "it's more likely that people who need long-term care will lose their homes and everything they have worked a lifetime to acquire, because they'll have to use their assets to pay for nursing home care" [Pear, 2005].

These issues are profound, complex, and will intensify. Attorney Marshall Kapp concluded that neither estate attorneys' Medicaid planning nor the government's attempts at recovery were ethically palatable [2006].

✂ *CONTINUE*

Yesterday's Soup?

After going days with little to eat, a homeless person asked an affluent woman to let him clean up her yard. After he finished, he asked, "I haven't had a decent meal in days. Do you have anything you could give me to eat?"

"Sure, but may I ask, do you like green pea soup with ham?"

"That would be wonderful," he replied.

"Even yesterday's leftovers?" she asked, to clarify.

"I'm not picky," he answered. "That sounds wonderful."

"Good!" she said. "Then come back tomorrow!"

In anticipation of the future economic crisis from the Alzheimer's epidemic, some countries require employees of companies or tax payers to purchase long-term care insurance. In the United States, individuals must find their own motivation to allocate a portion of their income for that purpose. A survey by the Charlton Research Company [2005] revealed that by a factor of two, people's most common fear is diminished mental capacity, not diminished physical ability (62% compared to 29%). Another survey question asked, "Have you made plans for the possibility of your getting Alzheimer's disease?" almost 9 out of 10 said, "No." So the most feared disease of losing one's mind is one that people rarely plan for.

Of great concern: Private long-term care insurance companies may have over-sold their capacity to fulfill their promise. Duhigg wrote [3-27-2007]: "Interviews by The New York Times and confidential depositions indicate that some long-term-care insurers have developed procedures that make it difficult—if not impossible—for policyholders to get paid.... In California alone, nearly one in every four long-term-care claims was denied in 2005, according to the state." The article mentioned Conseco, Banker's Life, Penn Treaty America, and John Hancock. It detailed how claims representatives intentionally sent wrong forms to wrong addresses and were not permitted to telephone to rectify "mistakes" so the company could deny paying claims to deserving patients for based on improper or delayed submission of "required paperwork." A second article [5-25-07] noted that Rep. John Dingell (Michigan), who chairs the Committee on Energy and Commerce, was demanding documents to begin an investigation into these "questionable practices" and wanted to know if other companies engaged in them.

If poor people remain poor as the middle class becomes poor by following the recommendations of The President's Council, that it is "morally correct" to spend all their assets on caring for those who are severely cognitively impaired instead of educating their promising young, what will be the result? The end of the middle class. When their lives have ended, they will have no assets to pass on to their children for whom funds for education were not provided. As the middle class disappears, so will the very fabric of what has made our democratic society great.

Combine the war on terrorism (or Iraq) with the war against "abandoning" our severely cognitively impaired dependent people, and we will eventually lose the quality of life as we now know it. In that scenario, Dr. McCue's use of the word "heroic" a decade ago may be too narrow for tomorrow's challenge. To quote him again: "Dying bravely is heroic, and a heroic death may be the most intense memory that we can pass to posterity" [1995]. Considering the economic challenges from Alzheimer's disease and other dementias, and the ways our political leaders are (not) planning on meeting them, a heroic death may be far more than an "intense memory." Yet individual choices to die heroic deaths—by forgoing the last years of life if cognitive impairment is severe—may not suffice to preserve our democratic society and its functional middle class. As a society, we may have to change our laws to presume (in the absence of Advance Directives), that people who have irreversibly lost their personhood and cannot appreciate the sacrifices being made for them, would want to choose "Permit Natural Dying."

Right now, we seem to have a choice. But when the incidence of dementia increases three-fold to 16 million by 2050 while the relative and absolute numbers of potential caregivers decrease, our economic and manpower resources will become overwhelmed. What we will do then? One fictional option was suggested in Christopher Buckley's "Boomsday." He noted that Social Security began when the ratio of working to retired people was 15 to 1. Now there are only 3 workers to 1 retired person. The result is that working people will find that most of their earnings from hard work will be diverted to support the older generation's retirement. So how can society solve this irresponsible Ponzi scheme? The hero in "Boomsday" suggests *Voluntary Transitioning*: in exchange for significant tax benefits they suggest that about 20% of 70-year-olds commit *mass suicide*. Although outrageous, this political satire's solution is grossly inadequate because the book underestimates the potential crisis, in part because it does not consider the effect of the Alzheimer's epidemic and escalation of other healthcare costs.

So the worst danger of The Council's report is that it espouses the *noble* quality of **equality** for all but urges a plan that will lead to greater **inequality**, speed up the demise of Social Security, Medicare, and Medicaid, and divert us from seeking solutions to one of the most challenging problems our society has ever had to face.

8. What motivated the Council to formulate these recommendations?

One need not be a psychiatrist to understand how difficult it is to let go of a relative whom you have dearly loved, as they suffer from severe dementia. The face and the body of this person, who perhaps gave you life, still seem here. David Brooks wrote in the New York Times, "As [Dr. Leon] Kass put it the other day, 'The much diminished mother I hugged on the day of her death was the same woman I'd been hugging all my life.'" This strong emotional sentiment is emphasized in The President's Council on Bioethics' report; for example, "Those who embraced or held her hand years ago and who do so again today are sure that they are embracing Margo"... and "This is true even (as in the case of dementia) when [her] reason and will [that is, her autonomy] have been compromised by disease." The Council's recommendation to extend existence is based on their stated premise: "It is this continuing **bodily presence** that is **fundamental to being human** and **that is the locus of all personal presence**." Belief in this premise is not universal, however. I favor the opposite premise, as stated concisely by Ronald B. Miller [2005]: "An intact mind is fundamental to personhood."

According to The Council, except when death is imminent, or when the treatment itself would present an extreme additional burden to the patient, caregivers must ask what they owe the human being in terms of what life remains, even though her life is so diminished. This act, The Council claims, is consistent with **basic family values** although they offer no proof since their argument is circular. Still, they generalize and glorify these values: "A society that sets its face against abandoning those whose lives are in decline has a better chance of being a society that thinks creatively about the trajectory of life and the bonds between the generations, of remaining a society in which **to live long** is also **to live well together**." {Emphasis added, since these phrases are discussed next.}

So The Council wants its readers to view its report as a virtuous expression of "family values." The Council's report fully recognizes the awesome economic and emotional burdens, which it describes with exquisite sensitivity. But then it asks us, as caregivers and as Proxies, to follow The Council's moral recommendations; to exercise restraint by not requesting our future caregivers and Proxies to perform in ways that are immoral by discriminating against our future disabled selves as we create our Advance Directives; and to provide "Best Care," instead of honoring the patient's previously expressed wishes. Sadly, The President's Council offers no solution to their addition to the enormous future challenges to our medical, economic, personnel, caregiver, and emotional resources.

It is easy to dispute The Council's stated ideal, "to live well together." Most patients with dementia must be institutionalized within three to five years after diagnosis, when their behavior becomes destructive and unmanageable. To "**live long**" costs approximately $100,000 per year—a sum that most Americans cannot afford. An increasing large percentage of Americans will therefore be required to pay a "**pre-death tax**"; that is, to spend down most of their assets to qualify for Medicaid (in California, MediCal) so that they or their loved ones can become eligible to be warehoused in what most people would consider to be low quality nursing homes for the demented.

With respect to advising caregivers to set aside a person's previously expressed end-of-life wishes, this quote of Povenmire [1998-1999] seems apt: "There is no interest so vital and personal to the individual as that of controlling one's own body. This interest is a fundamental precept of the common law and an essential element of the right to privacy protected under the United States Constitution."

The Council's report states as if it were universal truth: "Caring wholeheartedly for a frail patient or a disabled loved one is **incompatible with thinking that engineering their death is an acceptable** 'therapeutic option.'" Yet Michael Panicola, manager of ethics for SSM Health Care in Saint Louis, Missouri, summarized relevant Catholic ethics of 500 years when he wrote [2001], "Human life is a limited good subordinated to higher, more important spiritual goods (love of God and love of neighbor)," and "When medical treatment offers no reasonable hope of benefit in terms of helping one pursue the spiritual goods of life" such a decision is "not morally equivalent to killing oneself; it is a courageous choice by one to recognize higher, more important goods than the good of human life."

The President's Council on Bioethics report might merely have chosen to prioritize the virtues of caregiving and preservation of life over the explicit teachings of even a conservative religion, and over other interpretations of our Constitutional rights. However it is possible to view The Council's report as a strategic "slippery slope" initiative similar to other tactics that George Lakoff described in *Don't Think of an Elephant: Know Your Values and Frame the Debate* [2004], as furthering the need to retain the two-tier system that "the present American Economy *requires*," as explained further in *Moral Politics: How Liberals and Conservatives Think* [2002].

Before I elaborate on this less flattering way to view The Council's motivation, let me distinguish between the sincerity of the ethical positions taken by the individual members of The Council—which I do not doubt—and a possible agenda of politicians that may have influenced the selection of potential Council based on their known beliefs. I offer the following hypothesis only to be provocative, recognizing that politics is *not* my field of expertise.

✎ SKIP

Dr. Lakoff [2004] presented several examples; one is summarized here: An "education bill about school testing" was presumably invoked to improve the quality of education, but it could also have the opposite result. Testing schools can make it possible for the schools to be "punished for failing by having their allowance cut. Less funding in turn makes it harder for the schools to improve, which leads to a cycle of failure and ultimately elimination of many public schools. What replaces the public school system is a voucher system to support private schools [so] the wealthy would have good schools—paid for in part by what used to be tax payments for public schools."

Dr. Lakoff interprets the conservative position as based on the following belief [2004, *Page 32*]: "It is immoral to give people things they have not earned, because then they will not develop discipline and will become both dependent and immoral." For this reason, conservatives "are against nurturance and care... against social programs that take care of people" [*Page 8-9*]. This philosophy might also apply to Medicare. On May 1, 2006, the Trustees of the Medicare Program announced, "the health insurance system for the elderly will run out of money in 2018—two years sooner than predicted a year ago and 12 years sooner than had been anticipated when President Bush first took office." One of the trustees, Treasury Secretary John W. Snow, was quoted as saying that the programs "form the basis of a looming fiscal crisis for our nation as the baby-boom generation moves into retirement." [Goldstein, 2006]

If the *real goal* of testing schools is to eventually establish a two-tier system, "a good one for the 'deserving rich' and a bad one for the 'undeserving poor,'" [*Page 32*], then the presentation was **deceptive**. Lakoff suggests we consider if a similar is being applied to Medicare.

George Lakoff's perspective could provide a view of the moral/ethical guidelines that The President's Council on Bioethics proposed as conforming to the strategic "slippery slope" initiative. The Council's report directly appeals to positive aspects of identity and family values to influence current change while it omits serious consideration of the long-term consequences. Could the ultimate goal of the President's Council on Bioethics report be to destroy the "immoral" social programs of Medicare and Medicaid? If so, then implementing The Council's guidelines would lead to worse care of the vulnerable and needy—for all except the rich. The wealthy could use the money they saved in taxes from no longer having to fund Medicare and Medicaid, as well as from eliminating the death tax (estate tax), so they can more easily afford to hire private duty nurses on a 24/7 basis. This would be consistent with The Council's report stating [*Page 198*]: "Those with unlimited resources might owe their loved ones more in terms of medical care; those nations with greater wealth might owe their citizens more public assistance and support." What Lakoff wrote about the conservative stance would then apply: "Care for the aged and infirm are matters of individual responsibility. They are not the responsibility of taxpayers." [2004, *Page 84*]

To the extent that George Lakoff's style of skepticism is valid, we should ask more questions: Would conservatives encourage longer care of those who cannot appreciate such care, knowing that eventually, the result would be much less help from governmental programs to provide care for the poor elderly? If so, then like the plan to rate schools, if such a deception were consciously designed, would Lakoff and those who agree with his point of view characterize such behavior by the term "***betrayal***"?

❧ *CONTINUE*

Such a questions, while of paramount importance, will be left unanswered as it is speculative and beyond the scope of this book. Yet Lakoff urges us "to frame the debate" in positive terms. Warning that **the majority of people will support policies that are rationally NOT in their best interest**, he urges that we create competing positive frames designed to resonate with people's identity and values; in this case, to support the creation and implementation of Advance Directives. But before we create new arguments, let's analyze the power of The Council's stated position as it relates to identity and values.

The Council's values-based arguments

- I want to see myself and I want others to judge me as a devoted and selfless caregiver who respects the value and dignity of all human lives.

- My moral character respects the dignity of all human life, so I would never engineer ending the life of a person who loved me and to whom I owe so much.

- As a caring person, I would never abandon a vulnerable human being who needs my help just because I desperately needed relief from my role as caregiver, even if the role of caregiver became an extreme emotional and financial burden.

While applying such statements can ultimately lead to dangerous and destructive consequences, they resonate deeply with people's identity and values. This is thus an example of why the majority of people support policies that are rationally NOT in their best interest. Dr. Lakoff warns us to not believe the myths, "The truth will set us free," and, "If we just tell people the facts, since people are basically rational beings, they will all reach the right conclusions." To influence people's behavior, Lakoff insists on embracing the power of relating to people's identity and values. We cannot limit our argument to a logical explanation of why the opposing view is wrong and it expect it will suffice.

Consider this example of *not* following Lakoff's advice and imagine its impact:

Two logical, but not necessarily effective presentations of *true facts*

Doctors Casarett, Kapo, and Caplan [2005] argue that "it is illogical to require a higher level of evidence to withhold or withdraw Artificial Nutrition and Hydration (ANH) than would be required for other medical treatments or procedures that offer a similar risk-benefit balance." They offer this reason: it is "illogical [is] because it would impose certain restraints on liberty—the imposition of ANH without consent;" and furthermore, it is "not realistic" since it would "make it harder for surrogates to make decisions that reflect a patient's goals and preferences." The authors then propose five logical recommendations: 1) Pay physicians for the extra time it takes to discuss decisions about ANH; 2) stop reimbursing nursing homes at a higher rate for residents whom they administer ANH and stop citing them when their patients lose weight; 3) change state laws so surrogates are permitted to make these decisions; 4) encourage the creation of Advance Directives and permit a hierarchy of relatives or close friends to avoid conflict; and 5) use the POLST or a similar form to prevent changing the patient's preferences for treatment when moving to another facility or a hospital.

Will this well-reasoned and logical argument effectively overcome arguments proposed by The President's Council that relate strongly to identity and values?

Example two: my own oversight. I should have known better since I taught the psychotherapeutic technique of reframing to psychiatric residents. Yet I also forgot its importance as I impressed myself with these *true facts*:

- Here is how the law defines your duty as a designated Proxy: follow her wishes as previously revealed in discussions about end-of-life values and treatment preferences, and/or written in her Empowering Statements to My Proxy.

- This is your role as a **Living Will Advocate**: facilitate her written wishes.

- This is your role as physician: honor her Last Wishes.

- For patients whose end-of-life values and treatment preferences are not known, we must consider her *Best Interest* and ask: "Is there any compelling reason to believe she is not among the vast majority of 'reasonable people' who do NOT want to maintain their bodies in the state of severe dementia (or PVS)?"

9. How can we *reframe* our arguments and emphasize *positive values*?

How can we explain the virtues of serving as faithful advocates of patients' previously expressed end-of-life choices and relate to people's identity and values?

Values-based arguments to honor Advance Directives

- What greater human virtue is there, than to respond to the wishes of those you loved and who have loved you?

- When this special person to whom you owe so much nears the end of her life and few opportunities remain to demonstrate your love, that is when you must listen to and respond to her heart-felt requests. This is your duty even if she had expressed these wishes long ago, even if following her wishes will leave an emptiness in your life because you will miss her, even if her request is based on certain values that she holds dear but differ from your own values.

- For when someone is ill and can no longer make her own decisions, she depends totally on you to be her eyes and ears as you discuss her current condition and future prognosis with her doctors and others who care about her (including her attorney, counselor, family members, close friends, spiritual and religious advisors, and end-of-life consultant). After such discussions, it will then be your privilege and your responsibility to do her reflective thinking to make her decisions for medical treatment.

- To show your love, care, and respect, you must honor the trust she placed in you by making the decisions *she* would have made based on *her values*, not *yours*. You accepted this explicit role when you agreed to serve as her Proxy.

- Your last opportunity to honor her as a person, and her life, is thus very clear: do all you can to honor her Last Wishes.

The story below, a composite of several of my friends and their parents, strives to resonate with these values and identity.

Years ago, when still competent, Amy's mother asked her to serve as her Proxy. Since her mother declined to fill out what she referred to as a "morbid check list," which she doubted would have applied to her own parents, Amy insisted that they discuss her values and preferences, especially what kinds of situations she would not want her biologic existence to be maintained. Amy took notes as they talked.

To Honor My Mother's Last Wishes

Mother had been in the Permanent Vegetative State for two years. Two years without responding to my words, two years without hearing her voice. I had listened to the people who knew her best. I had consulted with all her doctors. I recalled the heart-to-heart discussions we had before she became ill. Yesterday, at home, I re-read for the umpteenth time, what she wrote about her values and wishes. Then I reflected deeply... Slowly, reluctantly, but finally, I arrived at a decision. —A most difficult decision. —An irreversible decision. I would have done anything to be certain that it was what she would have decided...

Today, I drove to the nursing home. I marched down the hall to her room with a mixed sense of determination and uncertainty. As always, I wanted to make contact, but this time the feeling was more intense than ever. I did not have a clear idea of what I would do when I arrived at her bedside. I opened the door and walked in. The two of us were alone. I looked at her in the silence. For a moment, I suspended my rational thought and just blurted out, as if she could suddenly have heard me and responded, "I think it's time. Do you agree? I've made the decision... As you asked... But tell me: please tell me... is it right? Is this the right time? Is this what you want now?"

My mother's body did not move. But I leaned forward, touched her shoulder, and looked into her face. Again I asked out loud, "Is this what you want?" As I stared at her face, I imagined what she would say... if by some miracle, she were suddenly granted one moment of lucidity... if for one moment she could hear me explain her current situation and prognosis and then she would tell me what she wanted. And then, after that impossible moment, she would return to her previous state, to live or die with the consequences of her *own* decision...

But she was still. So I continued to stare... I waited... I thought about how many dozens of times I had been with her like this. How many times I could say that... *I sat with her. I stood by her side. I held her hand. I stroked her hair. I cradled her head in my hands. I looked deeply and closely into her eyes. I implored. I cajoled. I begged. I tried everything I could to elicit any response, let alone any consistent response, beyond mere spontaneous reflexes.* *

Then I recalled how I felt some years back, when she had asked me to be her Proxy, when she deliberately and knowingly put me in this situation. I could not remember the exact words she used that day. But I could recall the intensity of my feelings.

I sighed. A weight had just lifted from my chest. I realized it was time to honor the trust she had placed in me, time to show her in this last way, time to respect her enough to honor her wishes. That would be the final way I could show my love.

I kissed her on the cheek, let go of her shoulder, and stepped back from the bed. It was time to look for her doctor, who had for weeks been waiting for me to make this decision. As I exited her room and walked down the hall, I imagined him asking me, "Why now?" How could I explain? What words could I use to describe how I felt as I made contact with my mother as she is... and with my mother as she was... as I recalled the feelings of our relationship and as I felt the responsibility of how I needed to show my love and respect? I sensed that it was time, but it was not logical. It was even beyond words. It was just a feeling, although a deep one. Nothing I could say would provide the doctor something to quote and to include in his final progress note in my mother's medical chart. —Even if he was among the few doctors who could understand.

So I decided it would be better just to say, "It's time."
And it was.

* Words in Italics from Jay Wolfson [2005], with permission.

୭ઓ

While this description of "Substituted Judgment" seem a bit sentimental, the story illustrates an ideal we all could strive toward: to honor the person that was, and the person that is, when we are privileged to be granted the opportunity to show how much we care by appreciating and advocating a person's Last Wishes.

Loewy [1998] quotes Eric Cassell as "taking a leaf from Nietzsche" as he argues "that life is a person's most personal piece of art, an artwork that all of us craft in our own entirely inimitable style. Schubert's *Unfinished Symphony* finished by Mahler" could "not ring true." Similarly, "substituting our own decision and completing their work of art in their stead would distort their life's intent: it would be... worse yet, in the style of Hindemith."

Now, let's reframe the recommendations to state how many individuals as well as society a whole could benefit, in terms that relate to identity and values.

If one of the main goals of this book was achieved, that people can create their Advance Directives with sufficient anticipatory trust that their Proxies would make sure that their wishes will be honored, then...

- People will be motivated to do advance care planning since they will have confidence that others will honor their Constitutional right to determine what happens to their bodies.

- People will not need to worry that they will be forced to endure unbearable suffering, total dependence on their caregivers, and prolonged indignity (in which state they will be remembered), or to survive so long that all their financial assets are spent in ways they consider wasteful.

- Patients with terminal or chronic illnesses can thus focus their energies on maintaining as high a quality of life and living by choice, as long as possible.

- Proxies and caregivers can be relieved of potential guilt from the burden of feeling that it is they who must make the ultimate decision.

- People in support groups can agree to serve as each other's Proxies, to respond with compassion and trust as they strive to honor each other's true wishes—which can be facilitated by asking for professional advice if and when needed.

- Policy makers including legislators can turn their attention to achieving the goal that every American has a right to good medical care, and if resources are determined to be limited, they can realistically respond by determining what is the fairest way to allocate those resources; that is, where they will help the most people who can most benefit from them.

- Treatment for individuals need not be continued if there is no hope for improvement—a policy consistent with the Hippocratic Oath, which forbids the medical profession from offering treatment when hope is not realistic.

- We can all recognize that the burden of disease is not limited to individual patients who have devastating diagnoses, but extends to family and to society.

- Our wealthy society can better appreciate the burden of disease from a global perspective and realize not only that the burdens of continued treatment can exceed the benefits on an individual basis, but can also consider allocating some of our resources to developing countries where they can do so much good.

- We can open for consideration two alternatives for the concept of "equality": A) That a person's soul resides in her body no matter how diminished, which must therefore be maintained at all costs, *versus* B) We must allocate our limited resources fairly so that needy human beings—including the poor, hungry, and sick in this and in other countries—can also benefit.

  While the magnitude of world health problems may seem overwhelming for us as individuals, there are actions that we can take as individuals and as groups of caring people that may begin to make a difference, for example...

- We can take the necessary steps to write carefully crafted Advance Directives that will increase the likelihood that others will honor our end-of-life wishes. We can follow this plan: Decide & Plan; then Authorize & Empower.

    1. Decide what you want in terms of end-of-life options and create an effective plan that takes present and future challenges into consideration.

    2. Authorize well-chosen Proxies who care about advocating your wishes. Empower them with *clear and convincing* supportive statements that can overcome the attempts of others who wish to impose their values to thwart your Proxy's efforts to honor your Last Wishes.

- When new challenges occur, as well as when your medical condition changes, revise your Advance Directive to discourage others from attempting to thwart your Proxy's efforts to honor your Last Wishes. On page 399 there are some examples of additions to an "Empowering Statement for My Proxy" as a result of the recommendations of the President's Council on Bioethics.

10. Conclusions

The President's Council on Bioethics takes a firm stand on the relative value of the four principles of medical ethics described by Beauchamp and Childress [2001]. More than denouncing **autonomy** as overemphasized, The Council's report characterizes *our* attempt to preserve our reasoned informed choices beyond the veil of incompetency from dementia as **discriminating against *our* future disabled self**. It casts doubt on whether *precedent autonomy* should ever apply if we become demented, even if our motivation to engage in advance care planning was precisely because we sought a durable mechanism to express our end-of-life wishes. The report argues that our present knowledge is inadequate to make decisions about our future treatment preferences for end-of-life treatment; therefore, we should NOT create **Living Wills**. While we may create a **Proxy Directive** to empower certain designated individuals to make our future medical decisions, The Council states that these individuals must first respond to their own moral judgment when such decisions need to be made, even if that requires our Proxies to set aside our previously articulated preferences. The Council's report thus casts a pessimistic view of advance care planning: neither Living Wills nor Powers of Attorney (Proxy Directives) are valid for patients with dementia, when primacy if given to The Council's moral views based on the philosophical theory of "human equality."

The Council's report does emphasize the virtues of two other principles of medical ethics: to maximize **beneficence** and to minimize **maleficence** by carefully weighing the proportionate benefit versus possible increase in suffering of proposed treatments for individual patients after taking into consideration, their current situation and future prognosis. Two corollaries of these principles, The Council insists, are that A) **we** (defined as loved ones, designated Proxies, caregivers, policy-makers, and society) can show that we care for demented patients only by doing all we can for whatever remains of their lives, no matter how diminished; and B) we must never consider doing "harm" by engineering the hastening of a patient's dying process—no matter how legal, how clearly written, how reasonable, how consistently previously expressed, or how widely held such a choice would be among "reasonable people."

The Council's report thus ignores this relevant ethical statement of the American Medical Association. Adopted a quarter of a century ago, it is still current today [E-2.20 Withholding or Withdrawing Life-Sustaining Medical Treatment; 1981 through 1994]:

The American Medical Association's Statement on Ethics

"The social commitment of the physician is to sustain life and relieve suffering.

"Where the performance of one duty conflicts with the other, **the preferences of the patient should prevail**."

The last principle of **social justice** (also called **social fairness**) extols the virtues of attempting to distribute fairly basic medical care. The Council's report considers this principle, but lightly. While it notes that resources are finite, the report fails to consider known ways to reduce the costs of long-term care that could be expanded, possible future sources of funds that will be needed, how other countries deal with rationing, or the present gross inequality of allocation of resources. Furthermore, The Council's report fails to acknowledge that if we follow their recommendations to extend the existence of demented persons who cannot consciously appreciate the sacrifices being made for them, the result will be significantly less funds available for poor both in America and globally.

As we die, we may experience many kinds of suffering: physical, psychic, spiritual, and communal. Many of us want the opportunity to leave our previously chosen legacies via Living Wills or Proxy Directives. Some of us will want to be remembered as "heroic" individuals who made the end-of-life decision not to waste valuable resources so that others can potentially obtain adequate medical care and advance themselves through education. While the problems of global poverty and inadequate medical care are enormous, the decisions of individuals about how much medical treatment they desire to prolong their inevitable dying may ultimately make a great difference.

Margaret Mead taught: "Never doubt that a small group of thoughtful, committed citizens can change the world. Indeed, it is the only thing that ever has." Similarly, each individual's commitment to consider **social justice** as they engage in advance care planning is an important beginning. Timing is obviously critical, and I would argue that The President's Council on Bioethics' report on "Taking Care" has taken a major step backwards. Hopefully, this book and others, and teachers and professionals in this field will function as mavens in the sense of Gladwell's *The Tipping Point* [2002] to get the message out before we reach an economic *sinking point*.

In conclusion, while The President's Council on Bioethics' report on "Taking Care" describes well the enormous challenge of long-term care for increasing numbers of patients with dementia, for many it will not serve well as a beacon of enlightenment. Instead, it provides a strong signal to warn those of us who want some control over the way we die, and/or are concerned about how scarce medical resources are allocated, to proceed with diligence in strategic planning, if we are serious about wanting to accomplish these personal and societal goals.

43. How Can I Put All these Strategies Together? and Which Documents Do I Need When?

Let's now turn to a fictionalized illustration that draws on many of the strategies this book explains. The story assumes that three reasonable changes in State and Federal law have occurred. The story of "Joyce" begins at age 16—when she is old enough to drive a "lethal weapon," but not old enough to be considered competent to sign an Advance Directive. Thus, her State provides her with a new form called, "Informing my parents (or Guardians) about my end-of-life wishes." The story continues with her State's Department of Motor Vehicles asking her to consider if she wishes to revise her Advance Directives whenever she renews her driver's license. Then, just before she turns 65, the Federal government provides her with a new notice to encourage her to consider creating a Proxy Directive or a Directive to Physician (Living Will), which is preferable to handing sick patients forms to complete as they enter a hospital, to comply with Medicare's funding requirements of the Patient Self-Determination Act. As of mid-2007, however, these three new forms or notices do not yet exist. The story below uses terms that are summarized and compared in a Table of *New* and Recommended Terms for Advance Care Planning that appears within the Glossary, which begins on page 457.

She revised her Advance Directives from age 16 to 86.

Joyce can hardly wait until she reaches the age of 16, when she can apply for her temporary driver's license. As she does, the clerk at the Department of Motor Vehicles hands her a new form entitled, **"Informing my parents (or Guardians) about my end-of-life wishes."** The clerk informs Joyce that a new law requires one of her legal Guardians (most likely, her parents) to sign a statement that can be detached from this form that indicates that she has completed the form, but the instructions state she can fill the form out any way she wants. [*This form does not yet exist.*]

Joyce checks the boxes to indicate she does not want machines to breathe for her, or for tubes to administer artificial nutrition and hydration—if, after the number of months she indicates in this box [___], two physicians have evaluated her and agreed that she has virtually no chance (or less than 0.01% chance) of recovery from her unconscious, PVS, or minimally conscious state. Like most families, Joyce and her parents use this opportunity to discuss the risks of automobile accidents, which are the most common cause of death for people in Joyce's age group. The form indicates that Joyce can change her answers at any time since the last option above her signature and date reads, "This form replaces any similar form I have previously signed."

As Joyce obtains her regular driver's license on her 18th birthday, the DMV clerk informs her that she must now complete an Advance Directive, which can be either a **Directive to Physician (Living Will)** or a **Proxy Directive**, or both. He hands her a brochure with brief descriptions of how these two Directives work. Like most people her age, Joyce prefers NOT to think about various end-stage illnesses and the options of withholding or withdrawing specific life-sustaining treatment. At this point in her life, the topic seems "morbid," so she merely names her father as her first Proxy and her mother as her second, since her brother is still a minor. She also checks a box "YES," in response to: "My Proxies DO know my wishes about continuing Food & Fluid, whether administered by oral or by artificial means." This Directive automatically revokes all previous forms, including, "Informing my parents (or Guardians) about my end-of-life wishes." The DMV also offers Joyce a new form entitled, **"Empowering Statements for My Proxy,"** which gives her the opportunity to add her own explanatory statements, and REQUIRES her to make this choice: "Do you want your Proxy's future decisions to OVERRIDE how other people interpret what you have written in this document or elsewhere?" Since Joyce has not thought much about end-of-life issues, she checks, "YES," and then sighs with relief that she does not have to think about this topic, anymore. (She has not yet created any other documents to override.)

Every time Joyce renews her driver's license, the DMV reminds her that she must either renew or revise her Advance Directive. At 23, and again at 28, she renews without much additional thought.

By the age of 33, Joyce is now married and has a young daughter, so when she renews her license, she designates her husband as her first Proxy, keeping her parents as second and third alternates. She makes no further changes at 38.

By the time she renews her documents at 43, Joyce has visited a nursing home at the request of her closest friend. Stacy's grandfather was suffering from Alzheimer's disease. Joyce was quite alarmed as she watched the nursing assistants force-feed the old man. So now Joyce decides to use check an option on the **Proxy Directive** that is different from the one she checked before. It states: "I specifically authorize my **Proxy to Refuse Food & Fluid**—whether administered through any type of tube or line that enters my GI tract or my circulatory system, or by assisted oral feeding by another's hand that requires that I swallow." She also explains her reasons using the form, **Empowering Statements for My Proxy**. This form provides Joyce the opportunity to give examples and explanations to state her wishes clearly and convincingly to make it less likely that others can effectively challenge her Proxy's authority. At this time, Joyce simply writes one sentence: "I do not want to be force-fed like Stacy's grandfather."

Five years later, after a few more visits to the nursing home, Joyce notes that Stacy's grandfather is still alive, that his dementia is more severe, and that he is now being fed by tubes. Joyce now writes down more details about her reasons for wanting to avoid prolonging a similar lack of dignity. She now lists several movies and books that have influenced her to make this choice. All this writing becomes her expanded form, Empowering Statements for My Proxy.

When she renews her license at 58, Joyce is now divorced, and her second parent (and last named Proxy) has died. She now names her brother as her first proxy and Stacy as her alternate. Although her daughter is very devoted, Joyce reasons that she may love her too much and feel too much guilt to let Joyce go if she had to act in the role of Proxy. After all, Stacy is still reeling from the guilt of refusing a feeding tube for her grandfather. So Joyce decides not to name her daughter as her Proxy.

At 63, Joyce has some medical problems, but none are life-threatening. A close friend died of breast cancer, but was not adequately treated for pain. That experience motivates Joyce to revise her Advance Directive: She changes her Proxy Directive by designating another friend's husband as number one. She trusts him to be her advocate because he knows her well, and since he is an oral surgeon, he knows how to relate to medical doctors. Joyce needs an alternate Proxy, but Stacy does not want to be her Proxy, and Joyce's brother has moved across the country. Joyce decides to designate an end-of-life professional advocate. Since this professional advocate does not yet know her values and preferences, Joyce complies with his protocol: First, she fills out several questionnaires, and then has a two-hour interview. Two weeks later, after considering her options further, she returns to his office, asks some questions, and signs the necessary documents. The professional advocate informs her that all her responses on questionnaires, all the notes from her interviews, and his narrative summary are incorporated into a document called Joyce's **Private Values and Treatment Preferences**. He will reveal its contents only if it becomes necessary to honor her end-of-life wishes. Joyce feels relieved since she is active in her church but does not agree with all her church's end-of-life guidelines.

Just before her 65th birthday, as Joyce completes the paper work to enroll in Medicare, she receives a notice in the mail that explains why she should complete a Proxy Directive, and/or a Directive to Physician (Living Will), if she has not already done so. Joyce feels that her current Proxy Directive will suffice. [*This notice does not yet exist.*]

At 73, Joyce's primary care physician sends her to a variety of specialists for managing her health risks, but Joyce still has no idea who will be her physician if she has a life-threatening illness. She reviews her Proxy Directive, her Empowering Statements for My Proxy, and her Private Values and Treatment Preferences, but makes no changes.

At 78, she has a follow-up visit with her professional end-of-life advocate since the health of her first choice Proxy, the oral surgeon friend, is declining. Joyce decides to designate the professional advocate as her first choice Proxy and signs another form that permits another professional in this professional group of advocates to be designated as her Proxy, if he is not available.

At 83, Joyce's internist refers her to a neurologist for symptoms of weakness and twitching in the muscles of her legs and arms. At the second visit, after many tests and a thorough examination, the neurologist explains, as gently as possible, that she is in an early stage of an ominous disease named after Lou Gehrig, ALS. He provides some reading material, refers her to the ALS Society for support, and asks her to return to his office in two weeks.

At that visit, the neurologist sits down with her and has a long talk about her disease. He explains that within a few years, her paralysis will become so profound that she will need to make a major decision. If she wants to remain alive, she will require medical technology to breathe and to speak (a mechanical ventilator and a computer). He also discusses the various ways she might otherwise die. She might suffocate from the weakness in the muscles needed to breathe, or she might drown in her oral secretions. Either way is likely to be associated with great anxiety unless she receives expert *Comfort Care*, such as hospice offers. Another way she might die is by aspirating some food into her lungs and contracting pneumonia—if she decides in advance not to treat infections aggressively.

For a while, Joyce's emotions seem like they were on a roller coaster. After a couple of weeks, she can review her life, appreciate the many years of good health she has enjoyed in the past, and be thankful that she still has some years left. These thoughts, and the discussions with her neurologist, help Joyce begin to accept her life's inevitable conclusion. She is impressed with her neurologist's knowledge, caring, and kindness, as well as his willingness to follow her choice of end-of-life wishes. At her next appointment, she engages in a focused discussion that leads to her creating a **Directive to Physician** (**Living Will**). She changes one statement in her Proxy Directive so that now, her Directive to Physician will OVERRIDE her Proxy's decisions. The effect of this change is to make her Proxy responsible for the more limited but still very important task of making sure that her last treating physicians will honor her previously expressed written wishes. (In effect, Joyce's decision-making Proxy has changed into a Living Will Advocate, who will now facilitate the decisions Joyce made with her physician.) Joyce gives copies of her Directive to Physician to her neurologist, her internist, her daughter, and her Proxy (the professional end-of-life advocate). She also gives them copies of her **POLST**, her **Physicians Orders for Life-Sustaining Treatment**, which her neurologist signed, in case he is out of town or she is rushed to the hospital in an emergency. That form prevents 9-1-1 calls to emergency teams or emergency departments from attempting to resuscitate her.

Joyce's Proxy still has a copy of her Empowering Statements for My Proxy, and this document still provides much useful information about her end-of-life wishes, however the document that will most determine her future care now, if Joyce cannot speak for herself, is her Directive to Physician.

Joyce receives excellent medical treatment, but her disease continues to progress. As her breathing becomes more difficult, she grapples with the option of mechanical ventilation. Joyce decides she would rather opt for **Physician-Aided, Patient-Hastened Dying**. Although it is legal in her State, there is some doubt whether her State regulatory bodies will continue to permit the prescription of medications that are listed under the Controlled Substances Act, despite the U.S. Supreme Court ruling that the 1970 Federal law did not apply. She is also concerned whether the U.S. Congress will soon pass a more restrictive federal law. So Joyce decides to ask for a prescription of barbiturates while it is still possible to obtain them. Her neurologist and her internist determine that she is terminally ill and that her judgment is intact (in other words, she possesses decision-making capacity and her request is voluntary), so her neurologist prescribes a prescription of lethal medications, which Joyce's daughter picks up from the pharmacy, after the mandatory waiting period of 17 days that started with Joyce's first request.

Joyce's intent is to wait as long as possible before taking the lethal medication. Now that she does not need to worry about experiencing a horrific death or becoming a prolonged total burden, Joyce continues to enjoy life as much as possible.

Five months later, when Joyce decides it is time to ingest the pills, she must face two new problems. Her state legislature passed a law so that it is no longer legal to use barbiturates to hasten dying. [*This has not happened in reality.*] Her neurologist informs her that he can prescribe a combination of medications that are not usually thought of as being lethal individually. Even more important, none of these medications are on the Federal list of Controlled Substances. The other problem is that one of her hospice nurses is known to be an outspoken opponent of Physician-Aided, Patient-Hastened Dying (Physician-Assisted Suicide).

Joyce's paralysis has progressed to the point where she can no longer feed herself. Although she can only say a few words at a time, Joyce states she cannot stop worrying about the hospice nurse. Could the nurse cause trouble by accusing her daughter of forcing her to ingest the lethal dose of medications? It is obvious to every visitor that Joyce needs to be spoon-fed. Could someone claim there is a conflict of interest? Trouble-makers could cite that her daughter will inherit what remains in Joyce's estate, and that amount would diminish if Joyce remained alive since she does not have long-term care insurance. All these considerations lead Joyce to insist on asking for a legal opinion.

The next day, an attorney visits. He informs Joyce that the law provides immunity for those who comply in good faith. He quotes a "Practice Tip" of Section 8.29 of Oregon's Death With Dignity Act [1997], that relates to "how much assistance is too much," which gives an example of "the family member or loved one who opens the bottle, places the pills in the patient's hand, advises the patient how many pills to take, and provides the necessary liquids." The lawyer reads, "Central to any inquiry will be whether the person in attendance *supported*, but did *not direct*, the patient's action," and then points out that the code does not define either the word "support" or "direct." [*As of April 2006, Oregon was the only State where "Physician-Assisted Suicide" was legal.*]

Joyce knows she will need total physical assistance so she asks him directly for his frank advice. He answers, "Given the *clear and convincing* documentation of your Last Wishes, it is not likely that a prosecutor would succeed in a jury trial, if he or she accused your daughter of forcing you to ingest the pills, based on an allegation made by the hospice nurse. However I recommend you not take the prescription of barbiturates, as special interest groups could make trouble for the physician who prescribed them, especially if your doctor can offer you an alternative."

Joyce thanks the attorney and states she will now consider her choices.

The next day, Joyce announces her decision, which is in effect an oral expression of her revised Living Will. She is competent now, and wants these stated wishes to be durable: "I want my final transition to be as peaceful as possible, without any serious worries, even if their possibilities are remote. As I die, I do NOT want to worry about possible legal actions against my doctor since he has been so good to me, or against my daughter who loves me so much. Even though I have been told that such allegations are extremely unlikely to succeed, the litigation itself could be a nightmare for them. I therefore have decided that the *BEST WAY* for me to say goodbye is to **Voluntarily Refuse Food & Fluid**."

In addition to her Living Will (**Directive to Physician**), Joyce completes two additional documents to reduce the risk that someone could sabotage her plan: **My Wish to Refuse Food & Fluid NOW**, and **I Wish to Decline Life-Sustaining Emergency Treatment**. She names as her Living Will Advocate, her daughter, who by this time, is at peace with her mother's ultimate decision.

Joyce's neurologist promises to provide her with adequate sedation for anxiety or discomfort. Actually, she needs very little medication before she drifts off peacefully. Joyce dies five days after beginning her **Refusal of Food & Fluid**, a few weeks before her 87th birthday.

Which Documents Do I Need When?

A. **Living Will**: If you know who your (last) doctor will be and you trust him or her... or you cannot identify an individual to be your Proxy whom you trust to exercise "Substituted Judgment"... or if your regional laws do not permit Durable Powers of Attorney for Health Care Decisions (as in Thailand), use FORM I (Living Will) instead of FORM IV (Proxy Directive). Recommended: Designate a Living Will Advocate and provide him or her with Empowering Statements, in the event the physician does not respond to "pieces of paper," which experience has shown are not self-enforcing. (If you prefer a Proxy Directive but cannot designate someone you already know, consider joining a Trusting Circle or contacting a professional organization to represent your end-of-life interests.)

B. **Proxy Directive**: If you cannot predict who your last doctor will be, or you do not have a trusting relationship with him or her, but you *can* identify an individual and alternates to serve as your Proxy and you do trust them to effectively exercise "Substituted Judgment," and your regional laws do permit Durable Powers of Attorney for Health Care Decisions, then use FORM IV (Proxy Directive) instead of FORM I (Living Will). Recommended: Provide your Proxy with "**Empowering Statements for My Proxy**." Optional: Private material and "working documents," which might be interpreted as inconsistent can be kept in a separate document called, "Private Values and Treatment Preferences."

Rational: A Proxy Directive has two separate functions: 1) to **designate** an individual; and 2) to **empower** that individual to make Typical challenges to Proxy's decisions are based on four arguments: 1) the specific current medical situation does not apply; 2) the decision is immoral; 3) the Proxy's decision is not in the patient's "Best Interests"; or 4) the Proxy is not acting in good faith. This book's strategy to minimize outside challenges by giving Proxies maximum power in the Proxy Directive and leaving specifics in a separate document that explains why you want specific decisions made on your behalf, and provides examples. (Empowering statements given to a Living Will Advocate will not have as much power since Advocates do not make decisions; they only facilitate your decisions.) If your situation or politics change, you can leave your Proxy Directive intact and just add additional statements to your "Empowering Statements for My Proxy." See example on page 399.

C. **Legal Alternative to Physician-Assisted Suicide**: If you are competent and you want to end your life now because of unbearable suffering, you need FORM II (I Wish to Voluntarily Refuse Food & Fluid NOW) and FORM III (I Decline Resuscitation/POLST).

D. If you are a minor, you can create a document called, "Informing my parents (or guardian) about my end-of-life wishes."

See also The Table of *New* and Recommended Terms in the Glossay, on pages 458-459.

44. *Why it is Better to Have Crossed Out and Rewritten Than to Have Never Changed at All?* and,

Can I Use My State's Free Form, or "Five Wishes"?

[FORM IV-a: *Empowering Statements for My Proxy To "Permit Natural Dying"*]

Regarding Forms Provided by Your State and the Internet

One size does not fit all. No matter what form you choose, you may need to modify it so it accurately reflects your specific end-of-life preferences. Why is it better to modify a form than to search for one that fits best? Because litigating attorneys sometimes challenge Advance Directives based on this theory: Your signature at the end of a long and complicated document does not necessarily imply that you fully understood and completely agreed to all of the form's individual terms. Forms where no action or little is required—such as leaving a space blank or checking a box—are easier to challenge.

In the shadow of the Terri Schiavo saga, sales of forms on the Internet reached record highs. Prices ranged from $5 to $39. Yet free forms were and still are available from most States and several organizations (some of these web sites are listed in this book's "Further Resources"). Still, do not assume that your "official" State form will be adequate.

Attorney Marshall Kapp, JD, MPH, FCLM, when he was at the Office of Geriatric Medicine and Gerontology, Wright University, categorized the sources of "legislatively induced harm" from State statutes—both in general and with respect to Artificial Nutrition and Hydration [2002]. He noted that some laws "lack linguistic clarity" or are open to "faulty interpretation" because of "poor, imprecise drafting of statutes... by failing to say clearly what their sponsors meant." They are "unintentionally and unwittingly interfering with patient autonomy and humane care because of inartful wording (often committed by attorneys with no grasp of the substantive clinical issues)." Other "statutes function exactly as their sponsors envisioned" whose intent was "making it more difficult for a person capable of making decisions to prospectively forego Artificial Nutrition and Hydration." Attorney Kapp concluded, "The practical impact of the law is determined by how it is perceived, rightly or wrongly, by those in the trenches, not by the elegant intellectual analyses engaged in by legal scholars and appellate judges."

What is the bottom line? Many forms may not prevent conflict, avoid delay, or assure that others will honor your end-of-life wishes. However, if you demonstrate your diligent thinking by explaining why you crossed out certain options, rewrote others, and added specific words and phrases—this alternative is quite acceptable. The extra effort will more precisely reflect what you want, and make it harder for others to challenge the final document. While you can add "Empowering Statements for My Proxy" to any standard form, make sure those statements do not contradict any statements in the primary form, or add a statement regarding which is to prevail in the event of a perceived conflict.

"Five Wishes" is one of the most popular forms, in part because faith-based organizations can purchase large quantities for as little as one dollar and because the form considers some humanistic and ceremonial aspects of dying. But the most important consideration is whether or not "Five Wishes" will set the stage for peaceful transitions. Below, I recommend some specific modifications.

How to Begin with a Popular Form
Such as "Five Wishes"

The non-profit organization, Aging with Dignity, who distributes "Five Wishes" states that this document *substantially* meets the legal requirements of Advance Directives in 36 States. (What they mean by "substantially" is discussed below.)

Almost seven million copies have been distributed. The form addresses certain aspects of end-of-life care that this book does not cover. For example, **Wishes 3, 4,** and **5** primarily address your *Comfort Care* (massage with oils, music, religious readings), how you want others to treat you (to display photos of children, for others to pray for you), and what you want your loved ones to know and remember (cherished memories, values, forgiveness). Yet without substantial crossing out and rewriting, conflicts and ambiguities could arise, and your Proxy might not be able to choose certain end-of-life decisions on your behalf.

❧ *SKIP*

Note: You do not need the 12-page form, "Five Wishes," in front of you as you read the following comments, some of which apply to other standard forms. Note that forms may use the term "Agent," "Health Care Agent," or "Proxy."

Attorney Charles P. Sabatino, Director of the American Bar Association's Commission on Law and Aging, comprehensively reviewed certain legal aspects of "Five Wishes" in the context of "the primary barriers in existing state legislation that inhibit the availability of national models of Advance Directives" [2005]. Mr. Sabatino noted two conflicting goals: one is to be user friendly for consumers; the other is to be accepted by doctors so that consumers can have confidence that their wishes will be honored. While your physician *may* accept what you have written regardless of what form you use, some doctors will not. If the form fails to comply with your State's requirements, the courts may not grant your physician immunity for following your instructions. Thus your form may not serve its primary purpose, to prevent legal battles among family members who disagree, for example.

Mr. Sabatino's article lists the specific States of concern in a long table where he labels some as "Probably Yes" to certain issues, and notes that others are only "substantially" in compliance. If the **Proxy Directive** conformed to State law, Mr. Sabatino considered "Five Wishes" as *substantially* in compliance, even if the **Living Will** was *not* in compliance because (in his words), these "statutes cover a far broader scope of health care decision-making than do Living Will laws. In addition, they permit the inclusion of any guidance the principal wishes to provide. As a practical matter, they can substitute for the Living Will and eliminate the need to rely on the separate Living Will statute as a basis for validity of the document."

My comments below reflect complete agreement on Mr. Sabatino's last point. Many of my suggestion have the goal of empowering the **Proxy Directive** (**Wish 1**) while attempting to eliminate (or at least minimize) potential conflicts with the instructions in the **Living Will** (**Wish 2**), or other sections of "Five Wishes."

General Comments about "Five Wishes":

A.   Attorney Sabatino's article did not cite any court case involving "Five Wishes." While that *might* be good news, it also means that use of the form has not been subjected to a legal test. We depend on appellate court rulings to set precedents.

B.   In the clinical arena, Hickman and others [Dec. 2005] stated, "Unfortunately, there are no published research studies to support the efficacy of 'Five Wishes' in guiding surrogates and health care professionals or in ensuring that wishes are honored" [*Page 29*].

C. The "Five Wishes" form includes this disclaimer: "It does not try to answer all questions about anything that could come up" (which speaks for itself). It also refers to "end-stage condition," which some clinicians consider too vague.

ᏚᎧCONTINUE

Modifying "Five Wishes" for Your Advance Directive:

1. **Wish 1** is a basic Proxy Directive. Like most standard forms (California is one exception), it does not provide the option to allow your Proxy's authority to become effective *immediately*. It also does not authorize your physician to ask an alternate Proxy to serve if your physician determines your acting Proxy has lost decision-making capacity. I recommend you consider adding these two phrases.

2.   The second bullet point states you "want your Agent" to "interpret any instructions I have given in this form or given in other discussions, according to my Health Care Agent's understanding of my wishes and values." While this statement might be circular, of greater significance is whether or not you want the words "to interpret" to mean that you authorize your Agent to OVERRIDE what others may interpret as your intent based on what you previously wrote. To be

certain about this important point, you could use the blank lines at the bottom of the *Page*, to write some words along these lines: "If there is a conflict between my Agent's understanding of my wishes and what others interpret as my wishes from the way I have filled this form by checking boxes or not, and leaving spaces blank or filled in; and from other discussions I may have had—then I want my Agent's decisions to be final; that is my Agent's decisions for me should OVERRIDE the interpretations of others." (As previously emphasized in this book, make this change only if you trust your Agent.)

3. If you have decided to authorize your **Proxy** to make all decisions about **Food & Fluid**: initial in the margin and cross out the word "artificially" prior to form's words "-provided food and water." Also: Cross out the third bullet point on *Page* 6: "I want to be offered food and fluids by mouth" to avoid possible conflicts. (Even if you cross out the entire point, "being kept clean" is covered in Wish 3.)

Write on the blank lines at the bottom of *Page 5*: "I authorize my Agent to make all decisions regarding administration of Food & Fluid, whether oral or by tubes or lines; that is, regardless of the route of administration," and "I have attached another document—**Empowering Statements for My Proxy**—that explains and illustrates how I arrived at my decisions." (The goal of this document is to meet the legal standard of *clear and convincing* of evidence—in case your State does, or will, require that level of proof.)

In commenting on the above suggestion, Mr. Sabatino [2006] stated that the Proxy "runs a risk of accusations of abuse and neglect. Also, nursing homes can face regulatory sanctions under federal law if they do not provide food and water by mouth to residents who are capable. A few states may have provisions similar to the one in Maryland law that says: 'A health care provider shall make reasonable efforts to provide an individual with food and water by mouth and to assist the individual as needed to eat and drink voluntarily.' MD Health General Code §5-611(d)."

My recommendations: Add to what you have written on the blank lines at the bottom of *Page 5*: "I am aware of the relevant State code, which in Maryland is Health General Code §5-611(d), but I authorize my Proxy to OVERRIDE it. I am also are aware of Federal law and will hold my nursing home harmless by following the decisions of my Proxy." (Ask an attorney in your State what Code or Statue is relevant to cite and what precise words to use.)

4. How much pain medication you want is indicated in the first bullet points of "**Wish 2**" on *Page 6* and of "**Wish 3**" on *Page 8*. (Only *Page 8* includes instructions that give you explicit permission to "cross out anything that you don't agree with.") The "Five Wishes" form states that you agree to an adequate dose of medications to not be in pain—even if the dose is so high that it makes you "drowsy or sleep more." I recommend adding these words to both *Pages* such as those on the standard form in California: "I direct that treatment for alleviation

of pain and discomfort be provided at all times, even if it hastens my death." This is consistent with the doctrine of **Double Effect** introduced by Catholics in the Thirteen Century and defined in the Glossary that starts on page 457.

5. If you "leave the space blank" on the bottom of *Page 7*, the "Five Wishes" form states "you have no other [medical] condition to describe" for which you choose to not continue "life-support treatment." Yet in addition to "close to death," permanent "coma," and "permanent and severe brain damage," other Living Wills typically list several other conditions. As a physician familiar with terminal illnesses, I *could* start my own additional list with the Minimally Conscious State, end-stage dementia, end-stage congestive heart failure, and terminal cancer. But even for myself, as well as your author, I do NOT recommend relying on such a list of diagnoses. Instead, I suggest you write on the blank lines at the bottom of *Page 7*, words similar to these: "Regardless of my specific diagnosis, I want my Proxy to consult with my treating physicians and to compare my current functioning and my future prognosis with what my Proxy knows about my values and preferences, to decide whether or not to withhold or to withdraw any medical treatment that has some potential to continue my existence." (These words are designed to avoid conflict due to being too general or too specific about diagnosis.)

Mr. Sabatino's comments on the above suggestion: "I like this. Indeed, it could substitute for everything in Wish 2."

6. You may wish to consider if there are any sections of the **Advance Directive that Grants My Proxy Maximum Power** that you wish to include; for example, the list of people you want your Proxy to consult before making life-or-death decisions. You may also ask your Proxy to sign a form that she or he agrees to serve as you wish, to make your Proxy Directive a two-way agreement, whose main purposes are, according to Mr. Sabatino, "to make sure that the agent knowingly accepts the responsibility and hopefully has read the document." (Note: this is required for your Proxy's authority to become effective in Michigan, North Dakota, and Oregon.) You may also want to waive your right to a court review (as explained in Chapter 3).

7. The second bullet point of "**Wish 3**" requests: "If I show signs of shortness of breath... I want my care givers to do ***whatever*** they can to do help me." {Emphasis added.} Mr. Sabatino and I agreed the following wording is better: "I want my caregivers to provide whatever palliative care is necessary to comfort me." Otherwise, the word "whatever" could refer to a wide range of options, from soothing music and holding hands, to the surgical implantation of a breathing tube through your trachea that is connected to a mechanical ventilator for ten years. You could also just cross out the words "shortness of breath" since such *Comfort Care* treatments should be routine, and you can allow your Proxy to make decisions about mechanical ventilation on your behalf; for example, consent to its short-term use to overcome an infection, but not maintain your indefinitely.

8. The last bullet point of "**Wish 4**" is: "I want to die in my home, if that can be done." Dying can always be done at home, but again, this decision might best be left to your Proxy to make based on your current condition. Your suffering might be so severe that you need a treatment option, such as terminal sedation, (palliative sedation) that is best performed in a clinical institution.

9. The remaining bullet points of "Five Wishes," including the kind of comfort, spiritual, and humane treatment you want, and your specific wishes about ceremonies and rituals, need no further comment.

10. I applaud the seventh bullet point of "**Wish 5**": "I wish for my family and friends and caregivers to respect my wishes even if they don't agree with them." (Contrast this statement with the recommendations of The President's Council of Bioethics' report on "Taking Care," discussed previously.)

Summary: "Five Wishes" offers a convenient way to express several non-medical end-of-life preferences, but its other content could be interpreted in ways that might not reflect your Last Wishes and may result in longer and more intense suffering. One option is to work diligently to modify "Five Wishes" to indicate your preferences. Another is to add what you like from "Five Wishes" to a form you create yourself that accurately expresses all your wishes.

Empowering Statements For My Proxy —To "Permit Natural Dying"

This book offers patient stories and legal cases, and cites movies and books to help readers decide what they want. Some people will supplement their personal experiences with this material to write their own narrative to explain their choices. Others will prefer the structured format of **FORM IV-a**, which suggests you review your answers and reconsider every item as you think about **personhood** and decide if you want to "**Permit Natural Dying**." (Of course, you can write a narrative and also complete this FORM.) Discuss these issues with your Proxies, physician, attorney, counselors, and family and friends. When signed, witnessed, and attached to your Proxy Directive (FORM-IV), **FORM IV-a** can guide and empower your Proxy to make the decisions that you would have wanted. If necessary, the document can also help your Proxy overcome outside challenges.

Why does the book present attachment **FORM IV-a** before **FORM IV**, the Proxy Directive? Because you need to know first what your Proxies must do before you select them. In that light, also see the **BASIC FORM: Why I Authorize My Proxy to Refuse Food & Fluid** on pages 236-239.

Note: Should you use a Living Will (Directive to Physician) instead of a Proxy Directive, change the word "Proxy" to "Physician" in the document and when completed, give the FORM to your Living Will Advocate.

Empowering Statements for My Proxy

*Directions: If you agree, **write your initials** on the blank. If you do not agree, **write "No."** To illustrate, here are my responses to two light questions:*

_No_ *1. For vacations, I prefer camping in a tent to cruising on a ship.*

_ST_ *2. For meals, I prefer prime rib at the Ritz to pizza delivered by Dominos.*

I feel these essential abilities are required for FULL PERSONHOOD:

____ A. To be **consciously aware** of my environment through my senses (to **experience** life). (*Write your **initials** on the blank line, or write "No."*)

____ B. To understand verbal communication and be capable of expressing my feelings and wishes; that is, to express my "**autonomy**." (*Your **initials** or "No."*)

____ C. To use reasoning to develop a purposeful plan; that is, to invoke my "**executive functioning**." (*Your **initials** or "No."*)

____ D. To express my **unique humanness** by remembering significant **events** of my life, by following my **values** when making decisions, and by interacting meaningfully in my **relationships**, and (if within my belief system) by appreciating a Supreme Being. (*Your **initials** or "No."*)

____ E. I agree with the above definition of **personhood**. (*Your **initials** or "No."*)

____ F. I can imagine myself in a state of moderate dementia and be capable of experiencing "child-like joy," however I still want my Proxy to consider the preferences I am making today as **durable** since they reflect my fundamental life-long values and my character. (*Your **initials** or "No."*)

I may lose some but not all of my personhood, as the 14 items below will describe. If these losses are *irreversible or progressive*, then I wish to indicate my preferences about receiving aggressive medical interventions and Food & Fluid (whether by mouth or by tubes)—*to keep me alive / prolong my existence*—by using the scale below. I have written a number from **1 to 5** next to each item:

1	2	3	4	5
I would still want to live/exist.	I'd probably still want to live/exist.	I am not sure.	I'd probably want to Permit Natural Dying*.	I'd want to Permit Natural Dying* (only *Comfort Care*).

* Permit Natural Dying means your caregivers **will** provide all methods of *Comfort Care* to reduce pain and thirst, but **will not** offer any medical intervention to maintain your biologic functioning including Food & Fluid by any route (oral or tubes). A peaceful transition from dehydration and/or the underlying disease usually occurs within 2 weeks.

THESE ARE MY PREFERENCES:

1. ___ I cannot recognize the people I used to love; (*Write in 1, 2, 3, 4, or 5.*)

2. ___ I cannot recall the essence of the person who I was, or the life that I led, in terms of its fundamental values or significant events; (*1, 2, 3, 4, or 5.*)

3. ___ I cannot communicate my wishes by words, by gestures, or by making consistent sounds; (*Write in 1, 2, 3, 4, or 5.*)

4. ___ I cannot indicate "Yes" or "No" by any means, even after a trial of technological assistance, if such a trial seems appropriate; (*1, 2, 3, 4, or 5.*)

5. ___ I am not aware of my environment through my senses and therefore cannot respond; (*Write in 1, 2, 3, 4, or 5.*)

6. ___ I cannot make meaningful plans to change my environment; (*1 . . . 5.*)

7. ___ I am totally dependent on others or machines for nurturance since I do not have the physical ability to eat or drink, OR I do not have the mental ability to know how to eat or drink, OR I actively resist people as they try to spoon-feed me by fighting them or by turning my face away from them or by clenching my teeth; (*Write in 1, 2, 3, 4, or 5.*)

8. ___ I seem extremely confused or scared, or to be living in a state of horror;

9. ___ I seem to harbor delusions that lead to behavior so dangerous that I could hurt myself or others unless I am physically restrained; (*1, 2, 3, 4, or 5.*)

10. ___ I seem extremely withdrawn, apathetic, despondent, irritable, or angry despite attempts to improve my mood by treatment including counseling and medications; (*Write in 1, 2, 3, 4, or 5.*)

11. ___ I am incontinent of urine or feces and so totally dependent that prolonging my biologic existence merely increases the chance that my loved ones, especially younger relatives, will remember me only in such a state of indignity; (*Write in 1, 2, 3, 4, or 5.*)

12. ___ I have such intense pain or unbearable suffering that relief can be achieved only by medications that sedate me so much that I can hardly be aroused; (*Write in 1, 2, 3, 4, or 5.*)

13. ___ The burdens of treatment to maintain my existence have become my, and/or my caregivers' overwhelming concern, even though there is almost no potential for benefit; (*Write in 1, 2, 3, 4, or 5.*)

14. ___ I seem unaware or unable to appreciate being alive and being cared for, yet my caregivers are making huge sacrifices on my behalf—by ignoring other enjoyable activities or responsibilities in their lives, by physical

exhaustion, by mental depression, or by draining their financial resources to the extent that my continued existence has become a hardship and/or is preempting the economic opportunities of my children and/or grandchildren, and/or precluding the use of my assets to benefit the poor and hungry of the world, as I would wish be done. (*Write in 1, 2, 3, 4, or 5.*)

I HAVE REVIEWED MY PREFERENCES by *reviewing my answers and I have ordered them based on their relative importance.*
To illustrate, here is how I ordered my preferences to the two light questions::

A _No_ *1. For vacations, I prefer camping in a tent to cruising on a ship.*

B _ST_ *2. For meals, I prefer prime rib at the Ritz to pizza delivered by Dominos.*

____ I reviewed the **14 irreversible** or ***progressive*** items above, and placed an "**A**" to the left of the one I feel is most important, a "**B**" next to the second most important, and so on for as many items as I wish. (*Your **initials** or "No."*)

Now I am CONSIDERING these three alternatives:

Alternative # 1: I want my life/biologic existence to continue for as long as medical technology makes it possible, so do not Permit Natural Dying!

Alternative # 2: I authorize my Proxy to Permit Natural Dying ONLY if I suffer from the following items: __, __, __, __, __, __,__, __, __, and __.
[You may write in any number of items BUT *realize that specifying any item* could make it possible for others *to challenge your Proxy's decisions* by arguing that an item does NOT describe your future mental/medical condition.]

Alternative # 3: I grant my Proxy full authority to Permit Natural Dying using this form only as a general guide after s/he *attempts* **to speak to people on the attached list:** (Such lists usually include close relatives and friends; and physicians, attorneys, counselors, and clergy.)

____ I have considered the three alternatives above. I have weighed how much I trust my Proxy versus how much I am willing to risk a conflict that might delay fulfilling my Last Wishes, I have made a choice of one alternative, which choice is indicated below. (*Your **initials** or "No."*)

My initials here and my signature below indicate my preference for Alternative (____ **1**), or (____ **2**), or (____ **3**). I have also **crossed out** the two numbers for the alternatives I do NOT want. Again, I prefer alternative: [____] (*Write in 1, 2 or 3.*)

X_____ **Date:** __ / __ / ____
(*Recommended: Sign in front of a notary or two qualified witnesses.*)

How To Reduce Potential Challenges Based on the President's Council on Bioethics' "Moral Paternalism"

How to add to your "Empowering Statements for My Proxy": These three additional statements arose from my specific concern about the restrictive potential of The President's Council on Bioethics' report, "Taking Care."

1.   While one of my criteria for selecting my Proxies is *their* high morals, I do NOT want my Proxy to judge the morality of *my* end-of-life decisions. I have already taken into consideration MY moral beliefs when I was competent as I completed my advance care planning. Refusing treatment is legal.

2.   I want others to consider the wishes I have previously expressed as DURABLE. I firmly believe that my life trajectory is determined by the continuity of my mind and not my body; hence, I want the decisions I made when my mind was competent to influence my Proxy in the future, if my mind can then no longer make medical decisions. It is for this precise reason that I created my Advance Directives. I hereby forbid others to argue otherwise. If others sincerely feel that I have made a mistake or oversight in describing my wishes, either in my writing or discussions—then I instruct my Proxy to inform them that I was and I am prepared to suffer the consequences. I recognize and accept the price of freedom, which has always been to suffer the consequences of making the wrong choice.

3.   Contrary to some of the moral views expressed in the President's Council on Bioethics, I DO believe that it IS not only acceptable but also in my "Best Interest" under some circumstances (which I have authorized my Proxy to determine) "to engineer" the hastening of my dying by refusing treatment. I do NOT believe this is the same as abandoning me or killing me. For example, I believe my existence should end even if my body is not terminally ill if I have lost all the human qualities of thinking, memory, and communication and my existence is characterized by suffering, indignity, and dependency. I have also instructed my Proxy to consider if maintaining my biological existence imposes huge economic and emotional burdens to my family and society, and if, given the scarcity of resources, these resources could better be used to help the poor and sick both in this country and around the world. These are some but not all of MY reasons for refusing what some people may call "ordinary care," which decision I authorize my Proxy to make on my behalf. For example, my Proxy may decide to Refuse Food & Fluid on my behalf.

(Note: To add statements to a document that you previously had witnessed or notarized, you should also have the addition witnessed or notarized.)

45. How Do I Create an Advance Directive That Grants My Proxy Maximum Power?

[FORM IV: Please Honor My Proxy's Decisions]

Cautionary Notes (see also "Disclaimers" in Chapter 1)

1. This **Proxy Directive** form is designed to stimulate discussion and/or to serve as a starting point to create an **Advance Directive** that will satisfy the law in your State. It is NOT a complete form. It is NOT ready for you to sign and to have witnessed by individuals who satisfy the criteria set forth in your State's statutes (laws), which criteria are often strict. (An alternative is often a Notary).

2. Before you decide to include some suggested wording below, consult with medical and legal advisors in your State about your specific situation and goals. They may suggest modifying some statements, including additional ones, and comment on including **Empowering Statements for my Proxy**.

3. This form is offered in the context of the strategies explained in the book, **The BEST WAY to Say Goodbye**, which in turn result from Dr. Stan Terman's understanding of the typically encountered end-of-life clinical challenges and the way courts have interpreted the relevant laws.

4. Consider this form if you trust your first choice Proxy and alternates and want to grant them maximum power, OR if you lack trust in the effectiveness of **Living Wills** that depend on your future doctor (whom you may not presently know) to interpret what you wrote in the way you intended, without further input from a decision-making designated Proxy.

   Consider instead creating a Living Will (**Directive to Physician**) if your doctor has given you a diagnosis of a serious terminal illness and agrees to care for you as long as you need it, and assures that your end-of-life decisions will be honored. (See the story of "Joyce" on page 383, and Living Will on page 259.)

5. There are other ways to balance the distribution of power between your Proxies, your doctor, and your Living Will, including the granting of "Leeway," which is yet another reason to discuss all options with your local, personal advisors.

6. Most States permit both a Living Will and a Proxy Directive. If there is a conflict between these two, State laws will determine which document overrides the other unless you specify otherwise. The form below empowers the Proxy.

7. This Advance Directive does not cover: your choice of a court-appointed conservator of a person; authorizations for organ donation; decisions about religious ceremonies, burials versus cremation, or autopsies.

8. Item 12, "Proxy's Acceptance & Agreement," is recommended to help establish your Proxy's legal standing and to document convincingly, your wishes A) for aggressive pain control, and B) for your **Proxy to Withhold Food & Fluid**.

Please Honor My Proxy's Decisions

1. Designation of Proxy and Alternates:

A) I _____ (your name) designate the following individual as my Proxy to make health care decisions for me:

Name: _____

Relationship: _____

Address: _____

Telephone numbers: _____

B) ALTERNATE PROXY (optional): **If** I revoke my Proxy's authority or if my Proxy is not reasonably *able*, not reasonably *willing*, or not reasonably *available* to make a health care decision for me—where "reasonably" is determined by the primary physician who is currently responsible for providing my medical treatment, **then** I designate as my first alternate Proxy:

Name: _____

Relationship: _____

Address: _____

Telephone numbers: _____

Note: This statement gives your primary treating physician the power to make such determinations as: "Your first choice Proxy does not possess the mental ability to make medical decisions." Or, "Your first choice Proxy is reluctant, hesitant, procrastinating, too far away, or just not responsive."

*If your first choice Proxy believes your physician's disqualification is in error, your first choice Proxy could demand to transfer your care to **another physician**, and this physician may be willing to continue to permit your first choice Proxy to remain as your decision-maker. If the second physician also* *wishes to disqualify your first choice Proxy, then your first choice Proxy could ask for a consultation from the **institution's ethics committee**.*

*If there is no ethics committee in your institution, as in many skilled nursing facilities, your first choice Proxy could contact the institution's **ombudsman,** or consult with an **elder law attorney**.*

If the second physician and the ethics committee agree, however, then perhaps it would be best for your second choice Proxy to assume the authority for making your medical decisions. While this protocol may seem cumbersome, obtaining these consultations is typically far more expedient than going to court.

C) SECOND ALTERNATE PROXY (optional): If I revoke the authority of my Proxy and first alternate Proxy, or if they both are not reasonably *able*, not reasonably *willing*, or not reasonably *available* to make a health care decision for me—where "reasonably" is determined by the primary physician who is currently responsible for providing my medical treatment, then I designate as my second alternate Proxy:

Name: _____

Relationship: _____

Address: _____

Telephone numbers: _____

2. Authorizations:

My Proxy is authorized to A) make all health care decisions for me, including decisions to **Withhold or to Withdraw Food & Fluid**—whether administered through any type of tube or line that enters my gastro-intestinal tract or my circulatory system, or by assisted oral feeding by another's hand that requires that I swallow—and to make all decisions regarding withholding or withdrawing of all other forms of potentially life-sustaining treatment; B) to choose a particular physician and health care facility; and C) to receive or to consent to the release of medical information and records, except as I state below:

Note: You may wish to RESTRICT your Proxy's authority; for example:

"I ALWAYS want to be provided with Food & Fluid by another's hand through my mouth, even if I fight my caregivers and I must be physically restrained as they try to feed me"; OR,

"I ALWAYS want to be provided Food & Fluid unless doing so increases my pain and suffering, or my body is physically unable to absorb Food & Fluid so that they provide no benefit, or I am currently in the process of dying."

[On the lines below, write your desired **restriction**, any other instruction you wish to substitute, or these words: "**No restriction.**"]

_____

_____

Note: The goal of the following *statement is to reduce your future physician's anxiety about a possible lawsuit or regulatory investigation. In our litigious environment, this statement should decrease your physician's fears so that he or she will neither increase nor prolong your pain and suffering:*

I authorize my Proxy to direct my physician to administer sufficient medication for pain relief or other suffering, even if there is a risk of my becoming addicted to those medications, and/or even if there is a possible but unintended side effect that the administration of such medications may hasten my death.

*[Note: **DO NOT LEAVE THIS LINE BLANK**. Either write, "**No restriction,**" or write whatever restriction(s) you prefer in this part of your authorization.]*

3-a. My Proxy's Authority Becomes Effective IMMEDIATELY. ___ *(Initials)*

OR

3-b. Alternative: *You can choose to have your Proxy's authority become effective only after ONE or TWO [indicate which] physicians or psychiatrists or psychologists [indicate which]—who are experienced in the assessment of decision-making capacity [indicate how much experience]—agree that you no longer have that mental capacity.* ___ **(Your initials either here OR in 3-a.)**

Please first read the explanation that follows; then either write the word "IMMEDIATELY," or state your of choices from 3-b. Also INITIAL above.

Note: As long as you possess the mental capacity to make medical decisions, you can always veto what your Proxy says; hence, there is no disadvantage to the "immediately" option. There are however five advantages to empowering your Proxy immediately:

A) You can learn how your Proxy tends to make medical decisions on your behalf. If you are not satisfied and you are still competent, you can remove him or her and designate another person to be your first choice Proxy. For example, you might discover that your Proxy imposes his or her values instead of being the champion of yours, or that he or she gets into power-seeking conflicts with your physicians that do not seem to resolve.

B) Your Proxy can learn about the specific duties and obligations of serving in the role of Proxy. This can be very important for individuals who have never before served as a Proxy, which is often the case when relatives are designated as Proxies. Better to learn without the stress of urgently needing to make a critical life-determining decision.

C) It is less of a hurdle for your Proxy to learn about your current medical condition by obtaining your medical records and by speaking to your doctors, since HIPAA privacy rules would not restrict your Proxy's access to them.

D) You may save critical time as well as some expense and possible controversy, which might even escalate to court hearings, by avoiding the requirement to establish that you have lost decision-making capacity.

E) Your energy and even your capacity to make medical decisions may fluctuate frequently during an illness (for example, if your temperature goes up and down, dramatically), and you may feel overwhelmed by the challenges of obtaining the best possible medical care, even though for some parts of some days, you can still make your own medical decisions. In such cases, you may find it very helpful to have a caring person serve as your collaborating advocate, which the "effective immediately" option permits.

Note: While about one-third of States explicitly permit your Proxy's authority to begin immediately, you should check with an attorney in your State to make sure this option is allowed. It may still be possible to honor this arrangement if all concerned agree, including doctors, relatives, and other interested parties.

*If your choice is 3-b rather than **IMMEDIATELY**, indicate **YOUR** specifics here:*

_____

_____

4. How my Proxy knows what I would want:

First, my Proxy shall make all reasonable attempts to determine what my current wishes are, rather than assume that I can no longer communicate. As long as I can indicate "Yes" or "No"—even if only by squeezing a hand, or by blinking my eye, I want all concerned to have the patience to ask me what I want. In other words, please "listen" to me even if I can only express myself one letter at a time. My Proxy may also decide to ask experts to employ **enhancement technology** (for example, muscle amplifiers and EEGs), if they seem appropriate. My Proxy may also consider using questionnaires similar to those that appear in the book, **The *BEST WAY* to Say Goodbye**, such as "Questions to determine if a brain-damaged person can consistently respond to his or her environment," and "A 'Yes' / 'No' conversation to make sure." If issues related to my Last Wishes were not previously asked and answered, then my Proxy might help me to create an additional document called **Empowering Statements for My Proxy**, and use any questions that seem appropriate from "A Guide for a Difficult Discussion," from this book.

Please also listen to me, even if I have been given a diagnosis of Alzheimer's disease or another dementia, or if I have suffered another kind of brain damage. Please do not assume that I cannot make such decisions unless a mental health professional with experience in evaluating decision-making capacity determines that I no longer possess that cognitive ability. As long as I can remember the relevant facts long enough to understand the alternative choices, appreciate their consequences, and use logical reasoning to express a consistent choice, I want others to honor my wishes. Also keep in mind that I may be capable of making certain kinds of decisions but not other kinds of decisions. For example, I may wish to change my first choice Proxy or the sequence of alternate Proxies for sound reasons, while I may not be able to make more complex treatment decisions based on specific hypothetical medical contingencies.

Note: Others may in the future challenge this document on the basis of whether or not you possessed the ability to make medical treatment decisions when you signed it. It is therefore prudent to attach the opinion of a mental health professional who has experience in performing evaluations on decision-making capacity after he or she interviews you, especially if you have a diagnosis that affects your ability to think or remember (cognition). Ideally, this evaluation should be close to the time you signed this form. Such a documented opinion may prevent future controversy, expense, and delay of honoring your wishes. Although most State laws assume adults were competent unless someone raised the issue when the document was signed, the argument that a life is at stake may persuade judges to hear the case.

Generally, my Proxy shall make health care decisions for me based on his or her knowledge of my values and wishes gained from our discussing my end-of-life treatment values and preferences. I fully understand that it is my responsibility to initiate such a discussion with my Proxy and alternate Proxies so that they learn this information. Otherwise, my Proxy will have to make end-of-life decisions based on the "Best Interest" standard.

Note: If you expect to have a long-term relationship with a particular physician, you should invite him or her to participate in the discussion of your treatment values and preferences, indicate that he or she has reviewed this document and has agreed to place the document in your medical chart.

Note: Even if your physician agrees as above, your Proxies must still accept the responsibility to present this document at the time and place (e.g., the hospital) where critical medical decisions must be made on your behalf—just in case this doctor and/or your medical chart are not "reasonably" available.

Note: It is your responsibility to inform all *your Proxies and other interested people about your end-of-life wishes. If your wishes are challenged, courts may hold your expression of end-of-life wishes to the high standard of proof called* **clear and convincing**; *hence, the following is highly recommended:*

I attach to this **Proxy Directive**, a document called "**Empowering Statements for My Proxy**" that may include several sections such as General Statements About Empowering My Proxy & Specific Statements About Refusing Food & Fluid (as on pages 236-239); Preferences About When to "Permit Natural Dying" (as on pages 395-398); and how to reduce other challenges (as on page 399). The suggested wording on how to interpret primitive reflexes, my answers to any questionnaire, and any other statement I have made, as well as any examples I have cited such as my feelings about movies, books, plays, or summaries of clinical and legal cases where the patient's wishes were or were not honored, are intended ONLY to guide my Proxy's decisions, NOT to set the bar for others to judge those decisions. I want to emphasize the importance of my wish that others NOT compare my Proxy's decisions with what I wrote in these attached statements. I trust my Proxy to interpret my wishes and I want others to honor those decisions. Conflict is more likely to Delay that granting of my Last Wishes. I trust that my Proxy understands my Last Wishes and has agreed to honor them. See also Item # 12, below.

5. Why I Do Not Have a Living Will (Directive to Physician):

My Advance Directive has no "Living Will," sometimes called "Health Care Instructions" or "Medical Treatment Directive," because I want to give maximum power to my Proxy to make health care decisions on my behalf, based on my future condition, prognosis, and the current state of medical science—all of which I cannot with certainty, predict at this time.

6. If I Decide that I Do Want a Living Will (Directive to Physician):

I still reserve the option to supplement this document with a **Living Will** (a **Directive to Physician**) in the future. If and when I do create such a document, then, unless I revoke this Advance Directive, all other statements herein, and all powers granted herein shall continue in effect.

7. If a Conflict Arises Between My Proxy's Decision and the Specific Instructions in my Living Will (Directive to Physician):

If I have created a Living Will, and an "interested party" interprets what I have written in this Living Will as being in conflict with my Proxy's CURRENT decision, then I want my Proxy's CURRENT decision to OVERRIDE what I wrote in my living will, and how they interpret what I have previously written elsewhere in this Advance Directive or in other relevant documents.

*[Important note: Do **NOT** include this statement unless you TRUST your Proxy.]*

8. I Wish My Proxy to Consult the Following People:

I have respect for certain people either because they know me well or they have knowledge or experience in the challenging area of making end-of-life decisions. Although I do not require my Proxy to consult with these individuals, nor do I insist that my Proxy follow their specific recommendations, I list their names as they may help ease the burden and help guide my Proxy's decision-making.

[Write the word "**NONE**" if no person in any particular category exists.]

A) My doctor(s): _____,

B) My attorney(s): _____,

C) My religious or spiritual leader(s): _____,

D) My counselor or social worker: _____,

E) These relatives: _____,

F) These close friends: _____,

G) My caregiver or hospice nurse: _____, and

H) My "end-of-life consultant": _____

who is a member of the organization called, _____.

(If the above named individual from this organization is not able, willing, or available, then my Proxy may consult another professional from this organization, as authorized by a supplemental form that is attached.)

I) Other individuals: _____ .

9. Individuals who I do not want to speak for me:

I Do NOT want the following people to speak for me in any role, whether as alternate Proxy, Surrogate, or court-appointed guardian, not do I want them to be notified about my Last Wishes. Unless these lines below are left blank, the names and the relationships of the people I do not want to speak for me are:

1. _____

2. _____

10. Regarding my right to have others review my Proxy's decisions:

I have [__] / have not [__] attached an additional form that my attorney has also signed, which waives my right to have my Proxy's decisions reviewed in a court of law.

I do [__] / do not [__] permit my Proxy to ask for opinions by religious leaders.

I do [__] / do not [__] permit my Proxy to ask for opinions by other individuals or committees, as indicated below:

_____

11. Regarding the confidentiality of my medical records:
I want my Proxy to have access to my medical records so I have signed the necessary State and Federal forms, including those required by HIPAA, regarding waiving confidentiality.

Signed: _____ Dated: __ / __ / __

Note: In most states, documents such as this become valid when signed and stamped by a Notary Public, some of whom make home or institutional visits. If you prefer to have your signature witnessed, check with the specific requirements of your State, which may be strict. (Your doctor, those who will inherit your estate, and the owner of your institution are typically excluded.)

12. Acceptance & Agreement: I accept & agree to serve as your Proxy:

[*Note: Item 12 is strongly recommended. Each Proxy should sign a separate sheet, but may do so at a time different from when you signed, above:*]

I have received a copy of the most recently revised Advance Directive of

_____ (the "requesting person"), dated, __ / __ / __ .

I have read and I understand this document, which designates me to serve as one of the Proxies to make medical decisions for the "requesting person,"

_____ when he or she no longer has the ability to make medical decisions,

OR

_____ immediately. [**Check one**.]

I agree to serve in the capacity of Proxy in good faith and to act consistently with the "requesting person's" desires, values, and preferences, based on my discussions with him or her, and the documents that he or she has or will provide to me. In so doing, I realize that I may have to put aside the particular medical decisions that I would have made for myself. Instead, I will try to make the decisions that I have come to appreciate that he or she would have made, which is called the **Substituted Judgment** standard of decision-making. I will try my best to consult with the people he or she has listed when I must make an end-of-life decision, although I realize I am neither obligated to do so, nor required to follow their advice.

If I must make a medical decision for which I do not have enough information about his or her desires, values and preferences, then I will make such medical decisions based on what is considered the **Best Interest** standard of decision-making.

I realize that as long as the "requesting person" has the ability to make decisions, he or she may make his or her own decisions and revoke the authorization of me as his or her Proxy. If I learn that he or she has revoked my authority as Proxy, or that he or she has revoked this Advance Directive, I will inform his or her current health care provider, if known to me.

Proxy's statement regarding values and convictions:

If I am called on to perform the role of Proxy for the "requesting person," my values and convictions will NOT prevent me from asking for either:

A) Sufficient medication to reduce pain, even if so doing may possibly lead to the unintended side effect of hastening death; or,

B) Refusal of Food & Fluid, even by manual assistance through the mouth, if the specific criteria previously described and discussed with me by the "requesting person" are, in my opinion, met.

Confirmation by the requesting person:

As the "requesting person," I initial here _____ to indicate that I DO |__| DO NOT |__| authorize my Proxy to ask for "A," above.

As the "requesting person," I initial here _____ to indicate that I DO |__| DO NOT |__| authorize my Proxy to ask for "B," above.

Signed: _____ (**Proxy**) Dated: __ / __ / __

Credit: While Dr. Stanley Terman takes full responsibility for the final form of this document, he wishes to acknowledge with appreciation, the valuable input and suggestions he received from Attorney Michael Evans, Dr. Ronald Baker Miller, and Attorney Charles Sabatino.

Conclusion

RESPECTING THE SANCTITY OF *MANY* LIVES

The greatest insult to the sanctity of life is indifference or
laziness in the fact of its complexity. —Ronald Dworkin

Should all patients—including the comatose who cannot feel pain, and the demented who cannot recognize their loved ones—be biologically maintained for as long as medical technology permits? Survey responses and individual choices in Advance Directives reflect the way most people answer: "No." How then should physicians respond? In 1984, the New England Journal of Medicine published "The Physician's Responsibility Toward Hopelessly Ill Patients" [Wanzer and others, 1984]. These ten authors stated that, if the prognosis of unconsciousness is known with a high degree of medical certainty, and the patient's and family's wishes are consistent, then "Naturally or artificially administered hydration and nutrition may be given or withheld... It is morally justifiable to allow the patient to die."

Is **Withholding or Refusing Food & Fluid** consistent with the *sanctity of life*? My answer is: Yes. Beyond that, such acts may respect the sanctity not just of *one* life but of *many* lives.[1] Ronald Dworkin book, *Life's Dominion* [1993] defined *sanctity* as the inviolability of human life based on its *intrinsic* character, as distinguished from usefulness to others or subjective experience. To respect the sanctity of **one** person's life requires that others respond in ways that are consistent with the integrity and dignity of the person's *character of life* taken as a whole. I suggest expanding the concept to the *sanctity of **many** lives* by embracing the fourth principle of medical ethics: Social justice recognizes that every human being has basic rights so the distribution of financial and medical resources should be fair.

----

1. Some religious leaders may object to comparing the cost of maintaining one life to potentially saving thousands of other lives based on the belief that every life is sacred. They may state it is not for man to judge which lives are more valuable. They may even consider the term, "sanctity of *many* lives," an oxymoron. Ronald Dworkin emphasizes that the intrinsic inviolable aspect of lives refers only to lives that already exist; it places *no* value on increasing the number of lives. I admit the term is a bit of a stretch but I resisted Michael S. Evans' suggestion to use instead, "distributive justice." I prefer *"sanctity of **many** lives"* as it may be provocative to the patient-centered paradigm that makes little or no allowance for the fact that the lives of others, for example African children, are also *sacred* but are rarely considered when making such decisions.

To illustrate that Advance Directives can be "moral documents" and respect the sanctity of *many* lives, I quote from my "Empowering Statements for My Proxy" section of my Proxy Directive. In following this book's advice to explain my choices, I will cite cases to illustrate: Terry Wallis, "Margo," and Bob Stern.

In 1984, Terry Wallis fell into a coma after his car crashed. Doctors predicted he would never speak again, but his mother never gave up hope. In 2006, Mr. Wallis said, "Mum" and "Pepsi." Although he could later utter short sentences, for clarity he still preferred to spell out words, letter by letter. His memory remained spotty, however, and he was paralyzed below the neck. For his continued existence, he remained totally dependent upon others to provide care.

After citing the case of Terry Wallis, my Advance Directive states:

While people of faith may cite this "awakening" as a reason to hold on to hope in support of not judging the value or the prognosis of any human life, statisticians note such recovery is extremely rare. Scientists may cast doubt on the initial diagnosis. For example, Ramsøy [2006] considered the case "a sensational awakening of the science surrounding this patient, not the patient himself."

My preferences: I do *not* want to be maintained in a coma for a long time—even if my doctors could predict with 99% certainty that I would recover to a level of functioning similar to that achieved by Terry Wallis after ten or twenty years. Instead of spending about $100,000 a year to maintain me in a comatose or related medical state, I would prefer those funds be used for more beneficial programs. One example is to prevent malaria that kills millions of African children under the age of five.

I realize that the mechanism to reallocate these resources is a problem not yet solved, despite the efforts of non-profit foundations such as The Bill and Melinda Gates Foundation [Specter, 2005]. Yet once the money is spent on people in comas, it can no longer possibly purchase 10,000 mosquito nets that have the potential to save or protect the lives of about 4,000 children. (Mosquito nets cost $10 each and are 40% effective.)

A second case is the much-discussed story of "Margo" [starting on page 356], which raises the question, What is the appropriate response of caregivers and health care providers if a demented patient is still happy but meets his or her other criteria for withholding life-saving medical treatment, and Food & Fluid?

After citing Margo's case, my Advance Directive states:

My preferences: I want to receive only *Comfort Care* if I contract pneumonia after my doctors have confirmed the diagnosis of irreversible progressive dementia. Even though I may *then* seem happy, as I write this statement I am more concerned about my subsequent life from that point on, and the many consequences of my disease. Another opportunity to let

Nature take its course may not come again for many months or years. Meanwhile, my dementia will continue to progress. It is likely that my mood would continue to change. Like many patients with dementia as my thinking ability diminishes, I might become scared, paranoid, horrified, delusional, depressed, apathetic, and/or withdrawn. I would also become an increasing financial and emotional burden to my loved ones. For these reasons, I have provided a separate list of behaviors to signal when my **Proxy should Refuse Food & Fluid** on my behalf [page 397]. But if I contract pneumonia or another life-threatening illness before I reach this behavioral state, then I want my Proxy to refuse aggressive medical treatment on my behalf.

I do NOT want anyone to override my Last Wishes by presuming he or she knows what my "Best Care" *is* in that moment. I do NOT want anyone to ask me *then* if I wish to receive potentially curative medical treatment. To explain: At that point, my incompetence would prohibit a fresh exercise of my autonomous right to make medical decisions. Hence, my *precedent autonomy* (the precise words I am NOW writing) would still apply. In other words, I want others to consider these Last Wishes as *durable*. I ask others not to interpret my present request of my Proxy as a cruel or discriminating act or one that lacks compassion for my future self. Instead, consider this example: Although I might have seemed happy *when* I contracted pneumonia, *were* I forced to receive antibiotic treatment and survived, in a few months my behavior could become so deranged that it would be dangerous for me to live at home. I might set a fire, or hurt myself and neighbors in other ways. At that point, I should be placed in an institution, even if I made clear and consistent demands to live in my own home again. Just as others should deny my request to live at home, they should deny my request for liquids, especially since *symptoms of thirst* are easily treated.

I must admit that, initially, my family found it difficult to accept my decision, so I provided these additional details, to explain:

1) The burdens of medical interventions are difficult to predict for patients who suffer from dementia. "A demented patient who is accustomed to one environment will have a much harder time adjusting to hospitalization and may need *restraints* in order to undergo even something as *simple* as intravenous *antibiotic therapy*" [Drickamer, 2006]. {Emphasis added.}

2) The presence of other serious medical conditions, called *co-morbidity*, can be quantified by such indices as the Chronic Disease Score [Boulos and others, 2006]) and Total Illness Burden Index [Steir and others, 1999]. For some diseases, such as prostate cancer, aggressive curative treatment significantly increases the risk of adverse outcomes, including death. The relative benefit can be compared by quantifying outcome as Quality of Life

[Bayliss and others, 2005].

3) Considered together, the above two points more than validate, they refine the proposal of Daniel Callahan's 1987 Pulitzer Prize-winning book, *Setting Limits, Medical Goals in an Aging Society*. Callahan used the gross criterion of age by suggesting "late 70s or early 80s" be a "cut off point" to consider NOT spending huge sums for medical treatment if the goal is to extend life. Yet when Callahan attempts the more difficult definition of what it means to be "a person," he suggests "we should give the benefit of the doubt to those who display [only] evidence of self-enclosed emotions" even if they have lost the other two qualities of personhood; namely, "the capacities to reason and to enter into relationships" [*his Page 179-180*].

As a person and psychiatrist, I respectfully disagree with Dr. Callahan. The subjective experience of emotions "in the here and now" without any appreciation of biographical history or future, without any ability to make decisions, and without any ability to relate to loved ones who can be remembered as such, would for me not be "a person" whose continued existence I would wish funds be spent to maintain. Also, I do not value emotions evoked by internal hallucinations that have no basis in reality. What reality do I value? The reality that my competent self appreciates now, as I contemplate these future possibilities that lead me to write these words.

4) Finally, although this book has strived to devise "an ironclad strategy for dementia" by **Refusal of Food & Fluid by Proxy**, it may be kinder to my caregivers if they do NOT treat my pneumonia when it occurs, instead of offering me treatment now and **Withholding Food & Fluid** later. To be clear, I am making the assumption that my Proxy will overcome all challenges to the honoring of my Last Wishes, in contrast with Bob Stern's lack of confidence that led him to decide to die prematurely as related on page 327. I am also predicting that my careful wording of my "Empowering Statements for My Proxy" will be adequate to eliminate my caregivers' guilt. Still, another year or two of caregiving would add to my loved ones' burden. It would affect them emotionally, financially, and socially.

Here I wish to note the sad story of my charming and gregarious friend. Being a young-in-spirit 85-year-old, I asked "Henry" to explain why, despite many attractive offers, he seemed uninterested in any romantic relationship. He answered, "For three years, I cared for my wife who had advanced Alzheimer's disease. I paid my dues. I would never want to go through that again. Nor would I would want any one else to have to do that for me."

My Advance Directive then explains (perhaps somewhat repetitiously):

I referred to the cases of "Margo" and Bob Stern to express my Last Wishes *clearly and convincingly*. I explicitly want others to consider them *durable*. I do NOT want others to override my Last Wishes by imposing their moral or clinical views of my "Best Care" or "Best Interests." I view my Advance Directive as a "moral document" and I consider my own experience of future enjoyment as a lower priority than these two goals: to lessen the burdens on my loved ones and to allocate fairly our world's scarce medical and financial resources. Compared to saving the lives of children under the age of 5, I would forego the limited pleasure of tasting ice cream and applesauce if I can no longer recognize and communicate with my loved ones, or remember who I am.

It was Ronald M. Dworkin who coined the term, "precedent autonomy." The Frank Henry Sommer Professor of Law, New York University and Quain Professor of Jurisprudence, University College London, wrote the book, *Life's Dominion* [1993], in which he argued, "Our opinions about how and why our *own* lives have intrinsic value influence every major decision we make about how we live" [*his Page 155*], and, "...It makes no sense to ask whether it feels worse to be permanently unconscious or wholly demented or dead. We must ask instead about the *retrospective* meaning of death or the diminution of life, about *how the last stage of a life affects its overall character*." {Emphasis added.} (I would add: ...and how others remember that life.) Professor Dworkin thus emphasized a standard to judge lives: "not just by reckoning overall sums of pleasure or enjoyment or achievement, but more structurally, as we judge a literary work, for example, whose *bad ending mars what went before*" [*Page 27*].

Dworkin wrote, "Someone who thinks his own life would go worse if he lingered near death on a dozen machines for weeks or stayed biologically alive for years as a vegetable believes he is showing more respect for the human contribution to the sanctity of his life if he makes arrangements in advance to avoid that, and that others show more respect for his life if they avoid it for him... he thinks dying is the best way to respect the inviolability of human life" [*Page 216*].

Dworkin distinguished among three values of life: *subjective, instrumental,* and *intrinsic*. The subjective relates to current experience. The instrumental relates to our utility to others. Dworkin believed the intrinsic value is what makes our lives inviolable and sacred. The moral obligation to *sanctity of life* imposes the responsibility that we should always consider with deep moral reflection, whether or not to hasten dying. [*his Pages 72-5*.]

Dworkin offered deep insight into the essence of the moral controversy over hastening dying. He focused on different kinds of *frustration* to explain people's divergent views about making end-of-life decisions. Some people believe that *frustration* of **human contribution** (what we humans can do) is most important. Others believe instead that *frustration* of **natural investment** (what Nature or a Supreme Being can do) is paramount. The first group is open to hasten dying if a patient's prolonged suffering is unbearable. The second group considers life as God's gift, which man is obligated to maintain as long as possible. Both perspectives embrace a *"sanctity of life,"* yet they mandate different actions.

With respect to the role of government, Dworkin asks, "Does a decent government attempt to dictate to its citizens what intrinsic values they will recognize, and why, and how?" This "legal question...is the deepest and most important Constitutional question raised by the abortion [and euthanasia] controvers[ies]" [*Page 117*]. Granted, the "State has an intrinsic interest in 'protecting human life,' [but this] might describe either of two goals... One is the goal of **responsibility**... the second is the goal of **conformity**. [These two goals] are not only different but antagonistic. If we aim at [moral] responsibility, we must leave citizens free to decide as they think right. If we aim at conformity, we demand that citizens act in a way that might be contrary to their own moral convictions, which discourages rather than encourages them to develop their own sense of when and why life is sacred" [*Page 150*]. Since (again), "Our opinions about how and why our *own* lives have intrinsic value influence every major decision we make about how we live" [*Page 155*], Dworkin warns: "**Making someone die in a way that others approve, but he believes a horrifying contradiction of his life, is a devastating, odious form of tyranny**" [*Page 217*, emphasis added].

According to Kevin Phillips, a former republican strategist and the author of *American Theocracy* [2006], religious fundamentalism was already on the rise in America before George W. Bush took office in 2001, although its influence has since accelerated to unprecedented proportions. The administration's position is reflected in The President's Council on Bioethics' report, *Taking Care: Ethical Caregiving In Our Aging Society* [2005]. The report *encourages* others to disrespect the Last Wishes of vulnerable incompetent patients, even if they were clearly and convincingly written when competent and with full appreciation that they were giving informed consent for limiting their *future* treatment. The Council's report takes the impassioned view that it is **immoral to create** an Advance Directive that requests letting Nature take its course by refusing future treatment because, in their opinion, it *discriminates* against a future *disabled* (*demented*) self. The Council's report also considers it **immoral** for Proxies, loved ones, caregivers, and health care providers **to respond** to such written requests. They thus insist (as discussed on pages 356 and 362), that if Margo were happy, we must treat her pneumonia, regardless of her previously written Advance Directives. Then, the report continues by arguing that treatment should not depend on a person's perceived mood or "well-being." In a November 2006 PBS TV broadcast, "Living Old," Dr. Leon Kass, chair of the President's Council for the *Taking Care* report, popularized his admonitions: "...for most of the decisions of long-term care, you can't write those things," and, "It's simply not true that we can know in advance how we ourselves will feel about many of these things."

So far, the doctrine of separation of power is working, albeit slowly. Florida's Supreme Court ruled that "Terri's Law-I" was unconstitutional in granting power to Governor Jeb Bush to reinsert her feeding tube. The U.S. Supreme Court later refused to reconsider evidence mandated by the U.S. Congress, which passed "Terri's Law-II." A Federal judge opined the law was unconstitutional. Yet State legislators who wish to coerce others to conform to their view of *sanctity of life* may still pass new laws. One agenda of the National Right to Life Committee is for States to pass laws that would make it illegal for physicians to **Withdraw artificially administered Food & Fluid**, even from patients whose doctors consider treatment is a far greater *burden* than a *benefit*. The only exception that would be allowed is if the patient, when competent, had created a legally valid written Advance Directive that *clearly and convincingly* authorized such withdrawal. As of mid-2006, at least 23 States were considering adopting the "model law" of the National Right to Life Committee. The goal: **to disqualify your loved ones and your personal physician** from making certain treatment decisions, possibly forcing you to maintain your biologic existence even if all who know you best agree that is *not* what you would have wanted and is *not* in your best interest. Example: The family of Raymond Schwaed watched helplessly for months as he suffered agonizing pain because the State of New York already has such a law. They learned too late that, in New York State, written Advance Directives must specifically authorize **Withholding of Food & Fluid** for family members to have the legal right to make such decisions [Davis HL, 2006].

Meanwhile, those who wish to Liberalize the law about ending-of-life options received another blow: In June 2006, one vote on a legislative committee blocked further consideration of California's proposed "Compassionate Choices Act," which could have created a law similar to Oregon's Death With Dignity Act.

Summary: Powerful political-religious forces combined with advances in medical technology have created an unprecedented situation where all of us have much more to fear. Others may force us to exist in a prolonged state of total dependency and indignity, or to endure unbearable pain and suffering, even when there is no hope for our recovery.

Fortunately, as individuals we still have one other choice. The 1990 U.S. Supreme Court ruling in Cruzan recognized our Constitutional right to refuse medical treatment even if it hastens dying. The Court also ruled that artificially administered Food & Fluid is "medical treatment." Hence, **Voluntary Refusal of Food & Fluid** by competent patients is *already legal*. Reports by lucid patients, observers, my own personal trial, and the medical literature consistently support the notion that **Refusing Food & Fluid** *will be peaceful* for most people. New laws are not needed for competent people to exercise this choice, which has this built-in safety factor: the act requires the continual resolve of the person who is refusing to eat and drink. For competent people, the challenge is to educate them so that they do not choose to die prematurely by illegal or violent methods. For people who are worried about impending dementia, on the other hand, the challenge is greater: their Advance Directives must incorporate diligently crafted strategies to overcome known and potential challenges so that they can **Refuse Food & Fluid by Proxy** (by a Proxy Directive) or **Withhold Food & Fluid by Physician** (by a Living Will). The American Dietetic Association [Maillet and others, 2002] and Doctors Truog and Cochrane [2005], among others, make *no* distinction based on whether Food & Fluid are administered by tubes or mouth.

In his fine, early review, Dr. Ira Byock [1995] employed this logic: If patients **Refuse ORAL Food & Fluid**, then they must also refuse "non-oral (enteral or parenteral) alimentation and hydration." Since the latter *is* medical treatment, they are therefore refusing medical treatment. Dr. Byock also noted, "it must be remembered that the decision to prevent malnutrition or dehydration is a *de facto* decision to have the person die of something else." While certain types of dying (slipping into a coma from liver or kidney failure, or the anesthesia provided by an adequate dose of barbiturates) are obviously peaceful, other ways of dying, including pneumonia, may not be as peaceful as **Ceasing all Food & Fluid**.

It is worth the effort to educate people about these strategies since the option to **Cease Food & Fluid** is potentially available to far more people than the option of Physician-Hastened Dying. Paralyzed or otherwise physically disabled people can **Refuse Food & Fluid** as long as they are competent. Effective Proxy Directives and Living Wills can potentially save years of indignity and dependency for millions of people in end-stage dementia and those with severe brain damage. Exercising this option has the potential to save many billions of dollars as it frees caregivers to proceed with their lives. At the same time, it allows health care providers to administer treatment to others who can appreciate and benefit from their efforts.

We must all die someday, but the choices we make *now* about how we die, both as individuals and as a society, will make an enormous impact on our future. Our country's future economic soundness and our quality of life in this and subsequent generations depend upon the attitudes and policies that determine how much freedom we are allowed when we wish to make our end-of-life decisions. I hope our individual and political attitudes change quickly enough so our society reaches a *tipping point* before it reaches an economic *sinking point*.

To add a personal note: My heart saddens when I hear stories about prolonged suffering as loved ones stand by feeling helpless, or when I learn about acts of premature mercy killing. (Consider another example in the Epilogue). I shudder as I view an instructional video on how to place a plastic bag over one's head to accomplish "self-deliverance." As a psychiatrist, the big "win" for me is to interview people in the early stages of dementia and if I determine that they still possess decision-making capacity, then I can ask some critical questions. (Other professionals can also make this assessment.) If the patient can clearly, convincingly, and consistently respond, they are entitled to feel a broad sense of satisfaction from having set the stage for good things that say volumes about their character. They will have informed their families exactly what they want and have spared them worry and guilt. If they make certain choices, the intensity and duration of their own *future* suffering, indignity, and dependency will decrease or be avoided. Having made these choices, they can then enjoy greater *current* peace of mind. Irrespective of their specific choices, I will feel privileged to have been part of a process where they felt free to exercise their preferences.

While some readers may not do so, I consider the world's limited resources as I formulate my end-of-life decisions since I view Advance Directives as "moral documents." I hope my efforts at diligent, strategic advance care planning makes my departure from this world not only legal and peaceful for me, but also leaves the world a better place having conserved resources that others truly need.

Certainly, it is a challenge to describe precisely the medical and mental conditions for which we would prefer to hasten dying rather than to prolong our suffering and indignity. It is also not easy to select individuals who will effectively advocate our end-of-life decisions after we no longer can. But the greatest challenge before us is to educate more people to write more effective Advance Directives. Such an effort can have far reaching benefits that span from the individual to the global, from the alleviation of one human being's suffering to the creation of a world that is a healthier place for all. When we appreciate the far reaching consequences of our Advance Directives, when we consider the tasks of creating and responding to Advance Directives as "moral documents," then the stage will have been set for us to responsibly honor the *sanctity of **many** lives*.

Epilogue

From Assisted Suicide (Really Murder?)...
to as Long and as Fulfilling a Life as Possible;
The Seven Principles of End-of-Life Decision-Making

New York City;
January to July 1995:

George Delury, former editor of The World Almanac, served four months in jail after he pled guilty to "assisting [the] suicide" of his wife, Myrna Lebov. During his four months of incarceration, he wrote a book, ***But What If She Wants To Die?*** [1997]. Reading the book impressed me with the depth and duration of the couples' love and devotion. Married for 22 years and in relationship for 27, the last six years were marked by the husband's spending 24/7 as his wife's full-time caregiver. He had become responsible for all her bodily needs as she became disabled by crippling multiple sclerosis. Yet I was also concerned about facts revealed for the first time in the book. Subtitled *A Husband's Diary*, the book documented the enormous burden of caregiving, which might have led to a misguided choice to die. At best, the decision seemed "premature"; at worst, "premeditated murder." Depending on where the truth lies along this moral continuum, perhaps a different question would be more appropriate: ***Was it Really He Who Wanted Her to Die?***

Myrna Lebov's multiple sclerosis was so severe that she needed a wheelchair to ambulate. She required four or more catheterizations to void urine every day. She was depressed and believed her ability to think would become so progressively impaired that at some point, she would *not* be able either to ask for her husband's help or to participate as required, to hasten her dying. Furthermore, if her husband became incapable of serving as her caregiver, she would be "condemned" to the "prison" of a nursing home for a decade or more.

My interest in this case piqued for *heuristic* purposes. I hoped it would provoke the discovery of an effective way to evaluate end-of-life decisions. I wanted to form an opinion about the nature of Mr. Delury's conduct: Were his actions morally (not legally) equivalent to assisted suicide or to murder? Did Delury's underlying motivation serve primarily his own needs? Were his personal needs so overwhelming that his behavior, whether conscious or unconscious, qualified as psychological coercion or *undue influence*? ["Undue influence" deprives a person of freedom of choice when another person inappropriately influences the vulnerable person's choice.] What alternatives could be offered to similar couples who crumble under the extreme burdens of caregiving for chronic illnesses?

The facts of the case were complex so I invited input from two co-authors: medical ethicist and physician Ronald Miller, and attorney and social worker Michael Evans. As we considered this case, The Seven Principles of Good End-of-Life Decision-Making emerged as a useful framework to structure opinions regarding any end-of-life decision.

This Epilogue presents the general Seven Principles and then illustrates how they can be applied to answer this specific question: Did George Delury and Myrna Lebov make a "good" **ending-of-life** decision? (I take responsibility for forming and writing this final opinion about Delury and Lebov.)

Delury's *A Husband' Diary* details the last few months of his wife's life as she and he decided to hasten her death. Delury frankly reveals his contemporaneous feelings as events unfolded, including both his loving and self-serving sides. In addition to many passages that reflect endearing devotion, he shares such remarks as, "You are sucking my life out of me like a vampire and nobody cares" [*Page 145 of his book*].

Delury admits his intense ambivalence. Here is what he wrote on May 5: "My problem: if she asks for the poison now but seems very depressed, should I comply? Is she still autonomous? If I comply, I may be serving my own interests more than hers. If I don't, she may be losing her last chance to make the decision. She's mentioned July 4 as 'independence day,' a possible suicide date, but at the rate her mind is declining, she may not still be a whole, autonomous person by that time. I believe I will comply—on the rationale (rationalization?) that I will be saving her from a fate worse than death. (What an ironic cliché in this context!)" [*Page 155*]. Delury then presents his opinion: "Myrna's mind was being ravaged by MS."

Delury's apparent candor when others asked him about his wife's decision to die may have increased his credibility. His openness was also reflected in a TV interview when he admitted that when his wife talked about wanting to commit suicide, he "did not want to talk her out of it." Perhaps his *apparent* openness facilitated the success of his defense attorney during plea-bargaining, as Delury received a sentence of 6 *months* rather than 5 to 15 *years*.

Attorney Michael Evans noted diligence as the couple approached their end-of-life decision: 1) They discussed the issue over a long **time** and in **depth**; and 2) Myrna **consistently** wanted to die by asking help to hasten her death. Yet additional criteria emerged making these two factors necessary but not sufficient. The Guideline on page 427 presents The Seven Principles of Good End-of-Life

Decision-Making. Of the additional principles, one seemed especially critical: Was Myrna **consistent** about WHEN, as well as about HOW she wanted to die?

Attorney Evans noted that the couple began discussing the promise of a hastened death in 1979 [*Page 129*], when Myrna began to experience "hitting the wall" from nerve exhaustion. This was 6 years *after* she received the diagnosis of multiple sclerosis and 16 years *before* she died [*Page 74*]. Over the course of her illness, her symptoms had a roller-coaster pattern of severity. She tried to maintain hope that her functioning would improve but at the same time, weighed the pleasures and losses of living to develop her personal criteria for deciding when she would no longer want to continue living. The *Diary* reveals that despite Delury's pledge to help her die, he refused when he considered her request as *not* prudent; for example:

1. April 8, 1995 [*Page 148*]: "In one breath Myrna said she wanted to die as soon as possible, and the next expressed astonishment at the idea she might not be alive next week."

2. April 17, 1995 [*Page 149*]: After her scooter chair broke and needed $750 to repair, "...she objected to the idea of paying for the Rascal's repair and said she wanted to check out [i.e., hasten her death] tonight. She seemed a little miffed and disappointed when I [Delury] said I wouldn't help on a spur-of-the-moment decision."

3. April 24, 1995 [*Page 152*]: "before she washed up for bed, Myrna said, 'I'm so scared. My mind is a mess. I want to die.' I [Delury] said, 'You're in a down period. Give it a week or two.'"

4. May 20, 1995 [*Pages 156-7*]: "Myrna said she wants to kill herself tonight. She was very serious, asking me detailed questions about how the process would be handled, how long it would take, whether I would make sure she is dead, how will I know, etc... Speaking of the poisonous concoction I've made, she said, 'That's a real solution.'...Later in the evening... she said over and over again that she wanted to die, but at the same time went over and over details that were generally trivial or irrelevant." She wanted so much to die at that point that I had to almost force her to wash up... Why didn't I urge it [death] on her? Because it was fruitless to urge her to do anything significant. But also it was not the pre-set date, which indicated that she was acting on the spur of the moment... and was so ambivalent and focused on trivia."

5. May 25, 1995 [*Pages 158-9*]: "After [relatives] left, Myrna spoke to me in great earnestness about killing herself. I told her I was very reluctant to help when she is dysphoric [depressed mood]... later [she began] speaking again about doing it tonight [and] what I would do to guarantee her death."

In contrast, the note of May 27, 1995 [*Page 159*] indicates an inconsistency: "Myrna's mood was erratic...assertive...forward-looking and without any indication that she wants to die...she suggested that I was the only one who wanted her to die." (The next day the couple went to see the Cirque du Soleil.)

6. May 31, 1995 [*Page 162*]: "Myrna surprised me by saying, 'I'm going to end it tonight or tomorrow night.' She is now trying to write a goodbye note to [her sister] Beverly. And apparently she did write a note. Months later, parts of the May 31 note were published after the D.A. released it to the press."

So six *Diary* entries provide evidence of consistency, about HOW Myrna wanted to die. Yet the entry of May 27, and certain other behavior such as insisting they attend the Cirque du Soleil performance, provide evidence against such consistency. But the six also support Delury's prudent refusal to help his wife die when he considered her request as "spur of the moment," or if her mood seemed "very strange" [*Page 162*]. The last entry refers to a note that clearly explained Myrna's motivation. It was found by the District Attorney's office on Myrna's word processor and released for publication nearly six months later. Addressed to her sister, Beverly, this note stated:

"My life is over. It's time to end it. I'm tired of bodily functions being my major concern, Peeing dominates my day...*still* have occasional accidents... worry a lot about having more. Even worse...a [bowel movement] in public, like in the swimming pool. Or on the bus... How helpless I've become! I can't cut my food, touch-type, wipe my ass, turn over in bed, travel by myself, etc... Translation: No freedom. I've been trapped in my life, with no escape—except suicide...I can't go on" [*Pages 175-6*].

About this statement Delury wrote, "the note was found on Myrna's word processing disk and was apparently never sent, because Beverly denied having seen it and questioned its authenticity" [*Page 175*]. Delury explained, "I would hope that the very plain language of the note would help authenticate it. I would not have put some of those words in Myrna's mouth" [*Page 176*].

Regarding the night Delury helped his wife die, he wrote: "I brought her a suicide note I had prepared in case she didn't do one herself... created on my computer, not on [her] word processor... She glanced at it and scribbled a signature as best she could" [*Pages 173-4*]. As the only witness, Delury reported Myrna's last spoken words prior to ingesting the lethal solution: "I am bored with my bodily functions and my mind is going. It's better to end it now, while I still can do something" [*Page 175*].

One point struck me as critically important. After he had paid for his crime by serving his prison sentence and could not be prosecuted again due to the Fifth Amendment's prohibition about "double jeopardy," Delury revealed in the *Diary,* the **true cause of his wife's death**. Compare these two accounts:

When questioned by police on the day of her death, as reported in the New York Times, Delury claimed that "he checked her at 5:30 A.M. and found 'no signs of life'" [James, 1995]. The New York Times published several entries from Delury's (not yet published) diary on December 12, 1995, including:

> "5:30 A.M. Slept through the alarm [referring to himself].
> It's over [referring to his wife]. Myrna is dead. Desolation."

In contrast, *But What if She Wants to Die?* reveals these additional details:

"Myrna has just consumed...about fourteen ounces of liquid, about half of what [he] had prepared" [*Page 175*]... "When I woke up later, much as I feared, Myrna was still breathing. I was confident that the solution would work sooner or later, but if it was later...I would be placing her [Gloria, the health aide] in an intolerable moral dilemma." She was "due to arrive at 8:00 A.M... I could not take the chance that Myrna could be 'revived' with who knows what kind of brain damage. I had promised her the suicide would be successful. So I steeled myself to do what I most feared doing, feared because of the probable psychological consequences and the legal questions if it were discovered. I went to the drawer where I had put some two-gallon plastic bags, put one bag inside the other, and picked up a piece of ribbon. I went to Myrna and, without changing her position on the bed, slipped the bags over her head and tied off the open ends at her throat with the ribbon... [Later] I took the bags off her head, cut them into shreds, and flushed them down the toilet with the ribbon" [*Pages 177-8*].

This complete account leads to these considerations: **Suffocation** by *Delury's* placing two plastic bags over Myrna's head while she slept, *not* an overdose by *Myrna's* "voluntary" act of swallowing, was the most likely the *proximate cause* of her death. [A "proximate cause" begins an event that would otherwise not have occurred.] Delury admitted that he had previously considered using the bags, and then feared their subsequent discovery so he took efforts to hide the evidence.

After his wife died, Delury rhetorically asked himself, "Am I a murderer? Or did I only carry a promise to completion?" [*Page 179*.] "It reminded me of the idea of ritual uncleanness and seemed to me to be related to simply having been instrumental in death" [*Page 178*].

The full account of Delury's act raises troubling questions. After reviewing the case, Dr. Ronald Miller asked: "If Delury had initially admitted the whole truth of using a plastic bag to the District Attorney, might he have received a longer sentence? (Instead of serving 5 to 15 *years*, he served 4 *months*.) Was Myrna Lebov's death assisted suicide, assisted dying, mercy killing, or murder? Why was Myrna's physician not involved? Might Myrna have benefited from hospice? Were her depression and her feelings of hopelessness treatable? Was the situation truly desperate, or only perceived to be so by either Myrna or Delury or both? Was either *unduly influenced* by the other? Did fear of financial destitution lead to premature action by Delury?"

I feel the most important question to answer is this: Did Delury have Myrna's explicit request to use the plastic bags? In general, I must ask: If Delury kept one secret, did he also keep others? Might he have misrepresented other information in *A Husband's Diary*? According to Myrna's angry sister, Beverly Sloane, who had been planning to "take Myrna to New Haven to visit family and old friends" [*Page 163*], the book is "full of lies, distortions and half-truths, all to bolster what Delury wants the world to believe" [letter to New York Times, 8-10-97].

The possibility of misrepresentation brings up this profound question: Was Delury's act selfless assisted suicide, or was it self-serving premeditated murder? To help decide, consider facts that may be relevant to the issue of *undue influence*:

Six months before she died, Delury wrote about a conversation he had with Myrna. **He** "decided that Myrna deserved a chance to make a choice before her mind was too ravaged to do so... so [**he**] pointed out that she was deteriorating rapidly; her body was close to useless; her mind was showing serious slippage; and her emotions no longer seemed consistently rooted in reality" [*Page 132*]. **He** then presented these dire possible predictions: A) Since **he** was exhausted from taking care of her without a break for nearly six years, **he** could collapse and die any time, in which case no one else would take care of her; B) Her sister would put her in a nursing home similar to the one in which her mother died. Myrna referred to that institution as "a prison whose best quality was that the inmates did not last long" where existing was "equal to being buried alive"; and C) With **her husband** gone, no one would help her die; hence, her prison sentence could last a decade or more [*Page 133*].

Around the same time, Delury depleted Myrna's financial independence. He cashed *her* $50,000 lump-sum check from *her* disability insurer. He explained that their finances were bleak due to tax liens; that it cost $145,000 a year to provide for her at home [*Page 157*]; and that it was very important she not lose her qualification for Medicaid [*Page 151*]. While these reasons are indeed factually compelling, they do not mitigate their emotional impact. Delury cashed Myrna's check against her expressed wishes, proving that Myrna had no control. Limited financial resources makes one feel more dependent. Dependency is depressing.

The grim "reality check" that Delury delivered to his wife contributed to Myrna's feelings of hopelessness and exacerbated her depression. Delury's rhetoric is thus circular: "**My** problem: if she asks for the poison now, and seems very depressed, should I comply? If I don't, she may be losing *her last chance* to make the decision" [*Page 155*]. Yet his presumption regarding "her last chance" may *not* have been correct. Furthermore, to keep open the option to hasten her dying, it was necessary to keep their plan secret, a hallmark of *undue influence*.

Delury wrote that the Cirque du Soleil outing occurred the day after "she suggested that I was the only one who wanted her to die" [*Page 159*]—a statement whose truth he admitted by writing, "I had the most to gain from her death," and by explaining, "Myrna's life had become a nightmare." Delury thus attempted to justify this remarkable argument: By her dying, his wife had less to lose than he.

Dr. Ronald Miller provides further insight into this couple's situation, one that is unfortunately not rare: "Myrna was neither terminally ill nor dependent upon life-sustaining technology. Yet she, like many others, might have considered her current life barely tolerable and *her probable future as totally intolerable.* Her fear of a bleak future made it harder currently to enjoy life. For Delury, the burden of caregiving was extremely demanding. Sacrificial giving becomes even less rewarding if the needy person becomes demented and can no longer recognize or appreciate her caregiver. This frustrating task can, and often does overwhelm elderly caregivers, both physically and emotionally."

Dr. Miller then asks: "Why don't we recognize the toll on the elderly caregiver, realizing that it may well be *we* who are called upon to serve? Why don't we have respite for those caring for relatives at home? For those less able, why don't we have clean, friendly, community-oriented nursing homes which are a pleasure to reside in and to visit?"

With respect to Myrna's better days, author Delury wrote: "The fact that Myrna could get out and enjoy something like the Cirque du Soleil might strike some readers as **reason enough for her to choose life**. And it might have been—if Myrna had **assurances that she could exit any time she wanted to in the future**. But Myrna lived in a society unwilling to grant such assurances, a society that makes no provision for dealing responsibly and openly with the possibility of chosen death. So, losing her mind and without recourse to any assistance but mine, **she was deprived of choices a less fearful society could have provided**. In short, the ban on assisted suicide and mercy killing can lead to **deaths that might otherwise be postponed**" [*Page 160*, emphasis added].

I resonate with Delury's criticism of society, but phrase the question differently: For people with chronic diseases such as Alzheimer's disease and other dementias that lead to profound indignity and dependency, why doesn't society provide a mechanism so that when they are competent, they can specify the precise level of impaired functioning... of suffering... of indignity... and of dependency... beyond which point they can be sure that their biologic existence will *not* be maintained?

The Epilogue's Summary and Perspective will offer possible solutions, but first let's consider "The Seven Principles of Good End-of-Life Decision-Making" and then use this conceptual framework to judge whether or not the *ending*-of-life decision that Delury and Lebov made was "good."

The Seven Principles of Good End-of-Life Decision-Making

1. Decide **WHAT** you want. For you, personally, what does *sanctity of life* mean?

- To live As Long As Possible (**ALAP**)?; or

- To Reduce Unnecessary Pain, Suffering, Indignity and Dependency (**RUPSID**)?

- If your choice is **ALAP**, the time frame is indefinite so no further specification is required. If your choice is **RUPSID**, precisely describe **WHEN**: it is easier to state a stage of a disease, but operationally better to describe the level of behavioral functioning.

2. Provide reasons that strive to be *clear* and *convincing* about **WHY** you want to make this choice, and give examples to justify these reasons. Use your own words, although you may consider citing examples from this book. For example:

- I want to follow the teachings of my religious leader;

- Quality of life is more important to me than duration of life;

- I prefer the unknowable experience of death to the known indignity and dependency of some states of severe physical and mental impairment; or,

- I want to conserve scarce medical and financial resources.

3. Anticipate **WHO** may **challenge** your wishes, and create an effective **strategy** to overcome the obstacles they may present. For example:

- State law in Texas allows ethics committees in hospitals to give patients' families 10 days notice that life-support will be discontinued. Therefore I provide a list of Catholic hospitals and possible sources for charitable contributions to keep me alive;

- The intense devotion of my spouse or child prevents him or her from carrying out the decisions I have chosen. Therefore I have designated certain end-of-life professionals to serve as my Proxies since I expect them to be more objective to make medical decisions on my behalf;

- My brother, a priest, believes that *my* redemptive suffering is not only necessary for **me** to enter Heaven but also for **others** to enter Heaven. I disagree so I have therefore added his name to my list of people whom I wish to exclude from participating in my medical or end-of-life decisions.

- I want funds from my estate to permit my grandchildren to attend college. Therefore I have described to my Proxy at what level of functioning I want

NO further aggressive medical treatment and want him or her to **Refuse Food & Fluid** on my behalf. (Alternate wording for Living Wills: I have described the level of functioning I want my future doctors to NOT provide aggressive medical treatment and to **Withhold Food & Fluid**); and,

- I know that "To Delay" can be equivalent "To Deny" the honoring of my Last Wishes if contested in courts of law. Therefore I have signed a form (after receiving advice from my attorney whose signature also appears on this form) to waive my legal right to a court review of my Proxy's decisions, and to request the disqualification of those named, from serving as "interested" petitioners in any court proceeding involving my medical or end-of-life decisions.

4. Establish that your JUDGMENT was SOUND when you created your Advance Directive as your DURABLE Last Wishes. Ask a mental health professional— preferably a psychiatrist or psychologist who has expertise in this field—to assess and describe your mental capacity to:

- **Understand** your choices;
- **Appreciate** the consequences of each choice—for you, and for others;
- Reach your decision by **logical reasoning** that was NOT influenced by **mental illness**; and
- **Consistently** express WHAT you want WHEN over time.

5. Professionals may need to establish that your decisions were **voluntary**:
- You were **informed** of all reasonably available choices;
- Your choices were NOT based on misunderstandings; and
- You were NOT subjected to subtle or direct pressure, or to **undue influence**.

6. SELECT, DESIGNATE, and EMPOWER certain individuals (and alternates) to encourage others to honor your Last Wishes if and when you can no longer make your own medical decisions. Use effective wording that may be modeled on that in **The BEST WAY to Say Goodbye**, as long as your local legal and medical consultants agree it is consistent with the laws that govern such designations in your legal jurisdiction. The person you designate will be:
- Your **decision-maker**, Proxy, or health care agent, if you use a Proxy Directive and may also be your first choice for a court-appointed individual, should that become necessary and the person is willing; or,
- Your **facilitator**, or **Living Will Advocate**, if you use a Living Will.

7. DISTRIBUTE and DISCUSS your Last Wishes and the documents that give them effect with those who love you, those who provide general care for you, and those who provide medical treatment for you (especially your physicians). For example:

- Check with your local legal advisors to make sure your documents are properly created and witnessed or notarized, so they will have legal effect;

- Give copies of your Proxy Directive to your first choice Proxy and all named alternates and end-of-life consultants;

- Make sure that your doctor, your Living Will Advocate, key members of your family, and end-of-life consultants all have copies of your Living Will;

- If you have given *oral* rather than written end-of-life instructions in a discussion with your physician, ask this doctor to give you a copy of what he or she wrote in your medical chart, and then distribute copies of these pages as the current document that represents your Living Will.

- Designate and notify all concerned about which end-of-life professionals are available for your Proxies and Advocates to consult, if they feel such consultations might be helpful; and,

- Leave clear instructions that no one should call 9-1-1, if that is your choice. Have your physician sign a document with "doctor's orders" that reflects your preference to decline emergency resuscitation and to refuse transfer to a hospital for aggressive care, just in case someone does call 9-1-1. (In some states, these instructions are formalized by a form called a "POLST," Physicians' Orders for Life-Sustaining Treatment.)

Did George Delury and Myrna Lebov's Decisions Satisfy the Criteria of "The Seven Principles of Good End-of-Life Decision-Making"?

1. **Myrna had decided WHAT she wanted, but not WHEN**. Clearly, she did not want to live as long as possible (**ALAP**); *eventually* she would want to reduce the amount of time in unnecessary pain and suffering, or indignity and dependency (**RUPSID**). Yet in the last weeks of her life her husband's *Diary* documented that she enjoyed movies, Cirque du Soleil, and Riverside Park. Hence, we are morally obligated to ask, or even explore: Would she have preferred a **later "WHEN"**? Clearly, Myrna was not yet at the point where she was forced to make the decision between the nursing home or dying.

2. **Myrna was** *clear and convincing* **about WHY**. She did not want "the living death" of a sentence in a nursing home, similar to what her mother had endured, and in her case, her time to serve would likely be much longer. Still, sick patients often "bargain down"; for example, Morrie (as related in *Tuesdays with Morrie*) stated he would not want to remain alive if he could no long wipe his own behind, yet he changed his mind when that time came. Athletes who state they would not want to live in a wheelchair sometimes find their calling in the law or in painting.

3. **Myrna did anticipate WHO might challenge her wishes**. Myrna may have believed that her sister Beverly would place her in a nursing home rather than pay for personal caregiving after her husband died. Delury presented only one other option, which Myrna may have believed: The only certain **alternative** to avoid nursing home placement was to die before her husband died. To keep this option open, Myrna may have agreed with her husband that it was necessary to keep secret the plan that she would someday ask for help to hasten her dying.

Comments:

1) Delury's prediction about the inevitability of nursing home placement may have been theatrically exaggerated, unconsciously biased, or intentionally self-serving.

2) Even if Delury's predictions about nursing home placement was likely, offering other options to Myrna might have given her hope that she could overcome this dreaded fear of events. (Other options are given below.)

3) The presence of a **secret pact** raises the **suspicion that undue influence** may be involved, although it does not prove it. Myrna's health aides had contact with her over several hours each day. Her successful concealment from them as well as from her sister implies that her concealment was maintained by her conscious and deliberate efforts.

4. **Was Myrna's JUDGMENT sound** as she expressed her Last Wishes? **NOT known.**

Considering *only* these two choices: 1) To hasten dying; *or*, 2) To endure a long placement in a nursing home, Myrna...

- **Understood** each choice;

- **Appreciated** the consequences of each choice to herself and to others;

Note: Independent verification of her understanding and appreciation appeared in the *content* of Myrna's letter to her sister, Beverly, which the District Attorney found on Myrna's word processor. The D.A. did not dispute the authenticity of this letter, but Beverly stated she never received this letter and she did question its authenticity;

- **MAY NOT have reached her decision logically without being influenced by a mental illness**. According to Delury, when his wife was in her "right" mind, she voiced the "realistic" wish to die, but when she was "euphoric" from mania, her stated desire to continue living did *not* reflect what she truly wanted. Delury thus formed the opinion that Myrna's psychiatric disorder explained why her **logical reasoning was impaired** when she expressed the desire to continue to live. Yet the opposite is also quite possible: Myrna may have wanted to live longer by postponing **WHEN** she would hasten her dying so that in the meantime, her real choice was to continue living; and

- **WAS consistent** in expressing her choice to not prolong her life under certain conditions (the **WHAT**), however,

- **WAS NOT consistent** with respect to **WHEN** she wanted to end her life. —A critically important point.

Comment: To my knowledge, Mr. Delury had no psychological or psychiatric training or experience, nor did he ask a qualified psychiatrist to render an opinion on these two critical questions:

1) What effect, if any, did changes in Myrna's mood have on her decision to live or die?; and,

2) Most important: **What was Myrna's true wish: to die now, or to die later?**

Myrna may have had mood changes from either manic depressive illness (since Lithium was prescribed) or from multiple sclerosis, or both. Still, if a psychiatrist had answered "Yes" to the two questions above, I would consider such an opinion treacherous. Why? Because if someone is ambivalent about living, all concerned should "Err on the side of life." As esteemed judges in several celebrated right-to-die cases have previously stated: actions that result in decisions to live are reversible; in contrast, actions that result in decisions to die are not. Patient's ambivalence, in my opinion, is a compelling reason To Delay.

Conclusion about decision-making capacity: Delury's interpretation is presumptuous since it serves as an outrageous justification for encouraging his wife to die prematurely. Furthermore, Delury was the self-appointed messenger to deliver the bad news that she had only two choices. The way Delury delivered this prediction made Myrna more depressed. This act may have influenced her to decide to hasten her dying. Had she been informed that there were other options, her mood might have been better and she might have maintained her resolve to postpone the time for asking to hasten her dying. Knowing other options existed could have thus led to her choosing to live longer, to avoid the tragedy of a premature death.

5. Was Myrna's decision **voluntary**? **Unlikely**. Had professionals investigated at the time, they could have rendered their opinions. However *no one asked them to do so*. Here is what we do know, in hindsight:

First, Myrna was **not fully informed** by her husband. He did not suggest that she could name alternative Proxies if he were not available. He did not suggest that members from the Hemlock Society could provide general support if she desired to hasten her dying after he had died. In the areas of alternate sources of financial support or of alternate places to live, however, Delury probably had little to offer.

When someone is given a *limited* number of choices and *other* choices are available, the individual's subsequent choice **cannot be voluntary**. Dr. Ronald Miller wrote, "When considering complex human problems of an ethical or moral nature, we should allow each individual to consider what he or she believes is best... Yet **what is best** is dependent: a) on being informed, and b) on what society has to offer."

Second, it is possible that Myrna's choice of **WHEN** she would hasten her dying resulted from subtle pressure... or worse, from **undue influence**.

Delury's book provides several descriptions of interactions with his wife that could be interpreted as his pressuring her to die. A few have already been mentioned; here are two more: Attorney Evans was impressed with the *Diary* note of June 9: Delury wrote about overhearing Myrna as she left a message on her niece's answering machine: "saying that 'Everything is wonderful now. Things are looking splendid,' etc. I blew up! Shouting into the phone that everything was just the same, it was simply Myrna feeling different. I told Myrna that she had hurt me very badly, not my feelings, but physically. 'Now what will [her sister] Beverly think? That I'm lying about how things are tough here?' I put it to Myrna bluntly—'If you won't take care of me, I can't take care of you.'"

I was impressed by the *Diary* entry of June 14. Delury wrote, "I told Myrna that 'I felt entirely alone and that no one was concerned about me.'" However after learning that "Beverly was ready to provide a vacation for me," Delury wrote, "It's amazing what a ray of hope will do for one's [e.g., *his*] energy." Referring to his energy, he wrote, "I've done more work today than in any day for the previous two weeks."

Delury admitted to having motivation that was adequate to pursue *undue influence*: If Myrna died, he would get his whole life back. In addition to financial relief, he would no longer would be trapped as her 24/7 caregiver. Perhaps Delury's mindset changed from ambivalence to determination after he experienced a week of living as a "free man" while he attended his niece's wedding. During that time, he may have reflected on what his life had become. While he previously had turned down his wife's requests to hasten dying, maybe now a hopefully shorter prison sentence seemed preferable to returning to a decade or more of providing daily care for her. Furthermore, he could use his time in prison to write a book. Yet Delury had no way of knowing for sure how long his sentence would be. Back then, Dr. Kevorkian had been accused of murder and was scheduled to stand trial for assisting suicide, but no jury had yet acquitted him based on his plea that he was only relieving pain. Therefore, Delury was taking an unknown risk.

Conclusion: Some themes support the theory of Delury exerting *undue influence* on his wife to decide to die **THEN**: the lack of fully informed consent, the question of veracity of the full account, the admission of his deep personal motivation, and keeping the plan a secret.

6. So... did Myrna select, designate, and empower certain individuals (including alternates) to advocate others to honor her Last Wishes? **NO.**

Myrna was given no other choices: no Guardian *Ad Litem* or conservator of a person, and no other friend or relative was empowered to speak for her... even though the issue was a matter of life-or-death.

It is critically significant that Delury simultaneously assumed many roles that the laws of most States keep separate because of the inherent conflicts of interest among these roles

Delury was Myrna's...

1. husband and primary companion;

2. financial partner and unilateral decision-maker in their community property;

3. primary caregiver;

4. (non-professional) provider of (partially) informed consent;

5. (non-professional) judge of her ability to make prudent decisions in the context of a (possible) psychiatric disorder and/or organic or reactive depression, whose mood changes may have influenced her decision to live or die;

6. co-creator and only witness to her (oral) Advance Directive—if in fact she did say, "I want to die now" the night she died;

7. only designated Proxy;

8. non-medical facilitator to hasten her dying;

9. (non-professional) "expert" who stated that she would eventually die from

the amount of lethal medication she was able to consume (see below);

10. probable unilateral decision-maker to invoke "Plan B," to use a plastic BAG to hasten her dying; and,

11. self-appointed explainer of her motivation as well as his own, by writing his book.

While certain roles would be presumed by the law such as #1, and in uncomplicated cases he would also be appointed as #7, and while multiple roles are not rare (for example one man can be father, brother, son, uncle, and so on), the multiplicity of roles and possible conflicts of interest of Delury exceed that of any case I have ever reviewed.

To clarify Item 9: Delury stated he was *certain* that his wife would eventually die from the amount of medication she managed to swallow. Yet medical scientists can never be certain which specific individuals will live or die after a given dose of toxic medication; they can only express the *probability*. For example, at a moderately high dose, 50% of a population will die and at a much higher dose, 90% will die. Scientists designate these doses LD-50 or LD-90, but no one can predict with certainty whether a given individual in a population will die.

Comments: Delury's book indicates that Myrna was concerned about being sure she would die, but it relates no previous discussion where Myrna asked to be suffocated by a plastic bag if the pills did not bring about a quick enough death. Yet Delury had previously stashed some plastic bags to use, in case that very scenario did develop.

Every psychiatrist knows individuals whose suicide attempts were not successful. For many patients, continued therapy and social support provide a path to live with renewed appreciation for those pleasures of life that still remain. While the percentage of such "appreciative" survivors may be lower for patients with chronic and challenging illnesses than for otherwise healthy psychiatric patients, it is still possible that had Myrna awakened, she might have concluded that "her time to die" had not yet come.

So... did Myrna select, designate, and empower certain individuals to serve as her advocate with the goal that others would honor her Last Wishes? **NO**: in every way, she depended *exclusively* on her husband.

Because of the multiple roles Delury assumed, Myrna was at the mercy of her husband. Myrna's sister stated there were NO discussions (that she knew about) to support Delury's claim that Myrna wanted to die.

7. Did Myrna distribute and discuss her Last Wishes and the documents that give them effect with those who loved her, those who provided general care for her,

and those who provided medical treatment for her (especially her physicians)? **NO**.

No such documents were created and Myrna relied on the will of her husband. He in turn took notes and relied on his memory regarding what his wife had indicated orally while she was alive. Other witnesses such as her niece and sister recalled **other** discussions and came to the different conclusion that Myrna did not want to die **THEN**. This dispute cannot be resolved.

One additional piece of evidence seemed to support Delury's position: the letter that the District Attorney found on Myrna's word processor. Since Delury did not present this letter to the D.A., it was assumed to be credible evidence. Delury also claimed not to know the password to her word processor. None of this proves that Myrna actually created this letter, however. Delury's diary indicated that he was aware that his wife was writing a letter to her sister on that date. So it is possible that Delury could have created the letter and left it on his wife's word processor for the D.A. to "discover," but there is no way to prove this.

Opinion based on The Seven Principles of Good End-of-Life Decision-Making: Did George Delury & Myrna Lebov satisfy them?

No; at best: Delury unintentionally facilitated the premature death of his wife because he did not provide her fully informed consent. He did not explore other possible options because he did not know they existed. Meanwhile, the extreme burdens of caregiving led to the draining of energy and financial resources. Delury thus unintentionally influenced his wife to decide to hasten her death **prematurely**.

No; at worst: Delury pressured his wife to agree to swallow a lethal dose of medication after he deliberately exacerbated her depression by engaging in several conversations in which he portrayed her future as exceedingly bleak and his burden of caregiving as so utterly exhausting, he could die at any time. By threatening her with the dismal alternative of placement in a nursing home, he thus exerted *undue influence* to encourage her to decide to hasten her death.

I considered one point extremely important: Myrna Lebov did not die from an overdose of medication that she (voluntarily?) swallowed. The proximate cause of death was suffocation: Mr. Delury placed a plastic bag tightly over her head as she slept. Delury did not admit this fact to the District Attorney prior to plea-bargaining in lieu of a trial.

Based on this more complete information there are two possibilities:

A) If Delury had promised his wife that he would end her suffering by assisting her suicide, and if he felt committed to the success of this goal but was worried that the health aid due to arrive the next day could abort the plan if Myrna was still alive at the time, then Delury committed **voluntary euthanasia**, on her behalf, as requested.

B) If Delury had a plastic bag ready to use but intentionally did not ask for his wife's fully informed consent to use it, just a few hours previously when she was still conscious, and if he suffocated her to end his being physically and financially trapped; that is, for his own personal gain—to recover his life—then the appropriate term for what Delury did is either **involuntary euthanasia** or **premeditated murder**.

   IUDICET LECTOR!   *(Latin for, "Let the reader decide.")*

Further reflections and a final note:

Why did Delury commit murder when there was another option? Why did he not simply leave his wife, if he wanted to free himself from **this trap**? While no one can know for sure, perhaps not even Delury at a deep or unambiguous psychological level, readers who wish to, may consider this psychodynamic hypothesis. (Here, I use the vague term "euthanizing" to refer to the act.)

Leaving his wife would have severely damaged Delury's self-esteem and left him with unresolved guilt from which there could be no redemption. How could the man face anyone after leaving his partner of almost three decades in an act of obvious selfishness? In contrast, by "euthanizing" her, Delury could assume the role of her "hero," a loving husband who was willing to risk a prison term of unknown duration so that his wife could be freed from **her trap** of increasingly impaired physical and mental functioning. By waving the flag of personal freedom and by blaming society for not providing a more humane way out, he could present himself to the world as a martyr. By writing a book, he could convince his readers (as he convinced himself) that "she really did want to die" **now**. By paying his "debt" to society with a sanctioned term of confinement in prison, he could thereafter be "redeemed," and ultimately, also be free of guilt.

This is the essence of my speculative reflection: To avoid the risk of being considered a selfish husband who left his sick wife to the care of others, Delury acted in such a way that he could portray himself as a martyr who sacrificed his own freedom to be her hero. He blamed society for limited available options, knowing that many would agree. But exactly what did Myrna want? Did his wife really ask him to assist her dying? We will never know for sure. Yet the known facts are uncomfortably consistent to supporting the dire opinion that Mr. Delury did murder his wife. ***Final note***: In June 2007, Delury committed suicide. He used an overdose of oral morphine and Fentanyl patches. The process of dying was long. EMTs tried to revive him and rushed him to a hospital. The former editor's last note was: "At age 74 it seems to me that I have lived long enough."

Summary and Perspective

The major theme of **The *BEST WAY* to Say Goodbye** is that when people are given the choice of *when* and *how* to die, they can, and often do, decide to live longer. Knowledge about the option of **Refusing Food & Fluid** can lead to avoiding illegal, violent, and **premature** dying.

As described in this book, the deaths of Janet Adkins, Judge Robert Hammerman, Bob Stern, and Myrna Lebov were all premature. Furthermore, the last months of their lives were plagued by depression, anxiety, and/or worry as they anticipated their respective futures were on inevitable courses toward increasing suffering and indignity, with no possibility of future escape unless they died before their trap doors closed.

Unfortunately, there are thousands of people with similar stories of premature dying, or who suffer from anxiety and worry in addition to their primary illnesses, during the final months of their lives.

I find Delury's account alarming. To me, it provides another reason to educate the public on **Refusal of Food & Fluid by Proxy**. I believe that, in July 1995, if Myrna Lebov knew this option was available in her future, she would have resisted her husband's attempts to persuade her to hasten her dying.

Unfortunately, the State in which Delury and Lebov lived, is still going in the opposite direction. New York requires explicit statements (usually written) that **Proxies** have been given authorization to **Withhold Food & Fluid**. In 1993, Assemblyman Richard Gottfried, D-Manhattan, introduced the "Family Health Care Decision Act" to change part of New York's law. Yet as of June, 2006, this Act has still not been passed. As mentioned previously, "Raymond Schwaed suffered agonizing pain in the months before his death, [since his] family did not have the legal right to make [medical] decisions about his care" [Davis HL, 2006].

Perhaps a jury would have found Delury guilty of second-degree murder if he had revealed his use of plastic bags. Some might still consider his act as self-sacrificing and noble. Yet some of the sentiments he voiced indeed seem valid:

Many people suffer from chronic diseases that include progressive dementia. Their future is realistically characterized by profound indignity and dependency. Society should provide a mechanism so that when competent, they can describe a certain level of impaired functioning, or pain and suffering, or indignity and dependency—beyond which they can legitimately demand that their biologic existence NOT be prolonged, and be assured that others will honor these wishes.

Competent people may choose among several criteria; for example, the point at which manually assisted oral feeding is observed to be forced, or when they can no longer recognize or communicate with loved ones. In contrast to the advice from The President's Council on Bioethics, that creating an Advance Directive that requests a **Proxy to Refuse Food & Fluid** is *discrimination against a future disabled [demented] self*, the law of the land and the community standards of the clinical practice of medicine agree that exercising this option is moral.

What is needed now is for more clinicians, attorneys, counselors, social workers, nurses, hospice workers, and spiritual and religious leaders to spread the word about this **legal peaceful choice**. I hope that non-professional people will form groups to provide mutual support for one another, groups where each member promises to serve as several others' effective advocates when "that time comes." I hope these Proxies can find willing end-of-life professionals with whom they can consult, as needed. Proxies are often asked to make difficult decisions about continuing or ending potentially life-prolonging medical treatment, yet many of them have never before been placed in that position of responsibility.

Professor Ronald Dworkin wrote that one way to judge a life is by its whole. In that sense, I offer this thought:

> *Our life is like a concerto.*
> *The final movement is one*
> *We all want to play*
> *As well as possible.*

Like childbirth, dying is sometimes a painful experience. If politicians do not let people choose Physician-Hastened Dying, then it is fortunate that there is another choice It is also fortunate that the method is peaceful as well as legal. While challenges continue to mount, they can be overcome by applying our present knowledge with diligent and strategic planning.

The authors of **The *BEST WAY* to Say Goodbye** hope we have presented the case for this ending-of-life alternative comprehensively enough so readers can decide if it is the *best* choice for themselves, and if their loved ones should consider it. While we have no choice about *whether* we will die, we do have a choice about *how*. If readers believe this way could also be *best* for others, then we hope they will spread the word so that those who do not yet know about this option can consider it while they are still competent as they engage in advance care planning. Otherwise, those in power may restrict their loved ones from making the decisions they would have chosen for themselves, or making decisions that would be in their best interest. Beyond that goal, who knows? It seems compelling to quote Margaret Mead again, as I did on page 382: "Never doubt that a small group of thoughtful, committed citizens can change the world. Indeed, it is the only thing that ever has."

Medical References and Legal Citations

(The Glossary has additional references and citations.)

Ahronheim JC, Mulvihill M, Sieger C, Park P, & Fries BE. (2005). State practice variations in the use of tube feeding for nursing home residents with severe cognitive impairment. *J Am Geriatr Soc 49*(2), 148-52

Ahronheim, J & Weber, D. (1992). *Final Passages: Positive choices for the dying and their loved ones.* New York: Simon & Schuster.

Ain, S. (2005, 25 March). Schiavo case creates ethical debate. Jewish bioethicists are split on feeding tube. *The Jewish Week*. Retrieved from http://www.thejewishweek.com/news/newscontent.php3?artid=10682

Alvarez, J. (2006, Aug 5). Brownback introduces a bill to prohibit physician-assisted suicide. *The Christian Post*. Retrieved from http://www.christianpost.com/pages/print.htm?aid=23506

Alzheimer's Association. (2005, 15 May). *About Alzheimer's disease statistics* (Fact Sheet). Retrieved from http://www.alz.org/Resources/FactSheets/FSAlzheimerStats.pdf.

Alzheimer's media releases, 2005, http://www.alz.org/Media/newsreleases/2005/122105.asp?id=529740

AMA 1996. E-2.20. Based on two reports: "Decisions Near the End of Life" and "Decisions to Forego Life-Sustaining Treatment for Incompetent Patients." Adopted June 1991. *JAMA 267*, 2229-2233 (1992); updated June 1996; current as of Aug 2006.

AMA policy E-10.01: fundamentals of the patient-physician relationship. Chicago: American Medical Association.

Andrews K, Murphy L, Munday R, & Littlewood C. (1996). Misdiagnosis of the vegetative state: Retrospective study in a rehabilitation unit. *BMJ 313*(7048), 13-16.

Angell, M. (1990, 23 July). The right to die with dignity. *Newsweek, 9.*

Arehart-Treichel J. (2004). Terminally Ill Choose Fasting Over M.D.-Assisted suicide. *Psychiatry News 39,* 15-51.

Aronson SG, & Kirby RW. (2002). Improving knowledge and communication through an advance directives objective structured clinical examination. *J Palliat Med 5*(6), 916-19.

Asbury Park Press. (2005, 9 June). Schiavo case inspired lawmakers seek to inform couples on living wills. *Associated Press*. Retrieved from http://www.app.com/apps/pbcs.dll/article?AID=/20050609/NEWS03/506090428/1007.

Asch DA, Hansen-Flasen J, & Laken PN. (1995). Decisions to limit or continue life-sustaining treatment by critical care physicians in the United States: Conflicts between physicians' practices and patients' wishes. *Am J Respir Crit Care Med 151:288-92.*

Attems J, Konig C, Huber M, Lintner F, & Jellinger KA. (2005). Cause of death in demented and non-demented elderly inpatients: an autopsy study of 308 cases. *J Alzheimers Dis 8*(1), 57-62.

Auriga Pharmaceuticals (10/2006). Aquoral spray. Patient insert. Norcross, GA.

Baca-Garcia E, Diaz-Sastre C, Basurte E, Prieto R, Ceverino A, Saiz-Ruiz J, & de Leon JA. (2001). A prospective study of the paradoxical relationship between impulsivity and lethality of suicide attempts. *J Clin Psych 62*(7), 560-64.

Back AL, Arnold RM, Tulsky JA, Baile WF, & Fryer-Edwards KA. (2005). On saying goodbye: Acknowledging the end of the patient-physician relationship with patients who are near death. *Ann Intern Med 142*(8), 682-85.

Bartholomew, K. (1994). *Doctor, Please Close the Door! A book on living wills, powers of attorney, terminal care, and the right to die with dignity.* Plantation: Distinctive Publishing.

Bayliss EA, Ellis JL, Steiner JF. (2005). Subjective assessments of comorbidity correlate with quality of life health outcomes: initial validation of a comorbidity assessment instrument. *Health Qual Life Outcomes.* Sep 1;3:51.

Bechhofer YG. (2005, 24 May). *Jewish ethical and legal sources on the treatment of terminally ill patients.* Retrieved from http://www.aishdas.org/rygb/medical.htm.

Becker, CB. (1990). Buddhist views of suicide and euthanasia. *Philosophy East and West, 40*(4).

Bell, M. (2005, 5 Aug). Guardians laud Michael Schiavo for fulfilling wife's wishes. *The Orlando Sentinel.* Retrieved from http://www.orlandosentinel.com.

Bernat JL, Gert B, & Mogielnicki RP. (1993). Patient refusal of hydration and nutrition. An alternative to physician-assisted suicide or voluntary active euthanasia. *Arch Intern Med 153*(24), 2723-28.

Betancourt JR, Green AR, & Carrillo JE. (2000). The challenges of cross-cultural healthcare. Diversity, ethics and the medical encounter. *Bioethics Forum 16*(3), 27-32.

Betancourt JR, Green AR, & Carrillo JE, Ananeh-Firempong O. (2003). Defining cultural competence: A practical framework for addressing racial/ethnic disparities in health and health care. *Public Health Rep 118*(4), 293-302.

Borenstein v Simonson. (2005). *NY Slip Op 25135.*

Boulos DL, Groome PA, Brundage MD, Siemens DR, Mackillop WJ, Heaton JP, Schulze KM, Rohland SL (2006). Predictive validity of five comorbidity indices in prostate carcinoma patients treated with curative intent. *Cancer* Apr 15;106(8):1804-14.

Bouvia v Superior Court. (1986). *179 Cal App 3d 1127, 225 Cal Rptr 297, Review Denied (Cal 5 Jun 1986).*

Braddock CH 3rd, Fihn SD, Levinson W, Jonsen AR, & Pearlman RA. (1997). How doctors and patients discuss routine clinical decisions: Informed decision-making in the outpatient setting. *J Gen Intern Med 12*(6), 339-45.

Bradley P. (2005, 7 Aug). "The difficulty is in deciding.." Torres and Schiavo cases raised different questions about the issue of life support. *Richmond Times-Dispatch.* Retrieved from http://www.timesdispatch.com/servlet/Satellit e?pagename=RTD%2FMGArticle%2FRTD_BasicArticle&c=MGArticle&cid=1 031784292540&path=!news&s=1045855934842)

Bramstedt KA. (2003). Questioning the decision-making capacity of surrogates. *Intern Med J 33*(5-6), 257-9.

Breitowitz R. Y. (1997). The right to die: A Halachic approach. *Jewish Law.* Retrieved from http://www.jlaw.com/Articles/right.html

Brockman B. (1999). Food refusal in prisoners: A communication or a method of self-killing? The role of the psychiatrist and resulting ethical challenges. *J Med Ethics 25*(6), 451-6.

Patricia E. Brophy v New England Sinai Hospital, Inc., N-4152 S.J.C. (398 Mass. 417, 430 (1986))

Buckley C. (2007) *Boomsday.* New York: Twelve, Hachette,Warner Books

Buckley T, Crippen D, DeWitt AL, Fisher M, Liolios A, Scheetz CL & Whetsine LM. (2004). Ethics roundtable debate: Withdrawal of tube feeding in a patient with persistent vegetative state where the patient's wishes are unclear and there is family dissension. *Crit Care 8*(2), 79-84.

Burdette AM, Hill TD, & Moulton BE. (2005). Religion and attitudes toward physician-assisted suicide and terminal palliative care. *J Sci Study Rel 44*(1), 79-93.

Byock IR. (1995). Patient refusal of nutrition and hydration: Walking the ever finer line. *Amer J Hospice and Pall Care* 8-13.

Callahan, D. (1987) *Setting Limits: Medical Goals in an Aging Society.* Touchstone Books. Also Georgetown U Press: Washington DC (1995)

Caplan A. (1995, 6 Apr). Must we all die with a feeding tube? Pope's directive undermines patients' medical rights. Retrieved from http://msnbc.msn.com/ id/4669899/.

Caplan A. (2005, 17 Feb). Movie asks the million dollar question. Film stirs controversy over life-and-death issues. Retrieved from http://www.msnbc. msn.com/id/6970787/.

Caplan A. (2005, 18 Mar). The time has come to let Terri Schiavo die. Politicians, courts must allow husband to make final decision. Retrieved from http://www. msnbc.msn.com/id/7231440/.

Caplan A. (2005, 31 Mar). What can we learn from the Schiavo case? Contentious battle offers Americans many important lessons. Retrieved from http://msnbc.msn.com/id/7289351/.

Casarett D, Kapo J, & Caplan A. (2005). Appropriate use of artificial nutrition and hydration--fundamental principles and recommendations. *N Engl J Med 353*(24), 2607-12.

Centeno C, Sanz A, Bruera E. (2004). Delirium in advanced cancer patients. *Palliat Med 18*(3), 184-94.

Center for Practical Bioethics. (2004). Examining new knowledge and controversies about serious disorders of consciousness. State initiatives in end of life care. Retrieved from www.practicalbioethics.org/SI_22.pdf.

Cerchietti L, Navigante A, Sauri A, & Palazzo F. (2000). Hypodermoclysis for control of dehydration in terminal-stage cancer. *Inter J Palliat Nurs 6*(8), 370-74.

Childs NL, Mercer WN, & Childs HW. (1993). Accuracy of diagnosis of persistent vegetative state. *Neurology 43,* 1465-7.

Clare AW. (1990). Psychological Medicine. In Kumer P &. Clark, M (Ed.), *Clinical Medicine* (pp. 965-1000). London: WB Saunders.

Cohen EN, Conner T, Cerminera K, & Tucker K. End of Life Legislation Chart. *MergerWatch*. Retrieved from http://www.compassionandchoices.org/documents/EndofLife_Legislation_Chart.pdf.

Colburn D. (2005, 17 July). Metro/Northwest. *Oregonian,* p. 1 & 10.

Colby WH. (2002). *Long Goodbye: The deaths of Nancy Cruzan.* Carlsbad, CA: Hay House.

Conservatorship of the person of Robert Wendland. *28 P 3d 151 (Cal 2001).*

Coombs Lee B. (2003). *Compassion in Dying: Stories of dignity and choice.* Toutdale, OR: Newsage Press.

Coombs Lee B. (2004, 21 Nov). *Perspectives on comfort and choice at the end of life* (lecture) at First Unitarian Universalist Church of San Diego.

Covinsky KE, Goldman L, Cook EF, Oye R, Desbiens N, Reding D, Fulkerson W, Conners, AF Jr, Lynn J, & Phillips RS. (1994). The impact of serious illness on patients' families. *JAMA 272,* 1939-1944.

Cranford RE. (1991). Neurological symptoms and prolonged survival: When can artificial nutrition and hydration be forgone? *Law, Medicine and Health Care 19,* 13-22.

Creque, SA. (Sept. 11, 1995). Killing with kindness. Capital punishment by nitrogen asphyxiation. *National Review.*

Cruzan v Director, Missouri Department of Health. (1990). *497 US 261, 302.*

Curlin FA, Lawrence RE, Chin MH, Lantos JD. Religion, conscience, and controversial clinical practices. N Engl J Med 2007;356:593-600.

Davis HL. (2006, 11 Jun) Life and death—who should make the choice? Retrieved from http://www.buffalonews.com/editorial/20060611/1028137.asp

Davis JJ. (1987). Brophy v New England Sinai Hospital: Ethical dilemmas in discontinuing artificial nutrition and hydration for comatose patients. *J Biblical Ethics in Medicine 1*(3).

Davis LL & Keller MH. (2004). *At the Close of the Day: A person centered guidebook on end-of-life care.* Rochester, WA: Gorham.

Davis MP, Walsh D, LeGrand SB, & Naughton M. (2002). Symptom control in cancer patients: The clinical pharmacology and therapeutic role of suppositories and rectal suspensions. *Support Care Cancer, 10*(2), 117-38.

DeBaggio, T (2002). *Losing My Mind. An Intimate Look at Life with Alzheimer's.* New York: The Free Press, Simon & Schuster; also Audio Works

Delury GE. (1995, 15 Dec). Excerpts from the diary of George Delury. *New York Times.*

Delury GE. (1997). *But What If She Wants to Die? A husband's diary.* Seacaucus, NJ: Birch Lane Press.

Descartes R. (1637, 2000). *Discourse on method and related writings.* New York: Penguin.

Ditto PH, Smucker WD, Danks JH, Jacobson JA, Houts RM, Fagerlin A, Coppola KM, & Gready RM. (2003). Stability of older adults' preferences for life-sustaining medical treatment. *Health Psychol 22*(6), 605-15.

Dorff EN. (1998, 2004). *Matters of Life and Death: A Jewish approach to modern medical ethics.* Philadelphia: Jewish Publication Society.

Drayer RA, Schaler JA, Ganzini L, & Goy E. (2003). Patients who refuse food and fluids to hasten death. *N Engl J Med 349,* 1777-9.

Drickamer MA. CHAPTER 4—LEGAL AND ETHICAL ISSUES Retrieved from http://www.geriatricsreviewsyllabus.org/content/agscontent/legal6_m.htm, in August, 2006 (original publication date not known)

Durham, Jr. WC. (1992) *Preparation for Life-Prolonging Decisions,* in *Encyclopedia of Mormonism.* MacMillan Publishing Company.

Duhigg C. (2007, 3-27 & 5-25) Aged, Frail and Denied Care by Their Insurers. & Congress Putting Long-Term Care Under Scrutiny. *New York Times.*

Dworkin RM. (1993). *Life's Dominion. An Argument about abortion, euthanasia, and individual freedom.* New York: Knopf; Random House: Vintage (1994).

Eagle, JM. (Director). (2002). *Alzheimer's: My mom, our journey.* (video)

Eddy DM. (1994). A conversation with my mother. *JAMA 272,* 179-81.

Eisenberg JB. (2005). *Using Terri: The religious right's conspiracy to take away our rights.* San Francisco: HarperSanFrancisco.

Elbaum v Grace Plaza of Great Neck, I. (1989). *148 AD 2d 244, 544 NYS 2d 840 (New York Appellate Division).*

Elgh E, Larsson A, Eriksson S, & Nyberg L. (2003). Altered prefrontal brain activity in persons at risk for Alzheimer's disease: An fMRI study. *Int Psychogeriatr 15*(2), 121-33.

Ellershaw JE, Sutcliffe JM, & Saunders CM. (1995). Dehydration and the dying patient. *J Pain Symptom Manage 3*(10),192-97.

Emanuel LL, Barry MJ, Stoeckle JD, Ettelson LM, & Emanuel EJ. (1991). Advance directives for medical care—a case for greater use. *N Engl J Med 324*(13), 889-95.

Evans DA, Funkenstein HH, Albert MS, Scherr PA, Cook NR, Chow MJ, Herbert LE, Hennekens CH, & Taylor JO. (1989). Prevalence of Alzheimer's disease in a community population of older persons: Higher than previously reported. *JAMA 262,* 2661-65.

Fagerlin A, Ditto PH, Danks JH, Houts RM, & Smucker WD. (2001) Projection in Surrogate Decisions about Life-Sustaining Medical Treatments. *Health Psychology 20*(3),166-75.

Fagerlin A & Schneider CE. (2004). Enough. The failure of the Living Will. *Hastings Cent Rep 34*(2), 30-42.

Feder S, Metheny R, Loveless RS, Rea TD. (2006). Withholding resuscitation: A new approach to prehospital end-of-life decisions. *Ann Intern Med 144,* 634-40.

Finucane TE, Christmas C, & Travis K. (1999). Tube feeding in patients with advanced dementia: A review of evidence. *JAMA 282,* 1365-70.

Fleck, LH. (1994, 24 Mar). Rationing: Triage for our country. *Insight on the News, 10*(12), 22.

Fried TR, Bradley EH, Towle VR, & Allore H. (2002). Understanding the treatment preferences of seriously ill patients. *N Engl J Med 346*(14), 1061-6.

Fromm, Erich. (1956, 2000). *The Art of Loving.* New York: HarperRow Perennial.

Frontline. (1992, 24 Mar). *The death of Nancy Cruzan.* Retrieved from http://www. pbs.org/wgbh/pages/frontline/programs/transcripts/1014.html.

Furlong v Catholic Healthcare West (St. John's Regional Medical Center). (2004, 22 Dec). Ventura County Superior Court; Case number B172067. *Cal App Unpub LEXIS 11667.*

Ganzini L, Goy ER, Miller LL, Harvath TA, Jackson A, & Delorit MA. (2003). Nurses' experiences with hospice patients who refuse food & fluids to hasten death. *N Engl J Med 349*(4), 359-65.

Ganzini L, Harvath TA, Jackson A, Goy ER, Miller LL, & Delorit MA. (2002). Experiences of Oregon nurses and social workers with hospice patients who requested assistance with suicide. *N Engl J Med 347*(8), 582-8.

Gert B, Bernat JL, & Mogielnicki RP. (2002). Physician involvement in voluntary stopping of eating and drinking. *Ann Intern Med 137*(12), 1010-11.

Giacino JT, Ashwal S, Childs N, Cranford R, Jennett B, Katz DI, Kelly JP, Rosenberg JH, Whyte J, Zafonte RD, & Zasler ND. (2002). The minimally conscious state: Definition and diagnostic criteria. *Neurology 58*(3), 349-53.

Gill-Thwaites H, & Munday R. (2004). The Sensory Modality Assessment and Rehabilitation Technique (SMART). A valid and reliable assessment for vegetative state and minimally conscious state patients. *Brain Injury 18*(12), 1255-69.

Gillick MR. (1999). Rethinking the role of tube feeding in patients with advanced dementia. *N Engl J Med 342,* 206-10.

Gillick MR. (2001, Feb). Artificial nutrition and hydration in the patient with advanced dementia: Is withholding treatment compatible with traditional Judaism? *J Med Ethics 27*(1), 12-15.

Gillick MR. (2004, 3 Aug). Terminal sedation: An acceptable exit strategy? *Ann Intern Med 141*(3), 236-7.

Gjerdingen DK, Neff JA, Wang M, & Chaloner K. (1999). Older persons' opinions about life-sustaining procedures in the face of dementia. *Arch Fam Med 8*(5), 421-25.

Gladwell M. (2002). *The Tipping Point: How little things can make a big difference.* Boston: Back Bay Books.

Goldstein A. (2006, 2 May). Trustee's report: Medicare will go broke by 2018. *Washington Post.*

Goodenough A. (2005, 18 Jun). Gov. Bush seeks another inquiry in Schiavo case. *New York Times,* sec. National.

Green AR. (2003). The human face of health disparities. *Public Health Rep 118*(4), 303-08.

Green AR, Betancourt J., Carrillo JE. (2002). Integrating social factors into cross-cultural medical education. *Acad Med 77*(3), 193-97.

Groopman J. (2007) *How Doctors Think.* Boston: Houghton Mifflin.

Gross J. (2003, 3 Aug). Striving for a gentle farewell. *New York Times.* sec. The Nation

Gross J. (2004, 16 Sep). Alzheimer's in the living room: How one family rallies to cope. *New York Times.* sec. Health.

Gross MD. (1998). What do patients express as their preferences in advance directives? *Arch Intern Med 158*(4), 363-5.

Guru V, Verbeek PR, & Morrison LJ. (1999). Response of paramedics to terminally ill patients with cardiac arrest: an ethical dilemma. *CMAJ 161,* 1251-4.

Haman EA. (2006). *Power of attorney handbook.* Naperville: Sphinx Publishing.

Hamel R, & Panicola M. (2004, 19 Apr). Must we preserve life? *America Magazine 190,* 14.

Hammes BJ, & Rooney BL. (1998). Death and end-of-life planning in one midwestern community. *Arch Intern Med 158*(4), 383-90.

Hanrahan P & Luchins DJ. (1995). Access to hospice programs in end-stage dementia: A natural survey of hospice programs. *J Amer Geriatr Soc 43,* 56-59.

Hardin SB, & Yusufaly YA. (2004). Difficult end-of-life treatment decisions: Do other factors trump advance directives? *Arch Intern Med 164*(14), 1531-3.

Harentiaux B. (2002). *VESTA* (Missoula Demonstration Project). Missoula: Life's End Institute, 515 W. Front Street, Missoula, MT 59802.

Hart DJ, Craig D, Compton SA, Critchlow S, Kerrigan BM, McIlroy SP, & Passmore AP. (2003). A retrospective study of the behavioral and psychological symptoms of mid and late phase Alzheimer's disease. *Inter J Geriatr Psychiatry18*(11), 1037-42.

Harvath TA, Miller LL, Goy E, Jackson A, Delorit M, & Ganzini L. (2004). Voluntary refusal of Food & Fluids: Attitudes of Oregon hospice nurses and social workers. *Int J Palliat Nurs 10*(5), 236-43. Discussion, 242-3.

Harvey, J. 2005. www.pbs.org/wnet/religionandethics/week830/perspectives.html.

Hastings Center. (1987). *Guidelines for the Termination of Life-Sustaining Treatment and the Care of the Dying*. Briarcliff Manor, NY: Hastings Center.

Hawkins NA, Ditto PH, Danks JH, & Smucker WD. (2005). Micromanaging death: Process preferences, values, and goals in end-of-life medical decision making. *Gerontologist 45*(1), 107-17.

Healy S, & McNamara E. (2002). Tube feeding controversial patients: What do dietitians think? *J Hum Nutr Diet 15*(6), 445-53.

Henig RM. (2005, 7 Aug). Will we ever arrive at the good death? *New York Times,* sec. Magazine.

Hickman SE, Hammes BJ., Moss AH. & Tolle SW. (2005) Hope for the future: Achieving the original intent of advance directives. Improving end of life care: Why has it been so difficult? *Hastings Cent Rep Special Report 35*(6), S26-S30.

High DM. (1988). All in the family: Extended autonomy and expectations in surrogate health care decision-making. *Gerontologist 28*(3, suppl), 46-51.

Hoefler JM. (1997) *Managing Death*. Bolder, Co: Westview Press. (See especially pages 90-91, 93, & 95.)

Hoefler JM. (2005). Retrieved from http://www.dickinson.edu/endoflife/Glossary.html.

Hoefler JM, & Neugebauer GP 3rd. (2006). Retrieved from http://www.dickinson.edu/endoflife/Religion.html.

Humphry D. (2002). *Final Exit: The practicalities and self-deliverance and assisted suicide for the dying.* 3d Ed. New York: Random House.

(In the Matter of: See last name, eg, Martin, O'Conner, Wendland, others)

Irving S. (2003). *Medical directives and powers of attorney for California.* 2nd Ed. Berkeley: Nolo Press.

Jacobs S. (2003). Death by voluntary dehydration: What the caregivers say. *N Engl J Med 349*(4), 325-26.

Jacoby MB, Sullivan TA, & Warren E. (2001). Rethinking debates over health care financing: Evidence from the bankruptcy courts. *New York University Law Review 76,* 375-418.

James G. (1995, 28 Dec). Papers tell of a wife's suicide plan. *New York Times.*

Jansen LA, & Sulmasy DP. (2002). Sedation, alimentation, hydration, and equivocation: Careful conversation about care at the end of life. *Ann Intern Med 136*(845-49).

    Responses to Jansen & Sulmasy from Sasser CG, Quill TE, Rousseau P, Gert B, Bernat JL, & Mogielnicki RP. *Ann Intern Med 133*(7), 560-65.

Jennett B. (2002). The vegetative state. *J Neurol Neurosurg Psychiatry 73,* 3556.

Kammoun S, Gold G, Bouras C, Giannakopoulos P, McGee W, Herrmann F, Michel JP. (2000). Immediate causes of death of demented and non-demented elderly. *Acta Neurol Scand Suppl 176,* 96-9.

Kapp MB. (2002). Regulating the foregoing of artificial nutrition and hydration: First, do some harm. *J Am Geriatr Soc 50*(3), 586-88.

Kapp MB. (2006) Medicaid Planning, Estate Recovery, and Alternatives for Long-Term Care Financing: Identifying the Ethical Issues. *Care Management Journal 7*(2), 73-78.

Kennedy P & Andreason D. (2004). Using human extra-cortical local field potentials to control a switch. *J Neurolog Eng, 1, 72-77.*

Keyserlingk E. (1984). Review of report: Deciding to forego life-sustaining treatment (President's Commission for the study of ethical problems in medicine and biomedical and behavioral research, 1983, Washington, DC) *Health Law Can 4*(4), 103-07.

Kirschner KL. (2005). When written advance directives are not enough. *Clin Geriatr Med, 21*(1), 193-209.

Kisken T. (2004, 12 Sep). Retrieved from Ventura County Star: http://www.venturacountystar.com/vcs/county_news/article/0;1375;VCS_226_3178169;00.html.

Koch T. (1998). *The Limits of Principle: Deciding who lives and who dies.* Westport: Praeger. (See page 33.)

Kolarik RC, Arnold RM, Fischer GS, & Hanusa BH. (2002). Advance care planning. A comparison of values statements and treatment preferences. *J Gen Intern Med 17*(8), 618-24.

Koopmans RT, Ekkerink JL, & van Weel C. (2003). Survival to late dementia in Dutch nursing home patients. *J Am Geriatr Soc 51*(2), 184-7.

Krakauer J. (2003). *Under the Banner of Heaven: A story of violent faith.* New York: Doubleday.

Kubler-Ross E. (1969). *On Death and Dying.* New York: MacMillan.

Kunz R. (2003). Palliative care for patients with advanced dementia: Evidence-based practice replaced by values-based practice. *J Gerontol Geriatric 36*(5), 355-9.

Lacey D. (2004). Tube feeding in advanced Alzheimer's disease: When language misleads. *Amer J Alzheimers Dis Other Demen 19*(2), 125-27.

Lakoff G. (2002). *Moral Politics: How liberals and conservatives think.* Chicago: University of Chicago Press.

Lakoff G. (2004). *Don't Think of an Elephant: Know your values and frame the debate--the essential guide for progressives.* White River Junction: Chelsea Green.

Landers A. (1995, 11 Nov). Doctors can't remove feeding tube. *Harrisburg Patriot*

Lanuke K, Fainsinger RL, & DeMoissac D. (2004). Hydration management at the end of life. *Palliat Med 7*(2), 257-63.

Lattanzi-Licht M, Mahoney JJ, & Miller GW. (1998). *The hospice choice.* New York: Simon & Schuster.

Li I. (2002, 15 Apr). Feeding tubes in patients with severe dementia. *Amer Fam Physician 65*(8), 1605-10.

Lipkin KM. (2006) Identifying a proxy for Health care as part of routine medical inquiry. *J Gen Intern Med* 10.1111/j.1525-1497.2006.00570.x; [Epub]

Limprecht E. (2004, 19 Nov). GPs paid peanuts for date. *Australian Doctor.*

Loewy EH. (2001). Terminal sedation, self-starvation, and orchestrating the end of life. *Arch Intern Med 161,* 329-332.

Lueck S. (2005). *Wall Street J. on line.* Retrieved from http://online.wsj.com/article/SB113512385722127936.html.

Lynn J. (1986). *By No Extraordinary Means: The choice to forgo life-sustaining food and water.* Indianapolis: Indiana State University Press.

Lynn J. (1991). Why I don't have a living will. *Law, Medicine and Health Care 19*(1-2), 101-04.

Lynn J. (2000). Learning to care for people with chronic illness facing the end of life. *JAMA 284,* 2508-9.

Lynn J. (2004). *Sick to Death and Not Going to Take it Anymore! Reforming health care for the last years of life.* Berkeley: University of California Press.

Lynn J, & Harrold J. (1999). *Handbook for Mortals: Guidance for people facing serious illmess.* New York: Oxford University Press.

Lynn J, Schuster JL, & Kabcenell A. (2000) *Improving Care for the End of Life.* New York: Oxford University Press.

Lynn J & Adamson DM. (2003). Living well at the end of life. Adapting health care to serious chronic illness in old age. Rand Corporation "White Paper," retrieved from http://www.rand.org/publications/WP/WP137

Machulda MM, Ward HA, Borowski B, Gunter JL, Cha RH, O'Brien PC, Petersen RC, Boeve BF, Knopman D, Tang-Wai DF, Ivnik RJ, Smith GE, Tangalos EG, & Jack CR Jr. (2003). Comparison of memory fMRI response among normal, MCI, and Alzheimer's patients. *Neurology 61*(4), 500-06.

Maillet JO, Potter RL, & Heller L. (2002). Position of the American Dietetic Association: Ethical and legal issues in nutrition, hydration, and feeding. *J Amer Diet Assoc 102*(5), 716-26.

Marco CA, & Schears RM. (2003). Prehospital resuscitation practices: A survey of prehospital providers. *J Emerg Med 24*(1), 101-6.

In re Martin. (1995). 450 Mich 204 [538 NW 2d 399, 409-11 & 399.]

McCann RM, Hall WJ, & Groth-Juncker A. (1994). Comfort care for terminally ill patients: The appropriate use of nutrition and hydration. *JAMA 272*(16), 1263-66.

McCue JD. (1995). The naturalness of dying. *JAMA 273*(13), 1039-43.

McIntyre A, & Zalta E. (2004). Doctrine of Double Effect. In *The Stanford*

Encyclopedia of Philosophy. Thomas Aquinas, Summa Theologica (II-II, Qu. 64, Art.6): http://plato.stanford.edu/archives/fall2004/entries/double-effect/.

McKenna MT, Michaud CM, Murray CJ, & Marks JS. (2005). Assessing the burden of disease in the United States using disability-adjusted life years. *Am J Prev Med 28*(5), 415-23.

McMahan J (2002). *The Ethics of Killing. Problems at the Margins of Life.* New York: Oxford University Press.

McNamara EP, & Kennedy NP. (2001). Tube feeding patients with advanced dementia: An ethical dilemma. *Proc Nutr Soc 60*(2), 179-85.

Meier DE, Ahronheim JC, Morris J, Baskin-Lyons S, & Morrison RS. (2001). High short-term mortality in hospitalized patients with advanced dementia: Lack of benefit of tube feeding. *Arch Intern Med 161*(4), 594-9.

Miller FG, & Meier DE. (1998). Voluntary death: A comparison of terminal dehydration and physician-assisted suicide. *Ann Intern Med 128*(7), 559-62.

Miller LL, Harvath TA, Ganzini L, Goy ER, Delorit MA, & Jackson A. (2004). Attitudes and experiences of Oregon hospice nurses and social workers regarding assisted suicide. *Palliat Med 18*(8), 685-91.

Mitchell SL, Buchanan JL, Littlehale S, & Hamel MB. (2004). Tube feeding versus hand-feeding nursing home residents with advanced dementia: A cost comparison. *J Amer Med Dir Assoc 5*(2, suppl), S22-9.

Mitchell SL, Teno JM, Roy J, Kabumoto G, & Mor V. (2003). Clinical and organizational factors associated with feeding tube use among nursing home residents with advanced cognitive impairment. *JAMA 290*(1), 73-80.

Mitchell SL, Teno JM, Intrator O, Feng Z, Mor V. Decisions to Forgo Hospitalization in Advanced Dementia: A Nationwide Study. *J Am Geriatr Soc 55*:432–438, 2007.

Monmaney, T. (1995, 9 Aug). Doctors often unaware of living wills, study finds. *Los Angeles Times,* A3, sec. Medicine.

Monteleoni C, & Clark E. (2004). Using rapid-cycle quality improvement methodology to reduce feeding tubes in patients with advanced dementia: Before and after study. *BMJ 329*(7464), 491-94.

Morita T, Shima Y, Miyashita M, Kimura R, & Adachi I. (2004). Physician- and nurse-reported effects of intravenous hydration therapy on symptoms of terminally ill patients with cancer. *J Palliat Med 7*(5), 683-93.

Morita T, Tei Y, Tsunoda J, Inoue S, & Chihara S. (2001). Determinants of the sensation of thirst in terminally ill cancer patients. *Support Care Cancer, 9*(3), 177-86.

Mower WR, & Baraff LJ. (1993). Advance directives. Effect of type of directive on physicians' therapeutic decisions. *Arch Intern Med 153*(3), 375-81.

Mueller PS, Hook CC, Hayes DL (2003). Ethical analysis of withdrawal of pacemaker or implantable cardioverter-defibrillator support at the end of life. *Mayo Clin Proc. Aug;78(8)*:959-63.

Murphy LM, & Lipman TO. (2003). Percutaneous endoscopic gastrostomy does not prolong survival in patients with dementia. *Arch Intern Med 163*(11), 1351-53.

New York State. (2005, Jan). *Form and Instructions for the New York Health Care Proxy.* Retrieved from http://www.oag.state.ny.us/health/Proxy_form.pdf.

Nuland S. (1994). *How We Die: Reflections on life's final chapter.* New York: Vintage.

O'Connor (1988, 13 Oct). On Behalf of Mary O'Connor, Appellant. Helen A. Hall and others, Respondents. *Court of Appeals of New York 72 NY 2d 517; 534 NYS 2d 886; 531 NE 2d 607.* Amended April 11, 1989.

Panicola, M. (2001). Catholic teaching on prolonging life: Setting the record straight. *Hastings Cent Rep, 31*(6), 14-25.

Panicola, M. (2001). Withdrawing nutrition and hydration. The Catholic tradition offers guidance for the treatment of patients in a persistent vegetative state. *Health Prog, 82*(6), 28-33.

Paris JJ. (1981). The six million dollar woman. *Conn Med 45,* 720-21.

Pasman HR, Onwuteaka-Philipsen BD, Kriegsman DM, Ooms ME, Ribbe MW, & van der Wal G. (2005). Discomfort in nursing home patients with severe dementia in whom artificial nutrition and hydration is forgone. *Arch Intern Med 165*(15), 1729-35.

Pasman HR, Onwuteaka-Philipsen BD, Ooms ME, van Wigcheren PT, van der Wal G, & Ribbe MW. (2004). Forgoing artificial nutrition and hydration in nursing home patients with dementia: Patients, decision making, and participants. *Alzheimers Dis Assoc Disord 18,* 154-62.

Patient Self-Determination Act of 1990. (1990). *Pub L No 101-508, 4206, 4751, 104 Stat, 1388.*

Pear R. (2005, 20 Dec). Budget Accord Could Mean Payments by Medicaid Recipients. Retrieved from http://www.nytimes.com/2005/12/20/politics/20health.html.

Phillips, K. (2006). *American Theocracy: The Peril and Politics of Radical Religion, Oil, and Borrowed Money in the 21stCentury.* Viking Adult.

POLST. (2005). Physician Orders for Life-Sustaining Treatment. Retrieved from http://www.ohsu.edu/ethics/polst/docs/POLST_nppi.pdf.

Ponsky JL, Gauderer MW, & Stellato TA. (1983). Percutaneous endoscopic gastrostomy. Review of 150 cases. *Arch Surg 118*(8), 913-4.

Pope John Paul II. (2004, 20 Mar). Life-sustaining treatments and vegetative state: Scientific advances and ethical dilemmas. (Speech/Allocution). Retrieved from http://www.vatican.va/holy_father/john_paul_ii/speeches/2004/march/documents/hf_jp-ii_spe_20040320_congress-fiamc_en.html.

Post S. (1995). *The Moral Challenge of Alzheimer's Disease.* Baltimore: Johns Hopkins University Press, in which Koch T. (1998) cited the original newspaper article that appeared in the 1993 *Cleveland Plain Dealer.*

Post S. (2001). Tube feeding and advanced progressive dementia. *Hastings Cent Rep 31*(1), 36-42.

Povenmire R. (1998-99). Do parents have the legal authority to consent to the surgical amputation of normal healthy tissue from their infant children? The practice of circumcision in the United States. *J Gender Soc Policy and the Law 7*, 87-123.

Prendergast TJ, & Luce JM. (1997). Increasing incidence of withholding and withdrawal of life support from the critically ill. *Amer J Resp Crit Care Me, 155*, 15-20.

Preston TA. (2000). *Final Victory.* CA: Prima publishing.

Priefer BA, & Robbins J. (1997). Eating changes in mild-stage Alzheimer's disease: A pilot study. *Dysphagia 12*(4), 212-21.

Printz LA. (1992). Terminal dehydration, a compassionate treatment. *Arch Intern Med 152*, 697-700.

Puchalski C M., Zhong Z, Jacobs MM, Fox E, Lynn J, Harrold J, Galanos A, Phillips RS, Califf R, & Teno JM. (2000). Patients who want their family and physician to make resuscitation decisions for them: Observations from SUPPORT and HELP. Study to Understand Prognoses and Preferences for Outcomes and Risks of Treatment. Hospitalized Elderly Longitudinal Project. *J Am Geriatr Soc 48*(5, suppl), S84-S90.

Quill TE, & Byock IR. (2000). Responding to intractable terminal suffering: The role of terminal sedation and voluntary refusal of food & fluids. American College of Physicians–American Society of Internal Medicine End-of-Life Care Consensus Panel. *Ann Intern Med 132*(5), 408-14.

Quill TE, Byock IR, & Nunn S. (2000). Palliative treatments of last resort: Choosing the least harmful alternative. *Ann Intern Med 132*(6), 488-93.

Raghavan K. (2005, 2 Aug). A plea for reason and a death with humanity. *The Daily Telegraph (Sydney, Australia).*

Ramsøy Z T. (2006) Welcome back, Terry Wallis? Retrieved from http://brainethics.wordpress.com/2006/07/10/ welcome-back-terry-wallis/

Reiman EM, Caselli R, Chen K, Alexander GE, Bandy D, & Frost J. (2001). Declining brain activity in cognitively normal apolipoprotein E4 heterozygotes: A foundation for using positron emission tomography to efficiently test treatments to prevent Alzheimer's disease. *Pro Natl Acad Sci 98*(3334-39).

Reiman EM, Chen K, Alexander GE, Caselli RJ, Bandy D, Osborne D, Saunders AM, & Hardy J. (2004). Functional brain abnormalities in young adults at genetic risk for late-onset Alzheimer's and other dementias. *Proc Natl Acad Sci 101*, 284-89.

Repenshek M, & Slosar JP. (2004). Medically assisted nutrition and hydration: A contribution to the dialog. *Hastings Cent Rep, 34*(6), 13-16.

Riemer J, & Stampfer N. (1994). *So That Your Values Live On: Ethical wills and how to prepare them.* Woodstock, Vt: Jewish Lights Publishing.

Rinpoche S. (1993). *The Tibetan Book of Living and Dying.* San Francisco: Harper.

Rocker G, Cook D, Sjokvist P, Weaver B, Finfer S, McDonald E, Marshall J, Kirby A, Levy M, Dodek P, Heyland D, & Guyatt G. (2004). Level of care study investigators: Canadian critical care trials group. *Crit Care Med 32*(5), 1149-54.

Roter DL, Larson S, Fischer GS, Arnold RM, & Tulsky JA. (2000). Experts practice what they preach: A descriptive study of best and normative practices in end-of-life discussions. *Arch Intern Med, 160*(22) 3477-85.

Ross LF, Clayton EW. Letter to Editor re Curlin. N Engl J Med 2007;356;1890.

Rousseau P. (2002). Careful conversation about care at the end of life. *Ann Intern Med 137*(12), 1009-10.

Royal Hospital for Neuro-disability. Coma, Vegetative State, and the Minimally Conscious State. Retrieved from http://www.rhn.org.uk/institute/cat. asp?catid=1268.

Sabatino CP. (1999). Survey of state EMS-DNR laws and protocols. *J Law Med Ethics 27,* 297-315.

Sabatino CP. (2005). National advance directives: One attempt to scale the barriers. *National Association Elder Law Attorneys Journal 1,* 131-64.

Schiff ND, Rodriguez-Moreno D, Kamal A, Kim KH, Giacino JT, Plum F, & Hirsch J. (2005). fMRI reveals large-scale network activation in minimally conscious patients. *Neurology 64*(3), 514-23.

Schmitz P & O'Brien M. (1989). Observations on nutrition and hydration in dying cancer patients. In Lynn J. (Ed.), *By No Extraordinary Means: The choice to forgo life-sustaining food and water.* Bloomington: Indiana University Press.

Schneiderman LJ. (1990). Exile and PVS. *Hastings Cent Rep 20*(3), 5.

Schneiderman LJ, Gilmer T, Teetzel HD, Dugan DO, Blustein J, Cranford R, Briggs KB, Komatsu GI, Goodman-Crews P, Cohn F, & Young EW. (2003). Effect of ethics consultations on nonbeneficial life-sustaining treatments in the intensive care setting: A randomized controlled trial. *JAMA 290*(9), 1166-72.

Schneiderman LJ, & Jecker NS. (1995). *Wrong Medicine: Doctors, patients, and futile treatment.* Baltimore: Johns Hopkins University Press.

Schulz R, Mendelsohn AB, Haley WE, Mahoney D, Allen RS, Zhang S, Thompson L, & Belle SH. (2003). Resources for enhancing Alzheimer's caregiver health investigators. End-of-life care and the effects of bereavement on family caregivers of persons with dementia. *N Engl J Med 349*(20), 1936-42.

Shannon TA, & Walter JJ. (2004). Implications of the papal allocution on feeding tubes. *Hastings Cent Rep 34*(4), 18-20.

Shepherd, L. (2006a). In Respect of People Living in a Permanent Vegetative State & Allowing Them to Die. Health Matrix: J Law-Medicine 16(2), 630-691.

Shepherd, L. (2006b). Terri Schiavo: Unsettling the Settled. Loyola U. Chicago

Law J. 37(2): 297-341.

Sieger CE, Arnold JF, & Ahronheim JC. (2002). Refusing artificial nutrition and hydration: Does statutory law send the wrong message? *J Am Geriatr Soc* 50(3), 544-50.

Silveira MJ, Rhodes L, & Feudtner C. (2004). Deciding how to decide: What processes do patients use when making medical decisions? *J Clin Ethics* 15(3), 269-81.

Silveira MJ, DiPiero A, Gerrity MS, & Feudtner C. (2000). Patients' knowledge of options at the end of life: Ignorance in the face of death. *JAMA 284*(19), 2483-88.

Silveira MJ, Buell R, Deyo RA. (2003). Prehospital DNR orders: What do physicians in Washington know? *J Am Geriatr Soc 51,* 1435-8.

Silveira MJ, Kabeto MU, & Langa KM. (2005). Net worth predicts symptom burden at the end of life. *J Palliat Med 8*(4), 827-37.

Simmons, PD. (2003). Religious beliefs and healthcare decisions: The Southern Baptist tradition. In P. Simmons (Ed.), *Religious Traditions and Healthcare Decisions.* Chicago: Park Ridge Center.

Singer PA, Thiel EC, Naylor CD, Richardson RM, Llewellyn-Thomas H, Goldstein M, Saiphoo C, Uldall PR, Kim D, & Mendelssohn DC. (1995). Life-sustaining treatment preferences of hemodialysis patients: Implications for advance directives. *J Am Soc Nephrol 6*(5), 1410-7.

Singer PA (2005, Sep-Oct). The sanctity of life. In *Foreign Policy*. Retrieved from http://www.foreignpolicy.com/story/cms.php?story_id=3159.

Slome LR, Mitchell TF, Charlebois E, Benevedes JM, & Abrams DI. (1997). Physician-assisted suicide and patients with human immunodeficiency virus disease. *N Engl J Med 336*(6), 417-21.

Smith WJ. (2002). *Culture of Death: The assault on medical ethics in America.* San Francisco: Encounter Books.

Smith WJ. (2003, Fall). Dehydration nation. *Human Life Review.* Retrieved from http://www.humanlifereview.com/2003_fall/article_2003_fall_smith.php.

Smith WJ. (2003, Oct). Waking from the dead. *First Things: A Monthly Journal of Religion and Public Life, v 36.*

Smith WJ. (2005, 24 May). The English patient. *The Weekly Standard, U.K.* Retrieved from http://www.cbsnews.com/stories/2005/05/24/opinion/main697526.shtml.

Smith WJ. (2005, 11 Apr). The legacy of Terri Schiavo: What we can do so this won't happen again. *The Weekly Standard, U.K.* Retrieved from http://www.findarticles.com/p/articles/mi_m0RMQ/is_28_10/ai_n13782019.

Smith, W. (2005, May). Never again. *Whistleblower, 39.*

Somogyi-Zalud E, Likourezos A, Chichin E, & Olson E. (2001). Surrogate decision makers' attitudes towards tube feeding in the nursing home. *Arch Gerontol Geriatr 32*(2), 101-11.

Southern California Bioethics Committee Consortium. (2005, 15 Jun). Hospital guidelines for reviewing healthcare treatment recommendations for patients who lack decision-making capacity and have no surrogates and no advance directives. [work in progress]

Soylent Green. (1973). Warner Bros.

Specter M. (2005, 24 Oct). What Money Can Buy. Healing Africa. *The New Yorker.* Retrived: www.michaelspecter.com/ny/2005/2005_10_24_gates.html

Stern S. (Director). (2004). *The Self-Made Man.* (video) Bernal Beach Films.

Stier DM, Greenfield S, Lubeck DP, Dukes KA, Flanders SC, Henning JM, Weir J, Kaplan SH. (1999) Quantifying comorbidity in a disease-specific cohort: adaptation of the total illness burden index to prostate cancer. *Urology* Sep;54(3):424-9.

Straw G, & Cummins R. AARP North Carolina End of Life Care Survey. 2003. Retrieved from: http://research.aarp.org/health/nc_eol.pdf

Sulmasy DP. (2000). Responses to letter. *Ann Intern Med 133*(7), 560-65.

Sunshine E. (2005, 8 Apr). Truncating Catholic tradition. Florida bishops avoid full consideration of ethical issues in Schiavo case. *National Catholic Reporter.* Retrieved from http://ncronline.org/NCR_Online/archives2/2005b/040805/040805k.php

Tabuchi H. (2007, 22 Jun). Hitachi: Move the train with your brain. Assoc. Press.

Teno J, & Lynn J. (1996). Putting advance care planning into action. *J Clin Ethics 7,* 205-13.

Teno J, Lynn J, Connors AF Jr, Wenger N, Phillips RS, Alzola C, Murphy DP, Desbiens N, & Knaus WA. (1997). The illusion of end-of-life resource savings with advance directives. SUPPORT Investigators. Study to Understand Prognoses and Preferences for Outcomes and Risks of Treatment. *J Am Geriatr Soc 45*(4), 513-8.

Terman SA. (1999, Feb). Kevorkian pushed the wrong envelope. *San Diego Physician, The County Medical Society Journal,* 10,15.

Terman SA. (1999, Summer). Healing from bedside harp playing--a psychiatrist's perspective. *The Harp Therapy Journal.* Retrieved from http://www.64peace.com/articles.htm#healing

Terman SA. (1999, 1 Apr). Learning from the judgments of Kevorkian. *San Diego Union-Tribune,* sec. B, 11.

Terman SA. (2001a). Determining the decision-making capacity of a patient who refused food and water. *J Palliat Med 15,* 55-60.

Terman SA. (2001b). Evaluating decision-making capacity in a psychotic breast cancer patient. *Primary Care Cancer 6*(45-8).

Terman SA. (2007). *Lethal Choice.* Carlsbad: Life Transitions Publications.

Texas Futile Care Law. V.T.C.A. *Health and Safety Code Sec 166.046.*

The AM, Pasman R, Onwuteaka-Philipsen B, Ribbe M, & van der Wal G. (2002). Withholding the artificial administration of fluids and food from elderly patients with dementia: Ethnographic study. *BMJ 325*(7376), 1326.

The President's Council on Bioethics. (2005). *Taking Care: Ethical Caregiving In Our Aging Society.* Washington: US Executive Office of the President. Can be retrieved from: http://www.bioethics.gov/reports/taking_care/index.html

Thompson T, Barbour R, & Schwartz L. (2003, 1 Nov). Adherence to advance directives in critical care decision making: Vignette study. *BMJ 327*(7422), 1011-14

Tierney MC, Yao C, Kiss A, & McDownell I. (2005). Neuropsychological tests accurately predict incident Alzheimer disease after 5 and 10 years. *Neurology 64*(1), 1853-59.

Tolle SW, Tilden VR, Drach LL, Fromme EK, Perrin NA, & Hedberg K. (2004). Characteristics and proportion of dying Oregonians who personally consider physician-assisted suicide. *J Clin Ethics 15*(2), 111-8.

Tresch DD, Sims FH, Duthie EH, Goldstein MD, & Lane PS. (1991). Clinical characteristics of patients in the persistent vegetative state. *Arch Intern Med 151,* 930-32.

Truog RD, Cochrane T. (2005). Refusal of hydration and nutrition: Irrelevance of the 'artificial" vs "natural" distinction. *Arch Intern Med 165,* 2574-76.

Tulsky JA, Fischer GS, Rose MA, & Arnold RM. (1998). Opening the black box: How do physicians communicate about advance directives? *Ann Intern Med 129*(6), 441-49.

Vacco v Quill. (1997). *521 US 793.*

van der Steen JT, Kruse RL, Ooms ME, Ribbe MW, van der Wal G, Heintz LL, Mehr DR. (2004). Treatment of nursing home residents with dementia and lower respiratory tract infection in the United States and The Netherlands: An ocean apart. *J Am Geriatr Soc 52*(5), 691-9.

van der Steen JT, Ooms ME, van der Wal G, & Ribbe MW. (2002). Pneumonia: The demented patient's best friend? Discomfort after starting or withholding antibiotic treatment. *J Am Geriatr Soc 50*(10), 1681-8.

van der Steen JT, Ribbe MW, Mehr DR, van der Wal G. (2004). Do findings of high mortality from pneumonia in the elderly make it the old man's friend? *Arch Intern Med 164*(2), 224-5.

van der Steen JT, van der Wal G, Mehr DR, Ooms ME, Ribbe MW. (2005). End-of-life decision making in nursing home residents with dementia and pneumonia: Dutch physicians' intentions regarding hastening death. *Alzheimer Dis Assoc Disord 19*(3), 148-55.

Volicer L, Seltzer B, Rheaume Y, Fabiszewski K, Herz L, Shapiro R, & Innis P. (1987). Progression of Alzheimer's type dementia in institutionalized patient: A cross sectional study. *J Applied Geront 6*(83-94).

Von Gunten CF. (2005, 25 Mar). The end of life. Values and principles should guide decision-making. *San Diego Union-Tribune,* sec. B, 7.

Waller A, Hershkowitz M, & Adunsky A. (1994). The effect of intravenous fluid infusion on blood and urine parameters of hydration and on state of consciousness in terminal cancer patients. *Am J Hosp Palliat Care 11*(6), 22-7.

Wallis J. (2005). *God's Politics: Why the right gets It wrong and the left doesn't get it.* San Francisco: HarperSanFrancisco.

Wanzer SH, Adelstein SJ, Cranford RE, Federman DD, Hook ED, Moertel CG, Safar P, Stone A, Taussig HB, & van Eys J. (1984). The physician's responsibility toward hopelessly ill patients. *NEJM 310*(15), 955-9.

Wanzer SH, Glenmullen J. (2007). *To Die Well. Your right to comfort, calm, and choice in the last days of life.* Cambridge: De Capo Press.

Washington v Glucksberg. (1997). *521 US 702.*

Webb M. (1997). *The Good Death.* New York: Bantam Books.

Weissman DE, & Block S. (2002). ACGME requirements for end-of-life training in selected residency and fellowship programs: A status report. *Academic Medicine 77*(4), 299-304.

Weller B. (2005, 5 Jan). A visit with Terri Schiavo: Very much alive and responsive. Retrieved from http://www.lifesite.net/.

Conservatorship of the Person of ROBERT WENDLAND, S087265, 28 P.3 d 151; 2001.

Westley D. (1995). *When It's Right to Die: Conflicting voices, difficult choices.* Mystic, Conn: Twenty-third Publications.

WGBH Educational Foundation. (1992, 24 Mar). *The death of Nancy Cruzan.* Retrieved from http://www.pbs.org/wgbh/pages/frontline/programs/transcripts/1014.html.

Whalen J. (2005, 22 Nov). Valued lives: Britain stirs outcry by weighing benefits of drugs versus price. Government arm finds pills for Alzheimer's too costly, angering patients, Pfizer. *Wall Street Journal, Eastern ed.,* sec. A, p. 1, 11.

Willing R. (2005, 4 Aug). Brain-dead Virginia woman dies after giving birth. *USA Today (New York),* sec. Nation. Retrieved from http://www.usatoday.com/news/nation/2005-08-03-torres-obit_x.htm?csp=34&POE=click-refer

Winberg H. (2001, 2 Apr). Physician-assisted suicide in Oregon: Why so few occurrences? *Medical J Aust 174*(7), 353-4.

Winter, SM. (2000). Terminal nutrition: Framing the debate for the withdrawal of nutritional support in terminally ill patients. *Am J Med 109*(9), 723-6.

Wolfson J. (Guardian *Ad Litem* for Theresa Marie Schiavo). (2003, 1 Dec). A report to Governor Jeb Bush and the 6th judicial circuit in the matter of Theresa Marie Schiavo. Retrieved from http://abstractappeal.com/schiavo/WolfsonReport.pdf.

Wolfson J. (2005). Erring on the side of Theresa Schiavo: Reflections of the Special Guardian *Ad Litem. Hastings Cent Rep, 35*(3), 16-19.

Zamrini E, De Santi S, & Tolar M. (2004). Imaging is superior to cognitive testing for early diagnosis of Alzheimer's disease. *Neurobiol Aging 25*(5), 685-91.

Glossary

The **Glossary** provides more information about key terms; for example, brain death, PVS, and MCS. The **Table** on the next two pages, "Recommended *NEW and STANDARD* Terms for Advance Planning," compares frequently used terms. [Items indicated by * were modified with permission, from James Hoefler's web site, 2005]. Citations are included. *New* suggested terms are Italicized.

The **GOAL** of this book: To **maximize the probability** that others will **honor** your end-of-life decisions (your **Last Wishes).**

Maximize the probability: To implement a proactive strategy so that your Last Wishes will be clearly interpretable, and will survive challenges by others instead of being either delayed or denied.

Honor: So others will faithfully respond to your end-of-life wishes.

Last Wishes: If you can no longer speak for yourself, these represent your preferences for medical treatment and other kinds of care (musical, spiritual, religious, and your wishes for ceremonies and so on), and who you would like to make medical decisions for you. The form can be written documents or audio/video recordings.

Advance Directive: {See **Table** on the next two pages.} Legal requirements vary greatly among States. California accepts what your doctor recalled you said in the form of what he wrote in your medical chart. Texas requires a specific form, and doctors may not have immunity even if the meaning is the same and the writing is *clear and convincing*.

Affidavit: A sworn statement in writing usually accompanied by an oath that it is true to the best of your knowledge, sometimes before an authorized notary, magistrate, or officer of the law.

Allocution: An authoritative or advisory address; lecture, speech.

*__Amicus Curiae Brief__: (Latin: "friend of the court"). Refers to reports offered by parties with special expertise who are not a party in the case.

*__Artificial Nutrition and Hydration (ANH)__: Any of several methods that supply sustenance to patients who are unable to take in food and fluids by mouth and swallow. (See PEG, NG, IV, below.) Since the only aspect that is artificial is the method of delivery, the suggested alternate term is **Artificially Administered Nutrition and Hydration (AANH).**

RECOMMENDED *NEW* and STANDARD TERMS for ADVANCE PLANNING			
Terms	**Purpose**	**Definition**	**Comments**
Advance Care Planning	Decide on your end-of-life treatment goals to exert control beyond your ability to make medical decisions. Success depends on your statements being *clear and convincing*.	Learning and effecting a plan that reflects your prudent end-of-life treatment decisions by creating documents so others will honor your Last Wishes.	The process leads to creating and/or revising written or recorded documents that are witnessed so they have legal effect.
Advance Directive for Health Care (AD)	**Advance Directives (AD)** contain specific instructions on the WHOs and WHATs to achieve your end-of-life treatment goals.	The written (or recorded) and witnessed documents that contain all your public instructions.	**AD = Directive to Physician** and/or **Proxy Directive**. (*Either one, or both*; see footnote below.)
Directive to Physician (DTP) = **Living Will (LW)**	**OPTIONAL*** part of an Advance Directive that expresses treatment preferences based on predicting specific future medical condition(s). Not self-enforcing. Physician's choice unless a Proxy functions as advocate.	Instructions to your physician. Usual format: **IF___ THEN ___**. "Living Will" no longer ONLY limits treatment; and sometimes means entire Advance Directive.	Most useful after receiving a diagnosis with a predictable trajectory. Informs your doctor and others. <u>Success</u> may depend on someone serving as your advocate.
Proxy Directive (PD) = **Durable Power of Attorney for Health Care**	**REQUIRED*** part of an Advance Directive that appoints & grants specific authority to your Proxy. Can state the degree of oversight you desire, regarding your Proxy's decisions.	Instructions that name & empower a sequence of people to make medical decisions for you if you no longer can. May possibly begin immediately.	Your instructions can state your Proxy's decisions will **override** statements in your Living Will, **ESMP** and **PVTP** (defined below), if there is a conflict.

RECOMMENDED *NEW* and STANDARD TERMS for ADVANCE PLANNING			
Terms	**Purpose**	**Definition**	**Comments**
Proxy **=** **Agent**	One or more individual(s) designated in your **Proxy Directive** to make your medical decisions.	Also called Attorney-in-Fact or Surrogate. (Exact meanings may differ in some States.)	Can state your Proxy should interact with others and perform other tasks.
Empowering Statements for My Proxy	*ESMP*: A *NEW* addition to **Proxy Directive** that anticipates challenges to specific preferences. Explains *why* you want to empower your Proxy to Refuse Food & Fluid on your behalf—if by oral and/or by artificial means.	Statements should strive to be specific and *clear and convincing* as the goal is to prevent others from challenging your Proxy's decisions by lawsuits, etc.	Explains & illustrates specific reasons for your treatment preferences. Success is preventing "third parties" from **delaying** or **denying** the honoring of your Last Wishes.
Private Statements about Values & Treatment	*PSVT*: A *NEW* separate document; NOT part of the public Advance Directive; revealed only if your Proxy decides it is necessary so others will honor your Last Wishes.	Any media (notes, questionnaires, recordings, etc.) that inform your Proxy/alternates well enough to make the decisions you would make, if you were competent.	Includes two kinds of statements: <u>specific</u> wishes you wish to keep private; <u>general</u> life and treatment values you would rather not offer as evidence.

* **Directive to Physician**: Optional for healthy people but strongly recommended for those with serious diagnoses. **Proxy Directive**: Required for all. If you know no one you can trust as your Proxy, consider designating an "end-of-life professional" as your advocate.

==================================

As Patient Permits (**APP**): Suggested term to avoid the *battery* of forced-feeding of patients who can only communicate non-verbally by offering Food & Fluid only if the patient willingly accepts.

Best Interests: A decision-making standard for incompetent patients based on assuming they would make the same choice as other "reasonable people" who were in a similar situation.

Invoked when no specific instructions are left in an Advance Directive and there is insufficient personal information to make such decisions on the basis of "substituted judgment." Often, the physician's opinion that further treatment would be **futile** is relevant, although in the United States, the presumption is to continue life unless there are compelling reasons not to do so, such as: "the degree of humiliation, dependence and loss of dignity probably resulting from the condition and treatment; life expectancy with and without treatment; the various treatment options; and the risks, side effects and benefits of each of those options." [In re Guardianship of L.W., 167 Wisc. 2d 53, 482 N.W.2d 60 (1992)]

*Brain Death (Death by Neurologic Criteria): The patient cannot breathe on her own; Pupils are fixed and dilated; the eyes do not move when the head is turned or when cold water is squirted into the ears; no blinking when the eye ball is touched; has no motor (even grimacing) response to intensely painful stimuli; does not gag or cough when irritated; absence of all reflexes; flat EEG. [Quality Standards Subcommittee of the American Academy of Neurology. Practice parameters for determining brain death in adults (Summary statement). Neurology. 1995; 45: 1012-1014. See also: Wijdicks EF. Determining brain death in adults. Neurology. 1995 May;45(5):1003-11.]

*Coma: A coma is an unarousable, sleep-like condition, similar to anesthesia that results from injury to the brain stem. A coma may last for an extended period of time, but is rarely permanent. Comas can resolve with the patient waking up to a normal life, or evolve into a persistent and then permanent vegetative state, or minimally conscious state that can also be persistent or permanent. Comas are sometimes rated by what it takes for the patient to open her eyes; to respond verbally; and by moving—which three areas are the basis for the Glasgow Coma Scale. [See: Contant CF Jr, Narayan RK. Chapter 74: Prognosis after head injury. *Pages* 1792-1812. IN: Youmans JR. Neurological Surgery, Fourth Edition, WB Saunders Company, 1996.]

Competence: The mental ability to understand problems and make decisions, as determined by a court of law. In contrast, Decisional Capacity (or Decision-Making Capacity) is a medical opinion. Both terms can and should only be applied narrowly to the specific task at hand; for example, a person may be incompetent to take care of his or her financial matters, but still retain "competence" to name a proxy to make his or her medical decisions.

Conservator: Judicially appointed guardian, with power of attorney over financial matters or health care decisions.

Death/Dying: The process of dying leads to the State of death; for example, the Coroner's answer to the Mayor of the Munchkin's question when he inquired about the Wicked Witch of the East (on whom Dorothy's house fell): She is "morally, ethically, spiritually, physically, absolutely, positively, undeniably and reliably..." as well as "really and sincerely" dead. [L. Frank Baum's, ***The Wizard of Oz***, 1900.] Back then in Oz, death simply meant the cessation of heart and lung functioning. Today, modern medical technology can prolong biologic existence after major organs have stopped functioning. The result has led to choices and conflict about which Mr. Baum could never have dreamed.

Decisional Capacity: The ability to understand, to appreciate, to use reason to form a decision, and to express it consistently, as determined by a clinician through one or more interviews. In contrast, "Competence" is a ruling determined by a court of law based on if individuals possess decision-making capacity. Both terms should be applied narrowly to the specific task at hand.

Declaration: a statement being offered as evidence in a legal proceeding.

Devastating Irreversible Brain States: Inlcudes these three diagnoses: persistent coma, Persistent Vegetative State, and end-stage dementia. Distinct from Dead by Neurologic Criteria, and Minimally Conscious State.

Do Not Resuscitate (DNR): An inappropriately short but often used term for **Do Not Attempt to Resuscitate** (**DNAR**) the functioning of the heart and lungs. Suggested alternate term: *Permit Natural Dying* (**PND**).

Double Effect: The doctrine that it is permissible to cause harm as a possibly foreseen, but not intended side-effect when the intent is to bring about a good result. It is not permissible to intend to cause this same harm to bringing about the good end. This principle allows a patient to receive enough pain medication to reduce suffering even if the foreseen but unintended side-effect is to hasten dying, but it is not permitted to give the patient so much medication that she will certainly die because there is no other way to treat the pain. The "natural and probable" result of the action is often argued to judge a doctor's subjective, internal, private thinking to infer **intent**.

Due Process: A constitutional limitation on the State or Federal government's ability to deprive a person of life, liberty, or property, which may be either Procedural or Substantive.

Procedural Due Process protects individuals from being deprived of their liberty or property, unless certain procedures are adhered to. For example, if an adult weighed 90 pounds and wanted to leave the hospital to **Refuse Food & Fluid**, before a doctor and hospital can force her to remain in the hospital and take in nourishment, they must prove that she suffers from the disease, anorexia nervosa.

Substantive Due Process protects individuals from being deprived of their liberty or property, unless the State can prove it has a legitimate basis for infringing on these rights. For example, the State of Missouri had a legitimate right to protect the life of Nancy Cruzan and therefore could insist on a level of proof that she wanted to express her right to refuse life-sustaining treatment by evidence that was *clear and convincing.*

Durable Power-of-Attorney: A Durable Power of Attorney enables the Agent to act for the Principal after the Principal is not mentally competent or physically able to make decisions. The Durable Power of Attorney may be triggered when the Principal has lost competence, or may come into effect immediately. Because it is durable, it is effective until revoked by the Principal, or the Principal's death. Can apply to financial or medical decisions.

Durable Power of Attorney for Health Care (Proxy Directive): {*See Table.*} The authority granted is called "durable" because, unlike some other powers of attorney, it lasts beyond the Principal's incompetence. If Terri Schiavo had granted the authority to her husband to discontinue life-support if she were determined to be in the Permanent Vegetative State, and then the Pope issued an Allocution that withdrawing life-support could be considered "euthanasia by omission," the later event would not change the durable authority previously given to her husband.

Empowering Statements for My Proxy **(ESMP)**: Statements which strive to be specific and *clear and convincing*; to prove what you wanted so that other third parties will not challenge your Proxy's decisions. This part of the DPAHC or Proxy Directive can anticipate challenges to the specific treatment preferences you desire. For example, if you wish to empower your **Proxy to Refuse Food & Fluid** on your behalf, it can explain and illustrate your reasons for this treatment preference so interested third parties will be less able **To Delay** or **To Deny** the honoring of your wishes.

Forms: Whether free from your State, from low-cost Internet sites, or from this book, you may need to modify them so they reflect your specific Last Wishes.

Gastrostomy: Feeding tube that goes through the skin directly into the stomach, also called a percutaneous endoscopic gastrostomy, **PEG** tube, which requires minor surgery to insert and to remove. If the tube goes through the nose to reach the stomach, it is called an **NG** tube, which is considered temporary.

*__Guardian Ad Litem__: Latin for "guardian at law" and refers in the medical decision-making context to a person who is appointed by the court to look out for the best interests of an incompetent patient. Must be a lawyer in some States. Often appointed to represent someone who may be at the center of a dispute, as opposed to two litigating advocates, who take opposing views. For example, Terri Schiavo's GAL was Jay Wolfson, DrPH, JD.

__Health Care Treatment Instructions__ or __Living Will__ or __Directive to Physician__): A statement or series of checked options intended to reflect the Principal's future wishes for the medical treatment that would be, or would not be, desired—based on predicting possible future medical and mental conditions.

__Hospice__ supports and cares for persons in the last phase of an incurable disease so that they may live as fully and as comfortably as possible. Hospice recognizes that the dying process is a part of the normal process of living and focuses on enhancing the quality of remaining life. It affirms life and neither hastens nor postpones death. Hospice exists in the hope and belief that through appropriate care, and the promotion of a caring community sensitive to their needs, that individuals and their families may be free to attain a degree of satisfaction in preparation for death. Hospice recognizes that human growth and development can be a lifelong process. Hospice seeks to preserve and promote the inherent potential for growth within individuals and families during the last phase of life. Hospice offers palliative care for all individuals and their families without regard to age, gender nationality, race, creed, sexual orientation, disability, diagnosis, availability of a primary care giver, or ability to pay. Hospice programs provide state-of-the-art palliative care and supportive services to individuals at the end of their lives, their family members and significant others, 24 hours a day, seven days a week, in both the home and facility-based settings. Physical, social, spiritual and emotional care are provided by a clinically-directed interdisciplinary team consisting of patients and their families, professionals and volunteers during the last stages of an illness, the dying process, and bereavement period. (Hospice Standards of Practice, National Hospice and Palliative Care Organization, 2000.)

__Informed consent__: A person's agreement to permit a specific medical treatment, after being fully appraised of the benefits and risks involved, and any treatment alternatives.

__Intravenous (IV) Line__: refers to the administration of medications or solutions (fluids) through a needle or tube inserted into a vein, which allows immediate access to the blood supply.

Killing versus Murder: To kill is simply to end a life by effecting physical death. Murder is the killing of another human being with malice and forethought. Malice is intent, without justification or excuse, to commit a wrongful act. ("Malice" is not synonymous with "ill-will", but rather refers to any wrongful intent as defined by the law.) Therefore, the act of smothering a terminally ill loved one who requests release from her unbearable suffering constitutes murder according to the law, while self-defense is killing but not murder.

Living Will (Directive to Physician): Though initially used only to limit medical treatment at the end-of-life, the term "Living Will" now refers to instructions that tell your physician what specific end-of-life treatments you DO want as well as do NOT want, based on predicting your future medical conditions. Almost 40% of States have Living Wills that can extend treatment as well as limit treatment. Some Living Wills include choices about *Comfort Care*, music and religious readings, photographs, the desired place to die, and what values or events they would like to be remembered for, spiritual needs, and ceremonies as well as choices about medical treatment. This book uses the term **Directive to Physician** to specifically mean *medical* preferences since the document is addressed to physicians who will hopefully respond to its written (or recorded) requests.

Each State defines its own terms so the health care instruction document has alternate terms such as "Living Will" and "Declaration" and many States do not use "physician," "health care," or "medical provider." Dr. Ronald Miller prefers "Treatment Directive" because more *or less treatment* may be desired.

Locked-In State or **Syndrome**: Patient retains consciousness, the ability to think, to see and hear, and to feel emotions BUT their voluntary muscles are severely paralyzed so they cannot communicate. The last muscles before complete paralysis are those that control vertical eye movements and blinking, which are sometimes used for limited communication. The end stage of ALS (amyotrophic lateral sclerosis) or Lou Gehrig's Disease is one cause of the locked-in state (which is not the same as the "Locked-in Syndrome").

Moral: Behavior conforming to principles of right and wrong, but relevant in the context of a particular belief system. For example, in war it is right to kill the enemy, even if you otherwise uphold the Ten Commandments. Nazis believed their mission to purify the human race was morally right.

Morality: Culturally dependent principles of right and wrong behavior.

Minimally Conscious State: The person is partially conscious with sleep/wake cycles; can either follow simple commands (even if inconsistent) or respond with gestures or "Yes" / "No" answers (even if not accurate), or can verbalize or demonstrate purposeful behaviors as a response to the environment (not reflexive). Examples of purposeful behaviors: appropriate smiling or crying, vocalizations of gestures in direct response to content of questions, reaching for objects in right direction, holding objects to accommodate for size and shape, appropriate moving of the eyes in visual pursuit or fixation. [Giacino JT, Ashwal S, et al. The minimally conscious state. Definitions and diagnostic criteria. Neurology. 2002; 58: 349-353.]

Patients in MCS can, in contrast to those in a coma or PVS, **sometimes** exhibits deliberate responsive behavior but it is not consistently correct. For example, a MCS patient may usually try to respond when asked a question, but will not be able to answer correctly six different obviously easy situational questions. Responses from PVS patients are reflexive. Comatose patients cannot respond at all. If a patient can correctly and consistently answer six out of six, then they are at a *higher level* of cognitive functioning than **MCS**.

Caution: Criteria may not apply to blind or paralyzed patients; more sophisticated methods of clinical evaluation may be needed.

Nasogastric (NG) Tube: Feeding tube that goes through the nose and down the throat to enter the stomach.

One-way Contract or Agreement: A "unilateral contract" is one where only one party makes a promise or requests another to perform in a certain way. Most Durable Powers of Attorney for Health Care Instructions do not require the designated Proxy to acknowledge that she or he agrees to take on the responsibilities as defined in the document, so they are considered unilateral agreements or requests, *not* legally binding contracts. However if the Principal asked for a signed acceptance of willingness to accept responsibility in the written document, then many attorneys would consider the document to be a two-way "agreement" (see below). Contracts typically require an exchange of promises in both directions such as a fee for providing a specific service.

Passive Euthanasia: Occurs when a patient dies because the medical professionals did not continue or initiate treatment necessary to keep the patient alive. Less emotionally charged terms could be used, such as: letting the patient die, letting Nature take its course, not prolonging the duration of dying, and **PND (Permit Natural Dying)**. In contrast, **active euthanasia** requires the physician to actively do something to cause the patient to die, which could be either voluntary (if the patient requests it), or involuntary (if unable to consent). In The Netherlands, involuntary euthanasia is restricted to following a protocol where there is no information about an incompetent patient for whom additional medical treatment is futile.

Permit Natural Dying (***PND***): An end-of-life choice that requests your caregivers provide all methods of *Comfort Care* to reduce pain and thirst, but will not offer any medical intervention to maintain your biologic functioning including Food & Fluid by any route (oral or tubes). A peaceful transition from dehydration and/or the underlying disease usually occurs within 2 weeks.

Private Statements about Values and Treatment (***PSVT***): {***See Table.***} Statements to inform your Proxy so he or she knows you well enough to make the decisions that you would make, if you were competent. This document includes two kinds of statements: those you want to be kept private, and others not designed for entering as evidence that will be revealed only if your Proxy decides it is necessary in the event of a challenge to honoring your Last Wishes. (See Substituted Judgment, below.)

Proxy: {***See Table.***} The person who is designated in your DPAHC or Proxy Directive to make medical decisions for you. Also called "agent", "agent in fact", "attorney-in-fact", or "surrogate".

Proxy Directive or **Durable Power of Attorney for Health Care**): {***See Table.***} Instructions that name (authorize) and empower a person ("proxy") or a sequence of people to make medical decisions for you when you no longer can, or, if you wish, immediately. These instructions also detail what oversight, if any, you want regarding your proxy's decisions. This particular authority is called "durable" because, unlike other powers of attorney, this authority lasts beyond the Principal's incompetence. Once your physician receives a copy of this document, it becomes a part of your medical record. (Different States use various acronyms for Durable Power of Attorney for Health Care, such as DPOAHC, PAHC, DPAHC, POAHC, PAHC, HCPOA, HCDPA, DPACHD.)

Sanctity of Life: Two definitions that can be mutually exclusive are: A) Life has intrinsic value since being "human" is a quality independent of functioning; therefore life should be preserved regardless of the patient's previously expressed wishes in terms of hope for improvement, unbearable suffering, dependency on others and medical technology for continued existence, or the financial and psychological burden on family and society. B) The respect for personhood in terms of specific qualities that characterize human functioning such as the ability to think, to remember, and to interact and communicate with other human beings and the environment, and to have the potential for a spiritual life. (See further discussion in the Conclusion, starting on page 411).

Sedation: treatment directed towards relieving the symptoms of anxiety and agitation, and sometimes insomnia.

*__Substituted Judgment__: The standard of decision-making that takes into account all that is known and relevant about the patient to attempt to make the medical decisions that the patient would have made, if still competent. The decision-maker thus attempts to "stand in the patient's shoes" with respect to making medical decisions.

One clear description of this standard comes from the New Jersey Supreme Court ruling In re Jobes, 108 N.J. 394, 529 A.2d 434 (1987), which is often cited by other courts. It instructs the surrogate decision-maker to take into account, "the patient's personal value system for guidance. The surrogate considers the patient's prior statements about reactions to medical issues, all facets of the patient's personality that the surrogate is familiar with—with, of course, particular reference to his or her relevant philosophical, theological, and ethical values—in order to extrapolate what course of medical treatment the patient would choose."

__Successor Proxy__: Also called "alternate proxy," this is a person named in addition to the Principal's first named proxy, who will serve as proxy in the event the person first named is unwilling, unavailable, or unable.

It is also possible for the Proxy Directive to empower an attorney-in-fact to choose alternate Proxies if the other Proxies are not willing, not available, or not able.

__Surrogate__: In general, a person appointed to act in place of another. Although often used interchangeably with "proxy" or "agent" a "surrogate for health care decisions" sometimes means a person the Principal named verbally to make decisions only during a specific hospitalization or only for a specified amount of time. It may also refer to family members in a specific sequence as provided by law, for patients who have left no written authorizing documents.

__Terminally Ill__: A prognostic term to describe patients who have fewer than six to twelve months to live under normal circumstances. Hospice benefits require the six-month definition as the Medicare criteria to be eligible for its benefit, but some patients live longer in part due to receiving excellent care. The six-month time period could also be considered the time by which one would expect one-half of patients to live longer.

__Terminal Sedation__: A better term is __Palliative Sedation__ since the goal of the pharmacological interventions is palliate (reduce) refractory symptoms in the terminally ill, by inducing/maintaining sedation as the option of last resort, and sometimes the patient does not recover consciousness before dying. See also __Respite Sedation__, page 110.

__Treatment Directive__: See Living Will.

Two-Way Agreement to Accept and to Agree: Living Wills and Proxy Directives are strictly not legal "bilateral contracts," where each party makes a promise to the other and thereby becomes obligated to perform a certain role. Yet the attempt to strive for such a contract can reduce future conflict. For **Proxy Directives**, if both patient and Proxy sign, it can help **establish legal standing** and **provide evidence of mutual understanding** of what the patient really wanted, when he or she was still competent.

Vegetative State, Persistent/Permanent: (While "vegetable" is derogatory and disrespectful of human dignity, "vegetative state" has been defined clinically and seems firmly entrenched.) A disorder of consciousness where the patient has no evidence of awareness of self or the environment; no ability to interact with others; no evidence of sustained, reproducible, purposeful, or voluntary behavioral responses to visual, auditory, tactile or noxious stimuli; no evidence of language comprehension or expression; intermittent wakefulness manifested by the presence of sleep-wake cycles; sufficiently preserved hypothalamic and brainstem autonomic functions to permit survival with medical and nursing care; bowel and bladder incontinence; variably preserved cranial nerve reflexes (pupillary, oculocephalic, corneal, vestibulo-ocular, gag) and spinal reflexes. **Caution: if patients are blind or paralyzed, patients may actually have higher brain functioning**. Also: patients' behavior may be ***assumed*** to be purposeful when it is actually reflexive so they may be given the diagnosis of MCS or higher when they are really in a Vegetative State. The Vegetative State usually emerges from a coma. Physicians usually wait three months to make a definitive diagnosis of PVS for patients who suffered a loss of oxygen to the brain, and one year to make a definitive diagnosis of PVS for patients who suffered mechanical trauma to the head. Although life expectancy for patients in a PVS is between two and five years, there are a number of cases where PVS patients are sustained on life-support for decades. It has been estimated that there are somewhere between 15,000 and 35,000 PVS patients being sustained in the U.S. at this time.

Ref: Council on Ethical and Judicial Affairs. (1990). Persistent Vegetative State and the Decision to Withdraw or Withhold Life Support. *JAMA 263*, 426-30.

Further Resources

Regarding the order of entries: The list begins with more important or more general resources, then reverts to alphabetical order, and ends with the organization with which the authors of this book are affiliated.

http://www.caringadvocates.org/links.html has additional links & updates.

Summary of State Bills Restricting End-of-Life Choices Introduced in 2005 & 2006
http://www.compassionandchoices.org/documents/EndofLife_Legislation_Chart.pdf

According to their web site, as of March, 2006, twenty-three states were considering new legislation. Some proposed laws would make it more difficult to remove a feeding tube from a permanently unconscious patient. Others would make it easier for politicians and organizations to tie up a case in court for years.

This web site was prepared for "MergerWatch" by Elena N. Cohen and Theresa Conner with the assistance of Kathy Cerminera and Attorney Kathryn Tucker of **Compassion and Choices**, an organization that is described below.

The President's Council on Bioethics. September 2005 Report: TAKING CARE: ETHICAL CAREGIVING IN OUR AGING SOCIETY. http://www.bioethics.gov

This web site has an extensive list of resources that begins with a "Thematic Bibliography" at http://www.bioethics.gov/reports/taking_care/bibliograpy.html, continues under "Sources of Information and Support" with Institutional, Governmental, and Private links to web sites (many of which also have extensive links), and finally lists "Web-Based Resources," which provide even more links.

The New York Times' free collection of articles about the theme of death and dying: http://www.topics.nytimes.com/top/news/health/diseasesconditionsandhealthtopics/deathanddying/index.html?8qa

American Academy of Hospice and Palliative Medicine. http://www.aahpm.org/

This web site has information and links of interest to professionals, & links for all.

American Hospice Foundation. http://www.americanhospice.org

This web site has information on how to locate a hospice in your community and an article worth reading before you do: "What to Expect and Demand of a Good Hospice," http://www.americanhospice.org/articles/consumerquestions.pdf.

American College of Trust and Estate Counsel; http://www.actec.org/

> This web site allows users to search for member attorneys who belong to this association since they counsel on preparation of wills and trusts, estate planning, and related issues.

National Academy of Elder Law Attorneys (NAELA); http://www.NAELA.org

> The field of "elder law" is broader than end-of-life issues, yet this web site offers basic information on Advance Directives and provides ways for visitors to search for lawyers who are members of the Academy.

> The site lists 14 States that require **mandatory forms**, 16 States (plus DC) that have strict **witnessing requirements**, and 2 States that prescribe specific phraseology for **wording instructions**. (Consider these numbers as a minimum.)

> NAELA poses five key questions to consider: 1. Who will serve as your Agent for Health Care and who will serve as the alternate? 2. Are there certain medical treatments or pain control measures you want or don't want? 3. Do you wish to take or refuse any medication that may reduce or eliminate the ability to communicate? 4. Do you have any particular directions regarding specific health care facilities, religious preferences, disposition of your body, donation of bodily parts for transplant or research, etc? 5. What directions will you provide related to end-of life decisions specifically regarding: if you can no longer eat, drink or breathe on your own; if you cannot function independent of machines; if you are confined to bed; or if you have no cognitive ability.

American Bar Association Commission on Law and Aging; http://www.abanet.org/aging

> The ABA Commission on Law and Aging of the American Bar Association is composed of lawyers in the field of law and aging who are dedicated to enforcing the rights of the elderly. There is a "Find a Lawyer" link on the main page.

> The Commission offers a comprehensive Advance Directive form as well as a "Consumer's Tool Kit for Health Care Advance Planning" to assist individuals in creating effective advance directives that reflect their wishes and values. The site also provides useful articles such as, "10 Legal Myths About Advance Medical Directives," by Charles P. Sabatino, J.D., Director of the American Bar Association's Commission on Law and Aging,

> In collaboration with the State of Marlyand, the ABA offers a guide, "Making Medical Decisions for Someone Else: A Guide for Marylanders," at http://www.oag.state.md. They hope that similar guides will be adopted by other States.

Lawyer Referral Service; http://www.ilawyer.com/

> For people in California, Houston, Texas, New York, Kentucky, Southern Indiana and Connecticut, this Lawyer Referral Service (iLawyer) asks users for brief descriptions of their legal needs and suggests qualified lawyers in their area.

State and County Bar Associations

> Each State and county bar association provide their own search tools for users to find lawyers in their area with the appropriate area of practice and expertise.

General links to find attorneys:

> www.findlaw.com   www.martindale.com   www.legalmatch.com
>
> www.lawyers.com   www.attorneylocate.com   www.attorneyfind.com

AARP; http://www.aarp.org; http://www.aarp.org/families/end_life/

> AARP was formerly the American Association of Retired People, yet only 44% of their 35 million *international* members are retired. AARP is a national nonprofit and nonpartisan membership organization for people aged 50 years and over, dedicated to enhancing quality of life through advocacy, information and service.
>
> The AARP has an active presence in every State and voices its opinion on national legislation, as well. They also conduct surveys on end-of-life issues. The "families/end_life/" web page offers an introduction to an estate-planning guide, a guide that explains financial powers of attorney, a self-help guide on the basics of creating a will, a list of web resources for those who are coping with the loss of a loved one, and a list of resources for professionals who help individuals coping with loss. Other articles address hospice, palliative care, and talking about final wishes with a loved one. The AARP offers extensive services and resources for professionals working with elders. Their address and phone number are: 601 E Street NW; Washington, DC 20049, and 1-888-OUR-AARP (1-888-687-2277).

Aging with Dignity; http://www.agingwithdignity.org or 1-888-5-WISHES (594-7437)

> Aging with Dignity is a non-profit organization that has, since 1996, focused on advanced care planning and distributing "Five Wishes," a document that now *substantially* satisfies the legal requirements of Advance Directives in about 37 States, and provides the structure to inform your family, friends, and doctors what kind of spiritual, musical, and ceremonial rituals you prefer.
>
> (In Chapter 12, *i-FAQ 41* provides detailed strategies on how to complete "Five

Wishes" so that it includes the relevant strategies to accomplish the end-of-life goal of this book, a "peaceful" and "legal" transition, if that is your choice.)

Alzheimer's Association; http://www.alz.org; 1-800-272-3900

The Alzheimer's Association is the nation's leading resource for anyone suffering from Alzheimer's disease or related dementias, their caregivers and loved ones. The Alzheimer's Association has over 81 chapters and 300 centers to help patients and loved ones cope with the many challenges of dementia.

Americans for Better Care of the Dying; http://abcd-caring.org

This organization aims to improve end-of-life care by learning which social and political changes will lead to enduring, efficient, and effective programs. It works with the public, clinicians, policymakers, and other end-of-life organizations to make change happen. Their goals are to: build momentum for reform; explore new methods and systems for delivering care; shape public policy through evidence-based understanding. Includes news, links, and excerpts from books by Joanne Lynn: Handbook for Mortals, and Improving Care for the End of Life.

American Medical Association, state and local societies: http://www.ama-assn.org/

These organizations can provide referrals to specialists in your area of need, including the new sub-specialty of **palliative care**. They can also refer you to hospices. The web site has links to their statements on medical ethics, http://www.ama-assn.org/ama/pub/category/2498.html. Information on advance directives for both patients and physicians can be found at http://www.ama-assn.org/ama/pub/category/14894.html. The AMA statement on end-of-life care can be found at http://www.ama-assn.org/ama/pub/category/7567.html.

Bet Tzedek, The House of Justice. http://www.bettzedek.org

Since 1974, *Bet Tzedek* has been providing free assistance to more than 100,000 people of every racial and religious background in the Los Angeles area. They were among the first to provide free Powers of Attorney for Healthcare. *Bet Tzedek* staff trains volunteer attorneys, who in turn, visit senior centers where each assists several clients.

Caring Connections; http://www.caringinfo.org

Caring Connections, a division of the National Hospice and Palliative Care Organization, is "a national consumer engagement initiative to improve care at the end of life." Caring Connections offers free resources on advance care planning, caregiving, pain control, financial issues, hospice and palliative care, and grief and loss. Caring Connections provides downloads of State-specific Advance Directives (Living Wills, Health Care Proxy). Caring Connections has a toll-free Hot Line,: 1-800-658-8898 and e-mail help: caringinfo@nhpco.org. National Hospice and Palliative Care Organization; 1700 Diagonal Road, Suite 625; Alexandria, VA 22314.

Compassion and Choices; http://www.compassionandchoices.org

The organization, Compassion and Choices, resulted from the union of "Compassion in Dying" with "End-of-Life Choices," two organizations dedicated to bringing attention to increasing the choices available to terminal patients. Compassion and Choices is dedicated to client service, legal advocacy, and public education. Its goals are to increase patient empowerment and self-determination with expanded legal end-of-life options. They provide free State-specific Advance Directive forms. Members may have their Advance Directive transferred to a wallet-sized CD-ROM for easy carrying. The professionals and volunteers at Compassion and Choices are also available to consult patients and families at Compassion and Choices, P.O. Box 101810, Denver, CO 80250-1810, or info@compassionandchoices.org, or 1-800-247-7421. Their client services staff can help those facing terminal illnesses to find a local hospice. They can speak to your providers about what to expect in the future, and if your current needs are not being met. They help you explore your end-of-life options including hastening dying if suffering becomes unbearable. Their web page, http://www. compassionandchoices.org/services/help.php, links to http://www.ltcombudsman. org/ that can help if you are concerned about the care of a loved one who is in a long-term care facility. If your loved one is in a hospital, they provide help when requesting medical records, speaking to the nursing supervisor or the hospital's risk manager or hospital administrator, and the hospital ethics committee.

Last Acts Partnership (See Caring Connections, above.)

Alan D. Lieberson, M.D., J.D.; www.preciouslegacy.com
Treatment of Pain and Suffering in the Terminally Ill (1999) An Internet book intentionally not copyrighted by its author (who wishes to be cited), that includes a 6000-word chapter entitled, "Voluntary Terminal Dehydration."

Midwest Bioethics Center—Caring Conversations; http://www.practicalbioethics.org

Caring Conversations is an initiative of the Midwest Bioethics Center to help individuals make their end-of-life wishes known to their family, friends and doctors. The goal of Caring Conversations is to focus attention on meaningful conversation between friends, doctors and loved ones that can lead to the most useful Advance Directives. In addition to advice and suggestions for initiating these difficult and emotional conversations, Caring Conversations provides free Advance Directive forms and a booklet to guide and assist their creation. 1-800-344-3829; The Midwest Bioethics Center for Practical Bioethics; Town Pavilion; 1100 Walnut Street, Suite 2900; Kansas City, MO 64106-2197.

Euthanasia Research and Guidance Organization (ERGO); http://www.finalexit.org
This is the web site of Hemlock's founder, Derek Humphry, who monitors an open web forum, org.opn.lists.right-to-die-request@lists.opn.org, where subscribers can note news and exchange views.

International Task Force on Euthanasia and Assisted Suicide; http://www.iaetf.org/
Contains articles in direct opposition to ERGO, above.

James Park created *The One-Month-Less Club* and offers books on the web such as "Safeguards for Life-Ending Decisions." www.tc.umn.edu/~parkx032/SG.html.

World Federation of Right to Die Societies; www.worldrtd.net/
Founded in 1980, this organization consists of 38 right to die organizations from 23 countries. It provides an international link to secure or protect the rights of individuals to self-determination at the end of their lives.

Caring Advocates; http://www.caringadvocates.org
Disclaimer: As its Executive Director, the author may benefit from this organization's activities.

Caring Advocates is a 501(c)3 non-profit organization that consists of a group of collaborating professionals from the fields of clinical medicine, psychiatry and psychology, law, social work, pastoral counseling, nursing, and medical ethics. They offer their combined knowledge, training, and experience in the areas of health care law and end-of-life ethics at three particularly critical times:

A) When individuals and families are discussing, creating, and revising their Advance Directives, the staff of Caring Advocates can offer advice.

B) When the designated Proxy must face challenging end-of-life decisions for loved ones about continuing medical treatment, especially if they are in persistently unconscious states or terminally ill with unbearable suffering, the staff of Caring Advocates can provide second opinions and support.

C) The staff advises clients on selecting appropriate Proxies to make medical decisions for them in the future. They facilitate forming and implementing "Trusting Circles," where members can agree to serve as each other's Proxies, seeking professional advice on an "as-needed basis." In special circumstances, clients can designate individual staff members of Caring Advocates or its affiliates in other States as one of their Proxies. Common reasons to join a "Trusting Circle" or select a staff member of Caring Advocates include: 1) To make sure a Proxy will be available even if the clients' relatives and close friends do not survive them, or happen not to be available, or are not well themselves. 2) To feel confident that non-related individuals have professional back up, or professionals themselves will be making the challenging decisions that the clients want without being influenced by strong emotions or experiencing guilt later. 3) To have professionals who strive to be well-informed about current health care law and end-of-life ethics, to articulate clearly and to argue effectively if necessary with those in power so that their Last Wishes are honored, instead of being denied or delayed by the challenges of others.

Caring Advocates professionals can also be asked to evaluate and provide a declaration of a patient's **decision-making capacity**; to evaluate family members and caregivers for possible **undue influence**; and to offer an opinion on the Proxy's decision-making capacity and the Proxy's behavior with respect to the patient's BEST INTEREST. Caring Advocates professionals can also be asked to help facilitate the stated wishes of a patient's Living Will, as a "Living Will Advocate."

Caring Advocates strives to make all the services of **Caring Advocates** available to those who cannot otherwise afford them. Its mission also includes educating the public and members of relevant professions on why Advance Directives must include *clear and convincing* documentation to empower their Proxies, and why Proxies should be granted the ultimate authority to make medical decisions, overriding the instructions in Living Wills. The staff thus provides continuing education programs to professionals; lectures and workshops to lay audiences; and distributes books, newsletters, audios and videos, by mail and by the Internet.

The website of www.CaringAdvocates.org includes links to other Internet sites, a "**Latest News**" section, a BLOG, and a Forum so visitors can share their views.

A related web site is www.ThirstControl.com. 1-888-THIRST-0 (888-844-7780)

Contact information: 1-800-64 PEACE (647-3223) or 760-431-2233; P.O. 130129; Carlsbad, CA 92009; info@CaringAdvocates.org.

About Dr. Ronald Miller and Attorney Michael Evans, who provided professional oversight

Ronald B. Miller, M.D., is Clinical Professor of Medicine Emeritus and founding Director of the Program in Medical Ethics Emeritus at the University of California, Irvine College of Medicine. He has devoted his professional career to the care of patients with kidney disease; to research and teaching in kidney disease, dialysis, and transplantation at Boston University and at the University of California, Irvine, where he founded the kidney division. For two decades, he has been intensely concerned with ethical issues, which he has taught to college and medical students and residents. He brings to Caring Advocates as Consulting Advisor, and to this book as a critical reader and contributor, many experiences including: He cared for patients with end-stage renal disease some of whom elected to discontinue the life-sustaining treatment of chronic dialysis. He served on the health care ethics committees of four hospitals and co-founded the Orange County Bioethics Network. He has written over 90 articles, two dozen of which deal with Advance Directives; end-of-life care; withholding, limiting, or withdrawing life-sustaining treatment; and physician-assisted suicide and euthanasia. In 1997, he was a co-signator of an *amicus curiae* brief to the U.S. Supreme Court on two cases concerning the right to physician-assisted suicide. He testified to the Senate-Assembly Health Committees' hearing on "California Stem Cell Research and Cures Act." He served on the Council on Ethical Affairs of the California Medical Association; and he testified to the California Assembly Select Committee on Palliative Care, the California Law Revision Commission on the Healthcare Decisions Act.

Michael S. Evans J.D., M.S.W., is an attorney and a social worker. He has been a member of the California Bar since 1970. For 13 years he was in private law practice that included litigation involving criminal defense, mental health commitments, and divorce. He taught at the graduate level in the School of Social Work, San Diego State University, and for six years at the University of San Diego Law School. He co-founded the Center for Professional Ethics and Law, a non-profit organization which among its projects, examined the impact of courtroom advocacy on the professional ethics of expert witnesses during litigation. He brings to Caring Advocates as Consulting Advisor, and to this book as a critical reader and contributor, many experiences including: He served as legal advisor to several right-to-choose-to-die organizations. He authored a model Advance Health Care Directive to broaden the range of choices available under California's Health Care Decisions Law. He helped draft model legislation to further expand end-of-life choices for Californians. He served on two bioethics committees in San Diego. He counseled individuals on creating and implementing Advance Directives to meet the varied challenges of making end-of-life decisions.

Why also a novel on end-of-life issues?

The answer is not the traditional one—some readers prefer to be *entertained* by a medical thriller while others prefer to be *taught* by a self-help book with memoirs, advice, and guidelines. If my writing goals are achieved, both books will entertain and educate. More substantively, each book attempts to solve two end-of-life challenges, making a total of **four practical end-of-life offerings**:

Lethal Choice shows **(1)** how technology can help a mentally competent adult who is **extremely impaired physically, even totally paralyzed, can hasten dying without direct help from others**. One reason so few people use Oregon's *Death With Dignity Act* (about three dozen a year), is that many patients are too ill to put the powder from pills mixed with pudding into their mouths and then swallow. If others offer help, they risk being charged with a felony. **(2)** The medical thriller asserts that **a combination of non-controlled prescription medications can effectively and peacefully hasten dying**. None of these medications are listed on the Schedules of the Drug Enforcement Act since individually, they are *not usually* considered lethal. This could be important if individual States impose strict restrictions on using controlled medications, now that the U.S. Supreme Court has affirmed that States have the "right" to determine what is, or is not, "legitimate medical use." The U.S. Congress could also pass new laws to amend the Controlled Substances Act of 1970. (Note: The novel does not reveal the names of these medications to prevent their misuse by patients who suffer from psychiatric illnesses.)

Beyond serving as a general guide to creating effective Advance Directives, where success is defined as setting the stage so that others will honor your Last Wishes, **The *BEST WAY* to Say Goodbye: A Legal Peaceful Choice at the End of Life (3)** details all aspects of the **peaceful legal alternative to Physician-Hastened Dying**. For competent adults, **Voluntary Refusal of Food and Fluid** is legal everywhere. **(4)** The book also describes strategies for competent adults to **plan for a future where they can avoid lingering in indignity and dependency of dementia**. They can trust that at a specific end-point of their own choosing, their designated Proxy can overcome potential challenges from others to honor their end-of-life decision to **Refuse Food and Fluid by Proxy**. This option also applies to those in the early stages of Alzheimer's disease, provided patients still have decision-making capacity (which ability should be documented). A diligently prepared set of documents should permit patients not only to refuse tube feeding, but also (if that is their choice) to refuse forced feeding at the hands of nursing assistants via the mouth, when restraints must be used, or when the process has become an unpleasant and unrewarding ordeal. Others have called this unique approach an iron-clad strategy for dementia.

Stan Terman's Professional and Personal End-Of-Life Beliefs

I can't remember who said it, but I'll never forget these exact words:

"I'd never want to die for something I strongly believed in ...because I might be wrong!"

More than believe, I *know* I will die. So let me turn this quote around with respect to process of dying itself: Why not die for something in which I *do* believe? After all, the risk incurred from being wrong would be relatively minor. So let me now consider *my* greatest fear:

Were I afflicted with dementia, I admit there is a possibility that I would become a *new person* who enjoyed the simpler things in life and thus considered *his* rare moments of partial lucidity as worth imposing the extreme burdens of *his* continued existence on *my* family and *my* society required by *his* continued care. (Note that I am distinguishing between this *new person,* to whom I refer as *his,* and *my present self.*) As a currently competent person, however, it seems far more important to me, as I view the overall character of my life, that *neither* **he** nor **I** (which ever the case may be) exist in the state of indignity from dementia for a prolonged period of time.

The reasons are deeply personal and intrinsic to my perception of myself, although they range from superficial to profound: My vanity wishes to avoid the likelihood that others will remember me in the state of indignity and forget my previous personality and accomplishments. My provincial selfishness wishes *not* to burden my family emotionally or financially. And my humanistic responsibility wishes *not* to drain the world's financial and medical resources.

Assuming that I would no longer appreciate the sacrifices being made on my behalf, and that they would provide me with virtually no benefit anyway (based on my current perception of "benefit"), I would not want to waste such resources if, considering the world as a whole, there is a possibility that a social mechanism could offer these same funds to the poor and needy who could indeed benefit; for example, children in developing countries who die of preventable diseases. Leaving part of my residual estate to a non-profit foundation is one individualized way to accomplish this goal. I hope our government's policy and law makers will provide additional mechanisms. Clearly, there is no chance of funds helping the poor and needy if the money is already spent.

So while I respect the argument that the previously stated Last Wishes when a person was competent may not apply after the process of dementia has created a *new person*, I neither personally nor professionally embrace that view. In this sense, I agree with some of the arguments presented by philosopher and law professor Ronald Dworkin, who wrote about "precedent autonomy," psychological continuity, and a single life narrative. He specifically addressed the first two principles of medical ethics when he wrote: "A competent person's right to autonomy requires that past decisions about how he is to be treated if he becomes demented be respected, even if they do not represent, and even if they contradict, the desires he has when we respect them, provided he did not change his mind while he was still in charge of his own life" [1993]. In other words, "Principles of self-determination would trump beneficence"; that is, **autonomy** would assume a higher priority than "best care" (**to benefit** the patient before us) as perceived by others when they have the power to make such decisions.

Patient autonomy and benefit are two of the four principles of medical ethics. The third principle is to **do no harm**, which can be applied at levels beyond those centering on the patient. I would ask, for example, does it "harm" the life of a mother if she almost completely devotes three decades of her life to feed and clean her child who is in a coma, hoping her child will wake up? Also, does it "harm" other people for the good acts the mother may have otherwise accomplished in her life? I believe the answers to both questions are, Yes.

Professor Dworkin champions autonomy; he views the expression of freedom as the highest goal of our Constitutional Liberty. I agree, but the compelling basis for my wanting to invoke **Withholding of Food & Fluid by Proxy** reflects my wish to emphasize the fourth ethical principle. **Social justice** requires fairness in the allocation of available resources for all people's basic needs. Throughout time, sages have consoled the dying and grieving by noting this reason for death: to allow new human beings to come into this world. If so, then the question that begs for an answer is, When do I decide to step aside? Part of my answer is encoded in criteria this book lists twice: on pages 263-264 and 397-398. Those pages list the limitations in functioning that for me, should trigger the "no aggressive treatment" and "**Withhold Food & Fluid**" options. Economist Professor Robert Frank phrased this sentiment simply and clearly: "Personally, if I were in such a state, I would not want anyone to spend a nickel to keep me alive. So by all means, save the money spent on late stage dementia patients and spend it instead on mosquito nets or something else in health care or education, which has the potential to do some real good."

Thinking about my priorities is necessary but not sufficient. I must also implement such decisions while still competent. It is my responsibility to plan in advance by creating diligently crafted, strategic documents, and by designating individuals who will effectively advocate my Last Wishes. I wish this not only for myself, but also for others. I hope to contribute by reducing suffering of terminally ill patients and their families. While I admit that I find end-of-life conundrums intellectually and spiritually intriguing, in part because so many disciplines have much to contribute, this is not the main reason I wrote this book.

Here now are some of my other personal and professional beliefs:

With respect to the role of religious and clinical professionals:

• I agree with religions that teach it is wrong to prolong inevitable dying.

• I fully endorse the goal and methods of **hospice** to do everything possible to make the transition of dying as comfortable and as meaningful as possible, and the efforts of palliative care medicine to reduce suffering, which should be offered both prior to and after admission to a hospice program.

• I do not believe that end-of-life suffering is *The* path to salvation. Instead, I believe that personal and professional caregivers should make every effort to reduce end-of-life pain and suffering.

• I believe physicians are in the best position to reduce patients' pain and suffering; to refer patients to hospice; to rule out depression and impaired judgment; and to explore why patients make requests to hasten dying.

• I believe professionals from other disciplines can help reduce suffering; including psychological counselors, social workers, religious and spiritual leaders, nurses, musicians, attorneys, financial advisors, and morticians, among others.

• I believe physicians should strive to be aware of their own personal, religious, and moral values so they can refrain from imposing them on their patients and their patients' families. Physicians should be willing to present options that they might not choose for themselves, in the spirit of providing fully informed consent.

• I believe that if physicians cannot comply with a patient's legal request, they must try to refer the patient on to another physician who may be willing to help.

• I feel it is cruel for powerful professionals to impose their own values on terminal patients and their families. —Or better said: On us, and on our families!

With respect to the needs and responsibilities of terminally ill patients:

• I believe that one of the greatest joys in life is to be heard and respected, and this is especially true for needy and vulnerable patients in the last chapter of their lives, when their most fundamental values are at stake. It is also the last opportunity for them to receive our kindness and our understanding.

• I believe we all should strive diligently to learn directly from the patient what she or he wants, and we should then try to honor those wishes.

• I believe patients let their relatives down if they do not take the time to diligently inform others about their Last Wishes; for example, if they wish to fund college educations for their several grandchildren rather than spend that sum of money on several miserable last months of their lives as they endure unsuccessful and burdensome medical procedures on Intensive Care Units.

• I believe that medical technology can be overused to maintain existence indefinitely, which the original inventors of these techniques had never intended.

• I believe the "right" to be treated indefinitely must be balanced with the "rights" of others in society to receive reasonable treatment with available resources.

With respect to other methods to hasten dying:

• I was professionally alarmed by the cavalier behavior of Dr. Kevorkian, who I believe ended some people's lives prematurely as he disregarded following even his own guidelines that called for thorough evaluations.

• I was personally repulsed by the original technique of the former Hemlock Society—to end their lives by suffocation using plastic bags. Now I worry about the dangerous "Peaceful Pill" should it become available to psychiatric patients.

• I am afraid to give physicians legal power to administer medications to end patients' lives. Although the term for this method is called *euthanasia*, which literally means "good death," it would be hard to establish absolute safeguards to make sure patients acts are always voluntary.

• I believe legalization of physician-aided patient-hastened dying in Oregon is helping a greater number of people than the few who choose to fill and then ingest a prescription of lethal medications. Many more patients are aware that they have a choice and therefore experience less anxiety and worry about having to endure prolonged suffering. Ironically, many will then choose to live longer.

• I appreciate why some patients prefer physician-aided patient-hastened dying to **Voluntary Refusal of Food & Fluid**. A few have contraindications based on their medical conditions; some have time constraints; others have a great psychological need to be in control. I have the most empathy for those who have inadequate health care insurance and no or limited access to *Comfort Care*.

• I have the impression from my limited experience that physician-aided patient-hastened dying may strain the doctor-patient relationship more than exercising the option of **Voluntary Refusal of Food & Fluid**.

• I refer readers to my position paper on efforts to legalize physician-hastened dying that is included in the back material of my novel, ***Lethal Choice***, where I propose a protocol to solve the *potential* problem of physician under-reporting, and I suggest ways to make sure that patients' decisions are truly voluntary. I also recommend informing patients about **Voluntary Refusal of Food & Fluid** (including its advantage of reversibility), to fulfill the condition of providing "fully informed consent."

With respect to the enormous future problem of Alzheimer's and other dementias (unless cures are discovered), and the role of **Withholding Food & Fluid**:

• I worry how society will be able to afford to maintain sixteen million brain-damaged patients by mid-century. Unless society's attitudes and policies change about how we treat end-stage dementia patients, the combination of financial, emotional and caregiving burdens will overwhelm society's resources.

• I feel it is inappropriate to force-feed people by mouth if they no longer understand how to eat or can swallow—especially if their prognosis is irreversible and the outlook is progressive decline, if they clench their mouths shut, if they turn away, or if they spit out the food. Similarly, I feel it is inhumane to restrain people's hands to prevent them from repeatedly pulling out their feeding tubes.

• I am impressed with **Refusal of Food & Fluid** as a humane and peaceful way to die that is available to many patients who have no other means to reduce the time they must endure suffering and indignity. I believe the method also offers opportunities for healing of self and of relationships, and that one of its most important advantages is that it permits competent patients to change their minds and continue to live.

• I am in favor of preserving our rights as guaranteed by the Constitution and reaffirmed by the U.S. Supreme Court that every competent adult has the right to refuse any unwanted medical treatment, which right can be expressed by designating a Proxy if the person no longer has the capacity to make medical decisions. While States have the duty to protect life, and the U.S. Supreme Court has ruled that States can set the standard for level of proof of what they patient would have wanted, I disagree with present or proposed State laws that would create unrealistic obstacles to Proxies to prevent them from refusing nutrition and hydration. I also disagree with those religious organizations that argue that tube feeding is not a medical treatment but ordinary and obligatory care.

• I worry about our personal freedom when politicians inappropriately use end-of-life issues as political footballs, when they consider new reactive legislation to restrict the Liberty of patients and their families to make personal decisions with their doctors, and when they explicitly adopt the beliefs of their religions to establish secular policies. I similarly worry about clinicians who impose their values on their patients and presume to know what is best for them.

With respect to my reasons for agreeing to have my written declaration submitted to Florida Judge Greer by the attorneys for Terri Schiavo's parents:

• I declined when asked, to give my opinion on the excerpts of the old video tapes that had been shown on TV so many times; however,

• I read the observations that attorney Barbara Weller made during her visit with Terri Schiavo, and wondered if there was a remote possibility that Terri Schiavo might have transcended beyond the Minimally Conscious State. If so, she might have been capable of indicating her preferences for further treatment and whether or not she wished to remain alive in her present state. Even though it was more likely that Terri Schiavo was still in the Minimally Conscious State or the Permanent Vegetative State (which would have made such communication impossible), I still predicted that my proposed bedside visit to perform an evaluation would have value. If Terri did not meet the consensus criteria of answering correctly six out of six situational questions [Giacino and others, 2002], if she could not use any combination of sounds or facial expressions to communicate even Yes or No, then the conclusion would have been that she could *not* communicate meaningfully. If the Schindlers could have accepted that conclusion from a professional brought in by their own attorneys, then perhaps they would have found it possible, or easier, to let their daughter go.

• When Judge Greer decided not to permit further clinical evaluations of Terri Schiavo, I did not disagree. —Not after so many years of thorough evaluations and re-evaluations. But had the Judge allowed further evaluations, I wanted to give Terri Schiavo every possible opportunity to speak for herself.

• I considered the subsequent reports that claimed that when Terri was asked if she wanted to live, she responded loudly with "Ahhhhhhh" and then "Waaaaaaaa." Her sister and others interpreted her response as indicating that she was struggling to say, "I want to live." Yet there were two other possibilities: She might have been beginning a different sentence with the same two words, "*I want* to die." More likely, her vocalization had no meaning, was not a response to the ultimate question, and was only a reflex. Yet if Terri could have consistently said either "Ahhhhhhh" or any other sound—once for "Yes," and twice for "No," then she might have been able to express her preferences. Back in March 2005, there was no basis for deciding how to interpret her vocalizations other than the neurological examinations that took place two years previously, and they supported the diagnosis of PVS. While there was no compelling reason to assume that her neurological condition had improved, that remote possibility could have been tested.

• I consider the results of Ms. Schiavo's autopsy as validating what happened. On June 15, 2005, Medical Examiner, Jon Thogmartin, announced that she died of "marked dehydration," not starvation; there was no evidence of abuse; her condition was "consistent" with being in a persistent vegetative state; her brain weighed less than half of expected; she was blind; she would not have been able to eat or drink had she been given food by mouth; and, no amount of treatment could have reversed her irreversible brain damage.

To sum up, I was willing to examine Terri Schiavo because I felt that every effort should be made to try to find out what the patient wanted—if possible; and because sometimes, unwanted results can eventually make it easier for loved ones to let go of the dying person. At this point, I hope the Schindlers can feel relief from the autopsy results and its conclusion that there was no hope for recovery.

About Dr. Stanley A. Terman

Stanley A. Terman is a board-certified psychiatrist who has dedicated nearly three decades of his professional life to relationship issues and end-of-life challenges. His degrees are **B.A.** (Brown University); **Ph.D.** (M.I.T.), **M.D.** (U. Iowa). Formerly on the faculty of the University of California, Irvine, he founded the nonprofit organization **Caring Advocates** whose staff of clinical, legal, and spiritual professionals helps patients and their families attain the goal of **peaceful transitions**.

In working with terminally ill patients and their loved ones, Dr. Terman regularly assesses the judgment and ability to make decisions of patients who wish to create strategic Living Wills and Powers of Attorney for medical or financial decisions. He also provides advice and support for individuals designated as Proxies when they are faced with the awesome responsibility to make an end-of-life decision for another. Having participated actively in three bioethics committees and consulted at the San Diego Hospice, Dr. Terman now lectures to professional and general audiences. A sample of topics includes: "Moral Paternalism and The President's Council on Bioethics," "The Sanctity of Many Lives," and "Does Hollywood Accurately Portray Alzheimer's disease?"

Dr. Terman believes educating people on the legal, peaceful choice to refuse food and fluid has potential to help far more people than expensive political campaigns to attempt to legalize Physician-Assisted Dying, especially since PAD cannot help millions of people avoid their greatest fear: progressive indignity and dependency from such devastating diseases as Alzheimer's.

Attorneys for Terri Schiavo's parents submitted Dr. Terman's declaration to Florida's Judge George Greer. Dr. Terman agreed to participate in the spirit of two beliefs he holds most dear: "We are morally obligated to honor a patient's previously expressed wishes," and "We should do everything possible to learn directly from the patient, what she or he wants."

Dr. Terman is currently creating a series of books, audio CDs, and DVDs in the series, **The *BEST WAY* to Attain Peaceful Transitions**. He also wrote **Lethal Choice**, a medical thriller based on a conspiracy theory of Physician-Assisted Suicide that explores end-of-life ethical principles.

Dr. Terman's family includes Sharon (his daughter); Elias and Alex (his sons); Alex's wife, Nadine; their son, Leo; and Emily and Lauren (Beth's daughters). He and his wife, Beth Gardner, live in Carlsbad-by-the-Sea with their two Pomeranian dogs, Priscilla and Bruno.